Women's Health
IN
COMPLEMENTARY
AND INTEGRATIVE
MEDICINE

A Clinical Guide

Women's Health
IN
COMPLEMENTARY
AND INTEGRATIVE
MEDICINE
A Clinical Guide

Tieraona Low Dog, MD
Director of Education
Program in Integrative Medicine
Clinical Assistant Professor
Department of Medicine
University of Arizona Health Sciences Center
Chair, United States Pharmacopoeia Dietary
Supplements/Botanicals Information Expert Panel

with
Marc S. Micozzi, MD, PhD
Director, Policy Institute for Integrative Medicine
Bethesda, MD

Editor, Medical Guides to Complementary and
Alternative Medicine
Bethesda, MD

With 20 illustrations

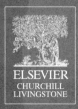

ELSEVIER
CHURCHILL
LIVINGSTONE

ELSEVIER
CHURCHILL
LIVINGSTONE

11830 Westline Industrial Drive
St. Louis, Missouri 63146

Notice

Knowledge regarding the proper use of drugs, herbs, and supplements is ever changing. Standard safety precautions must be followed, but as new research and clinical experience broaden our understanding, changes in use may become necessary or appropriate. Readers are advised to check the most current product information provided by the manufacturer of each product to be administered to verify the recommended dose, the method and duration of administration, and contraindications. It is the responsibility of the treating licensed practitioner, relying on experience and knowledge of the patient, to determine dosages and the best treatment for each individual patient.

This publication is not intended as a substitute for medical therapy nor as a manual for self-treatment. Readers should seek professional advice for any specific medical problems.

Neither the Publisher nor the authors assume any liability for any injury and/or damage to persons or property arising from this publication.

ISBN-13: 978-0-443-06639-9
ISBN-10: 0-443-06639-6

Publishing Director: Linda Duncan
Editor: Kellie White
Developmental Editor: Jennifer Watrous
Editorial Assistant: Kendra Bailey
Publishing Services Manager: Linda McKinley
Project Manager: Judy Ahlers
Design Project Manager: Bill Drone

Printed in the United States of America

Last digit is the print number: 9   8   7   6   5   4

From the midwives in the village to the physician in the clinic to the scientist in the research laboratory—this book is dedicated to all who work tirelessly to improve the health and well-being of women throughout the world.

TLD and MSM

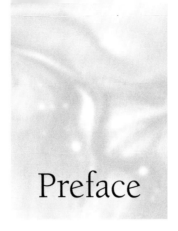

Preface

The landscape of complementary and alternative medicine (CAM) has changed dramatically since I started practicing as an herbalist in the desert Southwest 25 years ago. The marketplace has expanded at a pace that far outstrips that of research. With newspapers, magazines, and mass media providing a steady daily diet on the risks or benefits of a particular herb, nutritional supplement, or CAM practice, much misinformation abounds. The scientific data are confusing and contradictory, leaving patients confused and overwhelmed by their choices. Separating practices and products of possible benefit from those of poor quality or with little evidence of efficacy is a daunting task, especially for practitioners with limited time and minimal experience. This book was written to help health care providers become more conversant in offering informed guidance to women in their use of integrative treatment strategies.

Integrative medicine—the term being used by a growing number of practitioners who recommend both conventional and CAM therapies—describes an effort to offer patients the best of evidence-based treatments. If acupuncture reduces chemotherapy-induced nausea and vomiting, patients should be encouraged to seek the services of a trained acupuncturist. If calcium or chastetree berry safely reduces the symptoms of premenstrual syndrome, this should be conveyed to women as part of a treatment plan. If there is no evidence that essiac or shark's cartilage cures cancer, the public should be told in no uncertain terms, while practitioners gently guide patients to proven therapies. Each treatment must be judged objectively and not simply accepted, or rejected, because it is conventional or CAM. One day in the future I hope we discard these arbitrary terms and simply embrace the practice of *medicine,* in all of its unique forms. Until that time, the term integrative medicine most closely reflects my own philosophy.

This book takes an evidence-based approach to numerous practices and products used by women either to treat an illness or to enhance their health and well-being. Critical analysis of the scientific evidence is essential for clinicians, yet it is only part of the practice of medicine. Most women want to know what works so they can base their health care decisions on the evidence. But they also want to be treated with kindness, compassion, and respect by their health care provider. They want to be seen as whole human beings: as part of a family, community, faith, culture. Women want to be listened to and have their viewpoint considered.

The therapeutic relationship is a sacred one. Every patient encounter is an opportunity to sow the seeds of healing. As providers of health care, we must remember that we are healers first and foremost; we use science as our foundation so that we may effectively practice the art of medicine. For when the soul, not just the body, is nurtured and cared for, we enhance the lives of our patients and maybe even ... our own.

Tieraona Low Dog, MD
Corrales, New Mexico
May 2004

Acknowledgments

This book was birthed only through the generous mentoring, help, and encouragement I have received from teachers, colleagues, students, and friends over the many years. From the martial arts instructors who trained my body and disciplined my mind to the midwives, herbalists, and physicians who taught me the wonders and magic of the plants, medicine, and healing; I have been blessed by many in my life. There are a few, though, that I would like to specifically acknowledge: Arthur Kaufman, MD, and Alan Firestone, MD, whose passion for medicine inspired me throughout my medical training and beyond; Rosemary Gladstar, David Winston, David Hoffman, Michael Moore, Roy Upton, and Mark Blumenthal, whose love and commitment to herbal medicine has helped keep this noble tradition alive in the United States. There are those in the academic and scientific communities who have been mentors and friends along my journey: Fredi Kronenberg, PhD, Adriane Fugh-Berman, MD, Andy Weil, MD, Steven Strauss, MD, David Eisenberg, MD, Dennis Awang, PhD, and most especially the late Varro Tyler, PhD. My sincerest gratitude to Joseph Fins, MD, medical ethicist and physician, whose critical mind, uncompromising integrity, and unwavering friendship were invaluable as we co-wrote our minority statement for the White House Commission on Complementary and Alternative Medicine Policy. I would also like to express my deepest appreciation to Marc Micozzi, MD, PhD and the folks at Elsevier Publishing, without whom this book would never have made it to print.

A special thank-you goes to Viola Gutierrez, my delightful and infatigable assistant, who manages both my office and home with unerring aptitude; Jim Carnazzo, for his loving friendship; and most importantly, my children, Mekoce and Kiara, who are my most wondrous teachers and most delightful companions. Thank you for your patience, love, understanding, and support.

Tieraona Low Dog, MD
June 2004

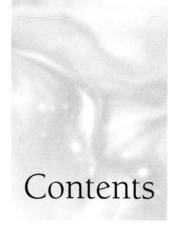

Contents

Section I
CURRENT CONCERNS ABOUT WOMEN'S HEALTH

Section II
REPRODUCTIVE BIOLOGY

Section III
THE NERVOUS SYSTEM

Section IV
MEDICAL CONDITIONS

Appendix
BOTANICAL PRODUCTS, 327

Women's Health

IN

COMPLEMENTARY AND INTEGRATIVE MEDICINE

A Clinical Guide

One

Current Concerns About Women's Health

The use of complementary/alternative medicine (CAM) and integrative medicine is widespread and on the increase among American adults, especially women. This fact underscores the importance of communicating with patients about CAM and integrative medicine. The results of a recent survey showed that two thirds of adults claimed use of CAM by the age of 33 years. The use of CAM is most widespread among post–baby boomers (7 of 10), with only 5 of 10 baby boomers and 3 of 10 preboomers turning to CAM. These trends may represent an openness to CAM on the part of baby boomers that relates more to the management of medical conditions more common among older Americans than to lifelong attitudes inclusive of "holistic" healing among younger Americans.

Two thirds of health maintenance organizations offered at least one type of alternative therapy as of 1999, with acupuncture, massage, and nutritional therapy the modalities most likely to be covered. The best predictor of CAM use is higher education, perhaps reflecting a greater amount of disposable income, as well as knowledge, awareness, and attitudes about CAM.

Regional variations are quite consistent, with one half to two thirds of respondents from such diverse areas as South Carolina, Northern California, Florida, and Oregon indicating that they use CAM. As many as half of all patients who use CAM do not tell their physicians that they are doing so, indicating that much work on the integration of CAM into the continuum of care remains to be done (see Chapter 1).

A high proportion of adults with cancer—80% or more, according to the findings of several surveys—use CAM. In one study, 40% of CAM users abandoned conventional care after turning to CAM. As many as 74% of patients with breast cancer said they used CAM, despite the relative effectiveness of conventional care. CAM use is also common among patients with neurologic diseases, psychiatric disorders, physical disabilities, psoriasis, and diabetes, among other ailments. The range of CAM modalities is reflected by the topics covered in this book.

In addition to the management of medical conditions, CAM therapies have gained increasing attention in the prevention of chronic disease. Although CAM is often considered a means of achieving a healthy lifestyle and preventing disease, much evidence exists to support the effectiveness of CAM in treatment. Increasing numbers of clinical trials of CAM are being conducted, whereas prevention trials are larger, longer, more costly, more complex, and, ultimately, rarer.

Obesity is increasingly recognized as a major contributor to chronic medical conditions and as a source of morbidity and mortality. Losing or managing weight is an important means of preventing disease. Controversy over the safety of ephedra has clouded the issue of herbal remedies in weight loss and has motivated efforts by Congress to enforce regulatory actions against all dietary supplements (see Chapter 2).

The role of dietary supplements in optimal health is increasingly recognized. A 2003 article by Fairfield and Fletcher[1,2] documented the importance of nutrition and provided clear substantiation of the role of dietary supplementation in light of the typical American diet and the nutrient composition of foods. The use of dietary supplements is already prevalent among older Americans, especially women.

References

1. Fairfield RH, Fletcher KM: Vitamins for chronic disease prevention in adults: scientific review, *JAMA* 287:3116, 2002.
2. Fletcher RH, Fairfield KM: Vitamins for chronic disease prevention in adults: clinical applications, *JAMA* 287:3127, 2002.

Communicating with Patients About Complementary and Integrative Medicine

This book is designed to serve as a bridge between two great bodies of knowledge. On one side is traditional Western medicine, with its basis in biomedical science. On the other is complementary/alternative medicine (CAM), with its emphasis on the whole person, often in subtle but profound ways that we are now only beginning to understand. Like any bridge, the one between these two approaches requires a firm foundation on each side of the span. The two forms of medicine share certain fundamental strengths: an internally consistent theoretical basis, extensive empirical evidence, and observable results. Beyond those broad commonalities lie differences in the specifics of philosophy, conceptual framework, techniques, and, sometimes, even objectives. Together the two great bodies of medical knowledge provide a vast array of healing possibilities. Whereas 80% of the world's population is confined to the limited range of health care options offered by local cultures, Americans have the unique and historical opportunity to integrate the best of the old and new healing practices of the Americas, Europe, Asia, Africa, the Middle East, and elsewhere.

In modern health care we have discovered that these different practices are not mutually exclusive and, indeed, they work well together. Eastern and Western systems, ancient techniques, and new therapies—all can be evaluated, selected, and combined in ways that greatly extend the spectrum of healing for an individual and for society.

As exciting as these choices are, knowing how or when to start making them is not simple. What criteria should be used to evaluate alternative/complementary therapies? When is it time to rely on traditional Western care? What about homeopathic remedies for insomnia or acupuncture treatments for chronic pain? Can St. John's wort and Prozac be used at the same time? Should you undergo therapeutic touch before, during, or after surgery? How can you design a lifestyle or care plan that comfortably combines conventional and alternative/complementary treatments?

This book will guide you through the process of understanding alternative/complementary therapies and how they can be successfully integrated with traditional Western care. It will help you learn how to draw on a larger repertoire of healing therapies and systems to get the full benefit of all the resources available from the world health community. Many people in the world rely on ethnomedicine, in which a local healer who has an ongoing relationship with the patient uses traditional methods to address the whole individual, encouraging the patient to take an active role in the healing process. These indigenous approaches—some of which are highly sophisticated systems that have been used effectively for centuries or even millennia—have often been dismissed by the conventional Western medical community as primitive. Throughout the first half of the 20th century, cultural biases made it increasingly difficult for Americans to appreciate the richness of other health care traditions. We were appropriately impressed by advances in surgery, antibiotics, and other lifesaving technologies developed by the medical-scientific community. Western medicine seemed to be leaving everyone else behind. Then, in 1972, while in Peking covering President Richard Nixon's visit, *New York Times* reporter James Reston underwent an emergency appendectomy. Reston's Chinese physicians used acupuncture for anesthesia during surgery and afterward for pain control, with excellent results. This became front-page news, introducing millions of Americans to the potential benefits of this ancient practice and launching a scientific and social debate that has continued to grow for three decades.

WHAT IS COMPLEMENTARY/ALTERNATIVE MEDICINE?

Broadly speaking, CAM is any therapy that is outside the American medical mainstream but is practiced by a significant number of people with observable results. Mainstream American medicine, or conventional Western care, can be defined as the allopathic approach—that is, the one used by physicians who hold MD degrees. It is also known as biomedicine because of its firm foundations in the hard science of biology. The term *alternative medicine* became part of the English language in the 1960s, when acupuncture and other Asian therapies first became known to mainstream Americans, who viewed them as an alternative, rather than as an adjunct, to conventional treatment. Many people, especially physicians, took exception to the term because of its exclusive, "either/or" connotation. A more accurate term, *complementary*, was adopted by some to describe those alternative therapies that were being used in conjunction with traditional Western medicine. As a means of combining this more accurate term with the more widely recognized original, the phrase *complementary and alternative medicine* was coined, then shortened to the acronym CAM. More recently, the term *integrative medicine* was coined, implying an active, conscious effort by patient and physician to incorporate alternative and allopathic treatments in a cohesive approach. In this book, the terms *alternative, complementary,* and *CAM* are used interchangeably to describe the therapies and systems drawn from other traditions that are now being used in conjunction with mainstream Western medicine. The plural term *alternative medicines* is used to emphasize that CAM is not a monolithic field but one that comprises many distinct traditions and approaches. The following criteria

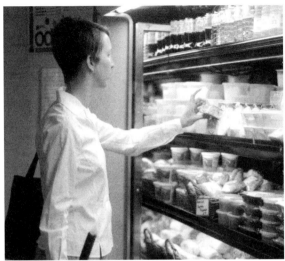

Figure 1-1 Self-healing and natural products are common themes through each chapter in this book. *(From Association of Women's Health Obstetric and Neonatal Nurses, Breslin E, Lucas V, eds:* Women's health nursing: toward evidence-based practice, *St Louis, 2003, WB Saunders.)*

were used to help determine which alternative medicines would be included in this book:

- The therapy is the product of an orderly, rational, conscious system of knowledge and thought about health and medicine.
- The approach has been sustained over many generations by many practitioners in many communities.
- Treatments have been widely observed to have definable results.

The goal of this book is to provide not the most comprehensive guide but the most useful one. The book does not include obscure therapies practiced by only a few individuals in isolated settings, therapies that have poorly defined theoretical underpinnings, or therapies that lack perceptible results. The complementary therapies described in this book were chosen on the basis of a significant body of rational, clinical, and scientific information and judgment; a history of results; and increasing integration into the American medical mainstream. This integration is largely a response to consumer demand, which has created a $50 billion alternative medicine industry, but it also reflects the recognition of new scientific findings that are expanding our view of health and healing.

Although each tradition carries it own rich history, benefits, and perspective, some characteristics are common to all of the therapies and systems presented in this book. They are oriented toward wellness and take into consideration the capacity for self-healing. Nutrition and natural products are also essential resources (Figure 1-1).

WHO USES CAM?

Some years ago, the *Healthy People 2000* report articulated national public health goals for the coming decade. Of the five flagship goals, two did not "add up": to increase average longevity and to increase the average number of years of healthy life span. A marked discrepancy existed between these goals of increased longevity and increased healthy life span, with the latter goal several years shorter than the former.

Today increasing concern exists that longevity should not outdistance healthy life span and mounting evidence that therapies classified as holistic, alternative, and complementary provide benefits. Most diseases and disorders are age related. Age is the largest single risk factor for most cancers and many chronic diseases.

The use of CAM is widespread and on the increase among American adults.[1] A recent survey showed that two thirds of adults claim use of CAM by age 33.[2] Furthermore, CAM use is most prevalent among post–baby boomers (7 of 10), with only 5 of 10 baby boomers and 3 of 10 preboomers turning to CAM. These trends may represent an openness to CAM that has more to do with the management of medical conditions than with lifelong attitudes inclusive of "holistic" healing.

In addition, two thirds of health maintenance organizations offered at least one type of alternative therapy as of 1999, with acupuncture, massage, and nutritional therapy the most likely modalities to be covered. The best predictor of CAM use is higher education, perhaps reflecting a greater amount of disposable income, as well as knowledge, awareness, and attitudes about CAM.

Regional variations are quite consistent, with one half to two thirds of respondents from such diverse areas as South Carolina, Northern California, Florida, and Oregon indicating that they use CAM. As many as half of all clients who use CAM say they have not told their physicians they are doing so, indicating that much additional work to integrate CAM into the continuum of care is needed.

A large proportion of adults with cancer—80% or more, in some surveys—use CAM. In one study, 40% of CAM users said they abandoned conventional care after turning to alternative therapy. As many as 74% of patients with breast cancer said they used CAM, despite the relative effectiveness of conventional care (see Chapter 15).

The use of CAM is also prevalent among individuals with neurologic diseases, psychiatric disorders, physical disabilities, psoriasis, diabetes, and other ailments.[3] The range of CAM modalities is reflected in the topics covered in this book.

In addition to their use in the management of medical conditions, CAM therapies have gained increasing attention in the prevention of chronic disease. Although CAM is often considered a means of achieving a healthy lifestyle and preventing disease, in fact the evidence supports the effectiveness of CAM in treatment. Increasing numbers of clinical trials of CAM are being conducted, whereas prevention trials are larger, longer, more costly, more complex, and, ultimately, rarer.[4]

Nonetheless, a 2003 article in the *Journal of the American Medical Association* documented the importance of nutrition and confirmed the role of dietary supplementation in light of the typical American diet and nutrient composition of foods.[5] The use of dietary supplements is already prevalent among older Americans.

HEALTH AND WELLNESS

Thirty years ago health in America meant freedom from symptoms severe enough to interfere with job performance and family life. Today health is perceived as a continuum. At one end is optimal wellness, with body, mind, and spirit functioning harmoniously and the individual flourishing; at the other end is a health crisis such as trauma or acute illness. It is at the crisis end of the spectrum that Western science, with its sophisticated, lifesaving diagnostic tools and interventions, has the most to offer. Alternative therapies are designed to enhance physical, emotional, and spiritual well-being in daily life so that an individual is less likely to become ill or be injured. When a medical concern or crisis arises, some complementary and alternative therapies may help address urgent needs, such as anesthesia or burn medication; all support recovery and healing.

All healing involves inner healing. People heal from the inside out. CAM invites the patient to be a full and active partner in creating conditions that promote a return to health. The mobilization of inner healing resources can involve one or many approaches, including such complementary practices as breathing exercises, herbs, and acupuncture, as well as mainstream medical interventions such as drugs and surgery. Part of the self-healing process involves learning enough about the options to make valid choices from among the many types of treatment available.

Every form of medicine monitors the body's energy in some way. Allopathic medicine measures the body's energy through the use of electrocardiography, electroencephalography, and electromyography. Asian and other healing traditions not only evaluate energy as an index to the body's condition but also manipulate energy flow to maintain and restore health. In these traditions, the emphasis is on the flow and balance of energy, implying a

---

Qi

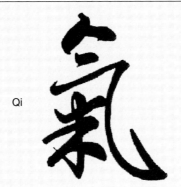

Qi

Chinese character for Qi. *(From Micozzi MS: Fundamentals of complementary and integrative medicine, ed. 3, St. Louis, 2006, Elsevier.)*

The Chinese character *qi*, which signifies the vital energy of the body, is a stylized drawing of steam rising from a bowl of rice. As the cornerstone of the Chinese diet, rice represents all food, even life itself. The portion of the character portraying rice depicts roots and stems, reflecting the individual's connection to the earth and all living things. The steam suggests that vital energy flows through us as naturally as steam rises from a bowl of rice.

dynamic interaction that is different from a static concept of matter. Known as *qi* (pronounced "chi") in China, *ki* in Japan, and *prana* in India, life energy is thought to flow through the body in deep rivers of energy known as meridians; when this flow is blocked or becomes stagnant, the body's organs can no longer function properly, and illness results. In Chinese medicine, an acupuncturist seeks to remove the blockage of *qi* by inserting extremely fine needles at critical points along the meridians. Other traditions, such as India's ancient practice of *ayurveda,* incorporate breathing, warm oil massage, and other techniques to stimulate the healthy flow of energy and relieve suffering.

The human body, as a physical entity and an energy system, evolves and exists in an ecological system. Years of evolution have resulted in a human organism adapted to draw nutrition from the plants, animals, and minerals that occur in its natural environment. In CAM, the potential long-term effects of many new artificial substances and processes, which may have been tested in accordance with biomedical criteria but not for their subtler interactions with the body as understood in alternative approaches, are a matter of concern. CAM practitioners believe that natural products enhance the body's energy and healing abilities more effectively, without the health risks associated with artificial components.

What is deeply rooted in nature cannot be uprooted.—*Lau Tzu*

The true focus of integrative medicine is neither the medical system nor the practitioner but the individual. Each person is viewed as unique, with highly individual resources capable of supporting the healing process. For example, a homeopathic physician treating five patients with the same condition might prescribe five different natural remedies because the physician would be aware, through extensive discussion and examination, of the details of each person's health history and health issues. With the needs of each individual determining treatment, practitioners and patients often go outside the realm of a single alternative medical system to draw on other practices. For instance, an osteopathic physician might also treat patients with acupuncture, a chiropractor might practice in an ayurvedic clinic, and an allopathic surgeon might include therapeutic touch in the care plan. Naturopathy, one of the most recent homegrown alternatives from the Western tradition, embraces a variety of therapies ranging from acupuncture to herbal medicine. This individualistic, eclectic approach complicates the work of conventional researchers and clinical practitioners, who find it very difficult to apply to alternative therapies such essential biomedical concepts as normalization, standardization, and generalization. But the consumer appreciates being treated as an individual, especially in the American culture, with its historical emphasis on individualism and freedom of choice. A growing number of Americans are no longer satisfied with a single, monolithic health care system, instead preferring to explore all their options and choose the ones that, in their opinion, offer the greatest possible health benefits.

In creating this text, we analyzed a wide range of individual therapies and healing systems to present the findings of a rapidly growing body of research into these practices and describe the foundations of each approach. The most widely used alternative practices, including herbs and aromatherapy, nutrition, Chinese medicine/acupuncture, the Indian practice of *ayurveda,* and chiropractic, are reviewed.

You can approach this book in several ways. You might read it from start to finish for the fullest possible understanding of the subject. Or you could start by exploring the particular medical problems, therapies, and systems that concern you most. Like alternative medicines themselves, this book is designed to be flexible, eclectic, and fine-tuned to meet individual needs.

References

1. Micozzi MS: *Fundamentals of complementary and integrative medicine*, ed. 3, St. Louis, 2006, Elsevier.
2. Kessler RC, Davis RB, Foster DF, et al: Long term trends in the use of CAM therapies in the US, *Ann Intern Med* 135:262-268, 2001.
3. Wooton JC, Sparber A: Surveys of complementary and alternative medicine usage. *Semin Integrative Med* 1:10-24, 2003.
4. Moon TE, Micozzi MS: *Nutrition and cancer prevention: investigating the role of micronutrients*, New York, 1989, Marcel Dekker.
5. Fletcher RH, Fairfield KM: Vitamins for chronic disease prevention in adults, *JAMA* 287: 3127-3129, 2002.

CHAPTER

2

Weight Loss Products

Obesity is an urgent and growing health problem in the United States. The U.S. Surgeon General reports that the risks of overweight and obesity may soon cause as much morbidity and mortality as does cigarette smoking. The prevalence of obesity in the United States is increasing to epidemic proportions. At present, more than 60% of Americans are overweight.[1]

Overweight and obesity are determined by measurement of body mass index (BMI), which is a measure of weight for height generally defined as weight in kilograms divided by the square of height in meters. A BMI of 25 to 29.9 in an adult indicates that the individual is overweight; obesity is defined as a BMI of 30 or greater (Table 2-1). The Centers for Disease Control and Prevention (CDC) has developed special charts to calculate BMI in children and adolescents. Overweight and obesity have been associated with a constellation of major risk factors and life habit risk factors that constitute a condition called the metabolic syndrome. The CDC estimates that one in five adults in the United States already has metabolic syndrome and this number is growing. Evidence indicates that metabolic syndrome is a major risk factor for cardiovascular disease and diabetes. The root causes of metabolic syndrome are poor diet, obesity, and sedentary lifestyle (Box 2-1).

In response to the staggering impact on the health of Americans, the Office of the U.S. Secretary of Health and Human Services has challenged both the public and private sectors to develop comprehensive efforts for controlling the obesity epidemic and improving physical activity levels in the U.S. population. Many consumers turn to a variety of diets and diet products in an attempt to manage their weight. Little evidence supports the benefit or safety of the large majority of these products and practices. The following discussion covers the most common dietary supplements promoted for weight loss.

DIETARY SUPPLEMENTS AND WEIGHT LOSS

Most dietary supplements currently used for weight loss are adrenergic stimulants or antiabsorptive agents. The adrenergic stimulants, such as ephedra, have been associated

Table **2-1**

Body mass index	
BODY MASS INDEX (WEIGHT/STATURE^2)	**WEIGHT STATUS**
Below 18.5	Underweight
18.5-24.9	Normal
25.0-29.9	Overweight
≥30.0	Obese

From http://www.cdc.gov/nccdphp/dnpa/bmi/calc-bmi.htm#English.

with adverse central nervous system and cardiovascular effects. The antiabsorptive agents appear to be safer than the adrenergic stimulants but can cause gastrointestinal side effects.

Ephedra *(Ephedra sinica, E. equisentina, E. intermedia)*

Ephedra, also known as ma-huang, was widely sold as a dietary supplement for weight loss and to enhance athletic performance in the United States until February 2004. Before its introduction in the West, Asian populations had used ephedra as an herbal remedy for asthma, cough, headache, fever, allergies, and congestion for more than 5000 years. Ephedra is the common name for three principal species: *Ephedra sinica, E. equisentina,* and *E. intermedia.* Asian species of ephedra contain varying amounts of pharmacologically active ephedrine alkaloids, mainly ephedrine and pseudoephedrine, whereas North American species (commonly referred to as Mormon tea) contain small amounts or are devoid of these alkaloids.[1] Ephedrine was first isolated from ephedra in 1887 by Japanese chemist N. Nagai but did not gain popularity in the West until K.K. Chen and Carl F. Schmidt published a series of studies on the pharmacological properties of ephedrine in

Box **2-1**

Diagnostic criteria for metabolic syndrome
Metabolic syndrome is a cluster of at least three of the following signs:
■ Abdominal obesity (waist circumference >102 cm [40 inches] in men, >88 cm [35 inches] in women)
■ Hypertriglyceridemia (>150 mg/dL)
■ Low concentration of high-density lipoprotein cholesterol (<40 mg/dL in men, <50 mg/dL in women)
■ High blood pressure (>130/85 mm Hg)
■ High fasting glucose level (impaired glucose tolerance [blood glucose > 110 mg/dL and <126 mg/dL] without diabetes)

the 1920s.[2] Research has shown that ephedrine stimulates heart rate, resulting in increased cardiac output, while constricting peripheral blood vessels, which leads to increased peripheral resistance and blood pressure.[3] Ephedrine relaxes bronchial smooth muscle, which explains its long history of use in the treatment of asthma.[3]

Efficacy. Ephedra has become one of the most controversial herbs on the U.S. market. Because so many questions have been raised with regard to the safety and efficacy of ephedra-containing products for weight loss and "energy enhancement," the government commissioned a review of the data to determine what action, if any, should be taken with regard to the sale of these products. The Rand Group conducted a meta-analysis of 20 trials of ephedra or ephedrine for weight loss. Of the 20 studies, only five tested herbal ephedra formulations as contained in products. Most of the studies were limited by methodological problems (particularly high attrition rates, which are typical with the use of weight loss products), and the reviewers noted that this might have contributed to bias. Nevertheless, their findings support an association between the short-term use of ephedrine, ephedrine plus caffeine, or dietary supplements that contain ephedra (with or without herbs containing caffeine) and a statistically significant increase in short-term weight loss compared with that seen with placebo. Both ephedra and ephedrine result in weight loss of approximately 2 lb per month more than that with placebo for as long as 4 to 6 months.[4]

The findings of the Rand Group review are reflected in another recent study, a randomized, double-blind, placebo-controlled trial of 167 subjects given a product containing 90 mg of ephedrine and 192 mg of caffeine per day as an adjunct to diet and exercise for 6 months.[5] The treated group lost 4.0 kg, compared with 0.8 kg in the placebo group. In addition to the weight loss noted in the treatment group, 23% of the treatment group withdrew after experiencing adverse effects, which included hypertension, chest pain, and palpitations. No participants withdrew from the placebo group. Translation of these fndings to to the general population of overweight Americans, many of whom may have undiagnosed hypertension or heart disease, should raise concerns.

Safety. The government-commissioned review of ephedra products also included a safety analysis based on controlled trials. The use of ephedrine, ephedra-containing dietary supplements, or ephedrine plus caffeine is associated with two or three times the risk of nausea, vomiting, psychiatric symptoms such as anxiety or change in mood, autonomic hyperactivity, and palpitations compared with placebo. However, the numbers of people treated in the clinical trials were quite small, thereby limiting a true estimate of risk. Therefore the Rand Group also reviewed 71 cases reported in the published medical literature, 1820 case reports provided by the U.S. Food and Drug Administration (FDA), and more than 18,000 consumer complaints reported to a manufacturer of ephedra-containing dietary supplements.[4]

Because most of the cases lacked appropriate documentation, only 65 cases from the published literature, 241 cases from the FDA, and 43 cases from the manufacturer were included in the analysis of adverse events. Reviewers found that sentinel events with prior ephedra consumption included two deaths, three myocardial infarctions, nine cerebrovascular/stroke events, three seizures, and five psychiatric cases. Sentinel events with prior ephedrine consumption included three deaths, two myocardial infarctions, two cerebrovascular/stroke events, one seizure, and three psychiatric cases. Approximately half of the sentinel events occurred in people 30 years of age or younger. An additional 43 cases were identified as possible sentinel events with prior ephedra consumption, and an additional seven cases were identified as possible sentinel events with prior ephedrine consumption.

Marketing. The marketing and promotion of ephedra/caffeine-containing products for weight loss and energy enhancement on the Internet has been a concern from a public safety perspective. Thirty-two products and advertisements were identified and systematically evaluated for deviance from truth-in-advertising standards. Of the 32 Web sites analyzed, 13 (41%) failed to disclose potential adverse effects or contraindications to supplement use. Seventeen (53%) did not reveal the recommended dosage of ephedra alkaloids. More important, 11 sites (34%) contained incorrect or misleading statements, some of which could directly result in serious harm to consumers.[6] Certain individuals, including those with heart disease, cerebrovascular disease, hypertension, diabetes, thyroid disease, and enlarged prostate, should *not* use these products. These supplements should not be taken by women who are pregnant or breastfeeding or by individuals taking certain psychiatric medications.

Summary. Ephedra is used in small doses in traditional Chinese medicine as, well as in Western herbal medicine, primarily for respiratory problems; this use does not appear to be dangerous. Virtually all adverse effects reported with ephedra have been associated with products intended for weight loss, exercise enhancement, energy enhancement, or recreational use, none of which is a traditional indication and all of which involve doses designed to increase metabolism.[7] Although some evidence indicates that these products can cause weight loss in the short term, the long-term safety and efficacy of ephedra with and without caffeine are unknown.

In response to the growing body of concern about the safety of ephedra products for weight loss, the FDA added Part 119 to Title 21 of the Code of Federal Regulations, entitled "Dietary supplements that present a significant or unreasonable risk." The full text of the rule (new Part 119.1) is as follows:

> Dietary supplements containing ephedrine alkaloids present an unreasonable risk of illness or injury under conditions of use recommended or suggested in the labeling, or if no conditions of use are recommended or suggested in the labeling, under ordinary conditions of use. Therefore, dietary supplements containing ephedrine alkaloids are adulterated under section 402(f)(1)(A) of the Federal Food, Drug, and Cosmetic Act.[8]

Bitter Orange *(Citrus aurantium)*

Citrus aurantium (also known as bitter, sour, or Seville orange) originated in China and seems to have entered the written record there by 300 BC. By about 100 BC, *C. aurantium* seeds appear to have reached Rome. The dried orange peel was traditionally used as a digestive tonic and flavoring agent. The German Commission E recognizes the use of dried *C. aurantium* peel for dyspeptic complaints and loss of appetite.[9] Many companies are substituting *C. aurantium* for ephedra in their weight loss formulations as a result of the unfavorable publicity of ephedra in the media. The use of *C. aurantium* will likely grow now that the ephedra ban is in place. *C. aurantium* is made from the dried outer part of the pericarp of the ripe or nearly ripe fruit.[10] It contains synephrine and octopamine, among other compounds, and has been reported in two studies to aid weight loss and in three to increase thermogenesis, at least to some extent.[11] Synephrine and octopamine are phenolamines found in sympathetic nerve fibers. Synephrine is similar to adrenaline, and octopamine is similar to noradrenaline (differing only in the number of hydroxyl groups on the aromatic ring).[12] Synephrine activates both α-adrenoreceptors and β_3-adrenoreceptors; both synephrine and octopamine inhibit production of cyclic adenosine monophosphate. β_3-Adrenoreceptor agonists are full lipolytic agents in rats, hamsters, and dogs but are less active in human beings.[7]

A double-blind, randomized, placebo-controlled, three-armed study of 23 subjects with BMIs of more than 25 kg/m^2 compared treatment, placebo, and no intervention as an adjunct to a 1800-calorie American Heart Association step I diet and a weight circuit training exercise program 3 days a week under the direction of an exercise physiologist.[13] The treatment product tested contained a daily dosage of 975 mg of *C. aurantium* extract (6% synephrine alkaloids), 528 mg of caffeine, and 900 mg of St. John's wort (3% hypericum) and was administered for 6 weeks. Outcome measures included weight, fat loss, and mood. Twenty subjects completed the study. Treated subjects lost a significant amount of weight (mean 1.4 kg) compared with the placebo group (mean 0.9 kg) and control group (mean 0.04 kg). However, the table in the article appears to indicate that the differences are significant compared with the baseline but not between groups. The amount of caffeine in this product is the rough equivalent of four cups of coffee or 10 cups of tea. The treatment group lost 2.9% body fat; no significant change was noted in the placebo and control groups. The researchers detected no significant changes in any group in a questionnaire profiling the subjects' mood states or in blood lipid levels, blood pressure, heart rate, electrocardiographic findings, serum chemistry values, or urinalysis. The treated group demonstrated a significant increase in basal metabolic rate, whereas the placebo group showed a significant decrease in basal metabolic rate; no change was noted in the no-treatment group. No side effects were reported. (NOTE: Although the trial lists the St. John's wort as containing 3% hypericum, it likely means the product was standardized to 0.3% hypericin. Assuming that the 3% hypericum reported in the study actually means 0.3% hypericin, the dose of St. John's wort in this product would be a therapeutic antidepressant dose.)

Small amounts of synephrine occur naturally in many citrus products. Human populations consume Seville, or sour-orange, juice without adverse effects. A crossover open-label safety study in 12 normotensive subjects ranging from 20 to 27 years of age was conducted to evaluate the cardiovascular effects of two doses of *C. aurantium* juice (8 oz, 8 hours apart). The test was repeated with water a week later. Blood pressure was measured every hour for 5 hours after the second dose of juice; systolic and diastolic blood pressure, mean arterial pressure, and heart rate were not significantly altered. It was estimated that the subjects consumed 13 or 14 mg of synephrine, comparable to a dose of phenylephrine in a decongestant-containing cold preparation.[14]

Pharmacokinetic data and safety studies have not been published on the high potency of synephrine-containing products. Any sympathomimetic agent in sufficient amounts can increase thermogenesis and cannot be presumed to be safe, especially in individuals with cardiovascular disease. *C. aurantium* extract has caused cardiac disturbances in animals.[14] Extracts available on the Internet contain between 4% and 50% synephrine, far greater than the amount that occurs naturally in the fruit and rind (0.25% to 2%). The extracts sold in weight loss products do not represent the traditional uses or doses of the crude herb. *C. aurantium,* known as zhishi or chih-shih in traditional Chinese medicine, has been used safely in the treatment of epigastric pain, constipation, and other digestive disorders for centuries. The safety accorded to crude preparations of bitter-orange peel cannot be extrapolated to weight loss products containing highly concentrated levels of adrenergic compounds.

Chitosan

As a dietary supplement, chitosan is claimed to control obesity and decrease serum cholesterol levels. Chitosan is a cationic polysaccharide derived from chitin in the exoskeletons of arthropods; the usual commercial source is the shells of shrimp and crab (necessitating caution on the part of individuals with shellfish allergies). Promoted as a "fat trapper," chitosan forms a positively charged gel in the stomach and binds negatively charged fats to its tertiary amine group; it also decreases normal cholesterol emulsification through hydrophobic binding. It becomes insoluble in the alkaline environment of the intestine, forming aggregates with fats and bile acids and interrupting enterohepatic recirculation.[15]

Clinical trials have shown a weight loss effect when chitosan was given with a hypocaloric diet for as long as 4 weeks, but a meta-analysis of these studies shows discrepancies in the data, suggesting that the studies are flawed.[16] A recent randomized, double-blind, placebo-controlled trial of 34 overweight volunteers (30 completed the trial) given 2 g/day of deacetylated chitin failed to show any difference between groups with regard to weight, blood pressure, cholesterol and triglyceride concentrations, or levels of vitamins A, D, and E or β-carotene.[17]

Because the premise of chitosan is that it traps fat in the bowel, leading to weight loss, this hypothesis was tested. A study was conducted to evaluate the effect of chitosan on fat absorption in 15 healthy men. Participants consumed no supplements during a 4-day control period, followed by two capsules of chitosan five times a day (4.5 g chitosan/day), 30 minutes before each meal, during a 4-day supplement period. All feces were collected from days 2 to 12. Oral charcoal markers permitted division of the feces into two periods. The two fecal pools were analyzed for fat content. With chitosan supplementation of 10 capsules/day, fecal fat excretion increased by 1.1 ± 1.8 g/day ($P = 0.02$), from 6.1 ± 1.2 to 7.2 ± 1.8 g/day. This level of fat excretion is not clinically meaningful and would have no measurable effect on energy balance.[18]

The safety of chitosan has been good in short-term animal studies. Only a few studies of chitosan have been conducted in human beings. In short-term trials of up to 12 weeks, no clinically significant symptoms have been observed with chitosan compared with placebo. Mild, transitory nausea and constipation have been reported in 2.6% to 5.4% of subjects.[15] If the product truly were a fat-antiresorptive agent, steatorrhea would be a concern. On the basis of the data observed to date, chitosan does not appear to offer much benefit to those trying to lose weight.

Hydroxycitrate (Derived from *Garcinia cambogia*)

Hydroxycitric acid is derived from the rind of the exotic Malabar tamarind (*Garcinia cambogia*), a citrus fruit. Animal studies have indicated that hydroxycitrate suppresses fatty acid synthesis, lipogenesis, reduces food intake, and induces weight loss. In vitro studies have revealed the inhibition of fatty acid synthesis and lipogenesis from various precursors. However, clinical studies have yielded controversial findings.[19] At this time, eight trials have been conducted to evaluate the effectiveness of *Garcinia*, or hydroxycitric acid, for weight loss. Five of the studies showed beneficial effects, two were published only as abstracts, and all had methodological shortcomings that could have introduced bias.

The most rigorous trial published to date was a 12-week, randomized, double-blind, placebo-controlled trial in an outpatient weight control research unit in New York of 135 overweight men and women ages 18 to 65 years with a mean BMI of 32 kg/m^2. Both groups consumed a high-fiber, low-energy diet and were given placebo or the active product (*G. cambogia* in a daily dose of 3000 mg containing 1500 mg of hydroxycitric acid) three times a day, 30 minutes before meals, for 12 weeks. Both groups lost weight, and no significant difference was detected between the two groups at the conclusion of the trial. Reported adverse effects were minor and not significantly different between the two groups.[20] Critics of this study point out that participants were not placed on a high-carbohydrate diet and since blood levels of hydroxycitrate were not monitored, it is unclear if enough of the active was absorbed to achieve a therapeutic effect. The amount of active ingredient used in the trial may also have been inadequate. Clearly, more research is needed in this area.

Caffeine-Containing Supplements

Many weight loss products contain botanicals that are sources of caffeine. Guarana seed (*Paullinia cupana*) and kola nut (*Kola nitida*) are often found in combination with ephedra and bitter orange. Green tea (*Camellia sinensis*) extracts are being promoted in the American marketplace as a natural product to aid weight loss. Although clinical trials have been conducted to examine the effects of caffeine on weight loss, they have usually involved caffeine in combination with other substances. When caffeine (200 mg/day) was added to an energy-restricted diet in a placebo-controlled, double-blind trial, it was no more effective than placebo in promoting weight loss.[21] Caffeine-chromium-dietary fiber combinations have not been found to cause greater weight loss than that seen in a control group.[22] Caffeine-ephedrine/ephedra combinations have been shown to cause greater weight loss than placebo, but adverse events are a concern (see previous discussion). Controlled studies have not shown fat loss in overweight individuals using caffeine in the absence of an energy-restricted diet.[23]

Although attention has been focused on caffeine, tea may have thermogenic effects that are not entirely the result of the presence of this alkaloid. A crossover study of 10 healthy men and involving the use of a respiratory chamber at the University of Geneva tested green tea extract on energy expenditure in fat oxidation.[24] On separate occasions, subjects were given green tea extract (50 mg of caffeine, 90 mg of epigallocatechin gallate), caffeine (50 mg), or placebo, which they ingested at breakfast, lunch, and dinner. Respiratory quotient, 24-hour energy expenditure, and urinary excretion of nitrogen and catecholamines were measured. Ingestion of green tea extract resulted in a significant increase in 24-hour energy expenditure (4%; $P < 0.01$) and a significant decrease in 24-hour respiratory quotient (from 0.88 to 0.85; $P < 0.001$) with no change in urinary nitrogen. Norepinephrine excretion was 40% greater during treatment with green tea than during administration of placebo ($P < 0.05$). Caffeine had no effect on energy expenditure, respiratory quotient, urinary nitrogen, or urinary catecholamines. No significant changes in heart rate were noted during the first 8 hours of assessment. One possible explanation for the additional thermogenic qualities is that flavonoids called catechins in tea inhibit the enzyme that degrades norepinephrine (which helps control thermogenesis and fat oxidation).[7] Mice made obese through the administration of a high-fat diet were treated with oolong tea for 10 weeks. Food consumption was not affected, but oolong tea prevented the obesity and fatty liver induced by a high-fat diet. Lipolysis of fat cells was enhanced, an effect found to be the result of caffeine; however, oolong tea extract inhibited pancreatic lipase activity, which would not be expected with caffeine.[25]

Chromium

Chromium is an essential trace element for mammals and is required for the maintenance of proper carbohydrate and lipid metabolism. In addition to its effects on glucose, insulin, and lipid metabolism, chromium has been reported to increase lean body mass and decrease body-fat percentage, which may lead to weight loss in human beings. The authors of several double-blind, placebo-controlled studies have reported on the effects of chromium supplementation and weight loss. Most studies revealed either a small effect or no effect at all.[26] Although chromium supplementation has been widely promoted as a way for athletes to decrease fat and increase lean muscle mass, after more than a decade of human studies with chromium picolinate, most of the findings have failed to demonstrate beneficial effects of chromium on the body composition of healthy individuals, even when taken in combination with an exercise program.[27]

Questions of safety have been raised with large doses or prolonged ingestion of chromium. Recent cell culture and in vivo rat studies have indicated that chromium picolinate generates oxidative damage to DNA and lipids and is mutagenic, although the significance of these results on human subjects taking the supplement for prolonged periods is unknown.[27]

Conjugated Linoleic Acid

Dietary supplements containing conjugated linoleic acid (CLA) are widely promoted as natural weight loss agents. CLA appears to produce fat loss and increase lean tissue mass in rodents, but the results from 13 randomized, controlled, short-term trials (<6 months) have yielded little evidence that CLA reduces body weight or promotes repartitioning of body fat and fat-free mass in human beings.[28]

Summary

Although some evidence indicates that ephedra/ephedrine, with or without caffeine, can increase weight loss over that achieved with a placebo, most products now being promoted as effective aids to weight loss do not deliver what they promise. More research is needed in the area of obesity; however, what is now known is that a diet rich in fruits, vegetables,

Box 2-2

Hints for a healthier diet

- Fill your plate with fresh fruits and vegetables. Fruits and vegetables are low in calories and fat and rich in nutrients, including cancer-fighting antioxidants.
- Use oil as the principal fat in your diet, reducing other fats such as butter and margarine.
- Keep saturated fat to less than 10% of your total calories.
- Add nonfat or low-fat yogurt to your daily diet.
- Eat whole grains and heavy, crusty bread. Avoid refined breads and cereals.
- Eat fish and poultry several times a week (if not vegetarian); limit red meat to a few servings per month.
- When dining out, look for dishes with plenty of vegetables and very little cream or cheese. Grilled fish with steamed vegetables and vegetarian pasta tossed in olive oil with a little Parmesan cheese are good choices.
- Avoid all-you-can-eat restaurants.
- For dessert, choose something that provides one serving of fruit (e.g., baked pears or apples with cinnamon, nutmeg, and a small amount of sugar, topped with yogurt). Limit sweets that are high in sugar and saturated fat to one serving a week.
- Emphasize the social aspect of eating. Meals are a time to get together, visit, and connect with friends and family.
- Moderate consumption of wine with a meal; one glass per day for women. (This is optional and should be avoided if you have a problem with alcohol.)

---

low-fat dairy products, lean meats, and whole grains in appropriate portion sizes, accompanied by daily physical activity, is one of the safest and most effective ways of managing weight (Box 2-2). Pharmacologic and surgical interventions may be appropriate for those who are morbidly obese but are generally not necessary for the overweight or mildly obese individual.

Obese individuals are often disheartened and depressed after multiple attempts at losing weight have failed or been short-lived. Many turn to unproven therapies and treatments, most of which are ineffective. Cycling on and off failed weight loss regimens ultimately can make weight loss harder (popularly called the "yo-yo syndrome"). Obesity is a chronic disease, like high blood pressure or asthma, except that many obese individuals have been the object of scorn because of the visibility of their disorder. Creating strategies for optimizing health, not necessarily achieving a "normal" body weight, is probably a more effective approach for health care providers. Losing just 10 to 20 lb can significantly decrease cardiovascular risk in obese individuals.

Physical activity is overlooked in many weight loss programs. Practitioners should encourage increases in all activities of daily living, not just going to the health club. Studies have shown that just walking 3 hours a week reduces a woman's risk of a heart attack by roughly 40%.

TOP REASONS TO EXERCISE FOR WEIGHT CONTROL & FITNESS

Exercise helps you maintain a healthy weight and fitness level. Cutting just 250 calories from the daily diet can help you lose half a pound a week—add a 30-minute brisk walk 4 days a week, and you can double your rate of weight loss. Regular exercise helps reduce abdominal fat, the type associated with the development of diabetes and high blood pressure.

Beyond individual responsibility, communities must become actively involved in ensuring that healthy foods are available for everyone, that safe environments are available for physical activity, that schools provide regular exercise programs for children along with healthy meals, and that workplaces are encouraged to promote healthy environments.

References

1. Caveney S, Charlet DA, Freitag H, et al: New observations on the secondary chemistry of world Ephedra (Ephedraceae), *Am J Botany* 88:1199-1208, 2001.
2. Tyler V: *Herbs of choice: the therapeutic use of phytomedicinals,* Pharmaceutical Products Press, 1994.
3. Hardman JG, Limbird LE, Gilman A, editors: *Goodman and Gilman's the pharmacological basis of disease,* New York, 2001, McGraw-Hill.
4. Evidence report/technology assessment number 76: Ephedra and ephedrine for weight loss and athletic performance enhancement: clinical efficacy and side effects. Available at: www.ahrq.gov. Accessed September 2003.
5. Boozer CN, Daly PA, Homel P, et al: Herbal ephedra/caffeine for weight loss: a 6-month randomized safety and efficacy trial, *Int J Obes Relat Metab Disord* 26:593-604, 2002.
6. Ashar BH, Miller RG, Getz KJ, et al: A critical evaluation of Internet marketing of products that contain ephedra, *Mayo Clin Proc* 78:944-946, 2003.
7. Fugh Berman A, Low Dog T: Dietary supplements for weight loss, *Alternative Therapies in Women's Health* 4:81-88, 2002.
8. Department of Health and Human Services, Food and Drug Administration: Final rule declaring dietary supplements containing ephedrine alkaloids adulterated because they present an unreasonable risk. Available at: http://www.fda.gov/OHRMS/DOCKETS/98fr/1995n-0304-nfr0001. pdf. Accessed February 2004.
9. Wichtl M, Grainger Bisset N, editors: Herbal drugs and phytopharmaceuticals, London, 1994, CRC Press, pp 94-95.
10. Evans WC: *Trease and Evans pharmacognosy,* 15th ed, London, 2002, Saunders, pp 266-67.
11. Preuss HG, DiFerdinando D, Bagchi M, et al: *Citrus aurantium* as a thermogenic weight-reduction replacement for ephedra: an overview, *J Med* 33:247-264, 2002.
12. Airriess CN, Rudling JE, Midgley JM, et al: Selective inhibition of adenylyl cyclase by octopamine via a human cloned alpha 2A-adrenoceptor, *Br J Pharmacol* 122:191-198, 1997.
13. Colker CM, Kalman DS, Torina GC, et al: Effects of *Citrus aurantium* extract, caffeine and St. John's wort on body fat loss, lipid levels and mood states in overweight healthy adults, *Curr Ther Res* 60:145-153, 1999.
14. Penzak SR, Jann MW, Cold JA, et al: Seville (sour) orange juice: synephrine content and cardiovascular effects in normotensive adults, *J Clin Pharmacol* 41:1059-1063, 2001.
15. Ylitalo R, Lehtinen S, Wuolijoki E, et al: Cholesterol-lowering properties and safety of chitosan, *Arzneimittelforschung* 52:1-7, 2002.
16. Ernst E, Pittler MH: A meta-analysis of chitosan for body weight reduction, *Perfusion* 11: 461-465, 1998.

17. Pittler MH, Abbot NC, Harkness EF, et al: Randomized, double-blind trial of chitosan for body weight reduction, *Eur J Clin Nutr* 53:379-381, 1999.
18. Gades MD, Stern JS: Chitosan supplementation and fecal fat excretion in men, *Obes Res* 11:683-688, 2003.
19. Jena BS, Jayaprakasha GK, Singh RP, et al: Chemistry and biochemistry of (-)-hydroxycitric acid from *Garcinia, J Agric Food Chem* 50:10-22, 2002.
20. Heymsfield SB, Allison DB, Vasselli JR, et al: *Garcinia cambogia* (hydroxycitric acid) as a potential antiobesity agent: a randomized controlled trial, *JAMA* 280:1596-1600, 1998.
21. Astrup A, Breum L, Toubro S, et al: The effect and safety of an ephedrine/caffeine compound compared with ephedrine, caffeine and placebo in obese subjects on an energy restricted diet: a double blind trial, *Int J Obes* 16:269-277, 1992.
22. Pasman WJ, Westerterp-Plantenga MS, Saris WH: The effectiveness of long-term supplementation of carbohydrate, chromium, fibre and caffeine on weight maintenance, *Int J Obes* 21:1143-1151, 1997.
23. Egger G, Cameron-Smith D, Stanton R: The effectiveness of popular, non-prescription weight loss supplements, *Med J Aust* 171:604-608, 1999.
24. Dulloo AG, Duret C, Rohrer D, et al: Efficacy of a green tea extract rich in catechin polyphenols and caffeine in increasing 24-h energy expenditure and fat oxidation in humans, *Am J Clin Nutr* 70:1040-1045, 1999.
25. Han LK, Takaku T, Li J, et al: Anti-obesity action of oolong tea, *Int J Obes Relat Metab Disord* 23:98-105, 1999.
26. Anderson RA: Effects of chromium on body composition and body weight, *Nutr Rev* 56:266-270, 1998.
27. Vincent JB: The potential value and toxicity of chromium picolinate as a nutritional supplement, weight loss agent and muscle development agent, *Sports Med* 33:213-230, 2003.
28. Larsen TM, Toubro S, Astrup A: Efficacy and safety of dietary supplements containing conjugated linoleic acid (CLA) for the treatment of obesity—evidence from animal and human studies, *J Lipid Res* 44:2234-2241, 2003.

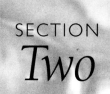

Reproductive Biology

Many women experience functional complaints related to the reproductive system through the phases of life. Integrative medicine offers approaches to help support the physiologic changes associated with premenstrual syndrome, menstrual cramps, and menopause.

Endometriosis is a pathologic condition of the reproductive system that may be addressed by integrative medical approaches.

This section presents chapters on the integrative medical management of premenstrual syndrome, menstrual cramps, endometriosis, and menopause.

Women are also concerned about more healthy and natural experiences with pregnancy, breastfeeding, and the postpartum interval. Chapters on integrative strategies during pregnancy, and on lactation, breastfeeding, and the postpartum period, provide a useful guide for the health of the mother and child.

3

Premenstrual Syndrome*

Premenstrual syndrome (PMS) is defined as a recurrent, cyclical set of physical and behavioral symptoms that occur 7 to 14 days before the menstrual cycle and are troublesome enough to interfere with some aspect of a woman's life. PMS is estimated to affect as many as 40% of menstruating women, with the most severe cases occurring in 2% to 5% of women between 26 and 35 years of age.[1] Although PMS has been recognized as a medical disorder for many years, its cause remains unknown and is heavily debated (Box 3-1). This uncertainty may explain the myriad of treatments that have been researched and are available in the marketplace.

Gonadal Hormones

A deficiency of progesterone or an abnormally high estrogen/progesterone ratio during the luteal phase has been a popular theory as to the cause of PMS for many years. However, studies of hormone levels in women with PMS compared with those in women without the disorder fail to support this hypothesis.[2]

Prolactin

Prolactin levels peak at the time of ovulation and remain high during the luteal phase. Prolactin excess may be associated with menstrual irregularities, diminished libido, depression, and hostility.[3] Some authors suggest that as many as 62% of women with menstrual disorders have some degree of increased prolactin.[4] Prolactin plays a role in breast stimulation and may be related to premenstrual breast tenderness. However, no consistent abnormalities in prolactin levels have been detected in women with PMS.[2]

Aldosterone

Aldosterone levels normally increase at the time of ovulation and remain high during the luteal phase of the menstrual cycle. This increase may be responsible for the congestive symptoms of PMS. Some women experience edema, breast swelling, abdominal bloating,

*This chapter is adapted from Chapter 45 in Rakel D: *Integrative medicine,* Philadelphia, 2003, Elsevier.

Box 3-1

Proposed causes of PMS

HORMONAL

Estrogen deficiency
Estrogen excess
High estrogen/progesterone ratio
Progesterone deficiency
Prolactin excess
β-Endorphin deficiency
Cortisol excess
Hypoglycemia
Reduced glucose tolerance
Thyroid abnormalities
Adrenal insufficiency

PROSTAGLANDINS

Prostaglandin excess
Prostaglandin deficiency
Essential fatty acid deficiencies

MICRONUTRIENTS

Pyridoxine deficiency
Vitamin A deficiency
Vitamin E deficiency
Magnesium deficiency
Calcium excess
Calcium deficiency
Potassium deficiency

FLUID AND ELECTROLYTE
IMBALANCE

Aldosterone excess
Vasopressin excess

High sodium/potassium ratio
Renin/angiotensin abnormalities

NEUROTRANSMITTERS

Serotonin deficiency
Dopamine deficiency
Norepinephrine deficiency
Low platelet MAO acitivity

HEREDITARY

Genetic risk

PSYCHOLOGICAL FACTORS

Beliefs about menstrual cycle
Co-existing psychiatric disorders
Poor coping skills
Poor self-esteem

SOCIAL FACTORS

Current marital/sexual relationship
Former marital/sexual relationships
Social stress
Psychosexual experiences
Cultural attitudes on PMS
Societal attitudes on PMS

weight gain, and headaches. Differences in absolute levels of aldosterone between symptomatic and asymptomatic women have not been found.[5]

Endogenous Opiates

Some researchers have noted an increase in β-endorphin plasma levels after ovulation. It is hypothesized that women with PMS have lower levels of these circulating endogenous opiates, or more sudden withdrawal, causing them to experience increased sensitivity to pain, as well as depression in some cases, in the luteal phase.[6]

A small trial was conducted to determine whether changes in peripheral β-endorphin levels during the periovulatory phase were associated with PMS symptoms. Twenty-one women with PMS and 10 control subjects were enrolled. All participants were in generally good health, with a history of regular menses for at least six cycles and no psychiatric illness. The day of the luteinizing hormone (LH) peak was called day LH-0. β-Endorphin and LH levels were measured with the use of a radioimmunoassay. Blood samples were obtained between 8 and 10 AM daily for 8 days, beginning on the 10th day of the menstrual cycle, for one cycle. β-Endorphin levels were lower throughout the periovulatory phase in the patients with PMS; the greatest differences were noted on LH days 0 and 4.[7] However, a 1998 study of 10 patients with PMS and 10 control subjects failed to show any differences in levels of β-endorphin, adrenocorticotropic hormone, cortisol, or testosterone after sampling of the subjects' blood over one complete menstrual cycle.[8]

Vitamin B$_6$

Vitamin B$_6$, or pyridoxine, is required for the metabolism of amino acids, carbohydrates, and lipids. The active forms of this vitamin are necessary coenzymes in the decarboxylation of 5-hydroxytryptophan to 5-hydroxytryptamine and dopa to dopamine. Pyridoxine deficiency is associated with increased levels of prolactin and low levels of serotonin and dopamine.[9] Pyridoxine deficiency can lead to depression, peripheral neuropathy, and mood changes. Vitamin B$_6$ has been subjected to numerous trials over the years. The evidence supporting pyridoxine deficiency as a cause of PMS symptoms is reviewed later in this chapter.

Magnesium

Although serum levels of magnesium are often normal in women with PMS, researchers have noted lower levels of magnesium in the red blood cells of women with the disorder.[10] Calcium and dairy products may interfere with absorption of magnesium, and refined sugar increases its urinary excretion. Magnesium deficiency can reduce dopamine and thyroid activity (with a resulting increase in the prolactin level) and lead to depression, mood changes, and muscle cramping.

Hypoglycemia

The body appears to be more sensitive to insulin during the luteal phase, leading some researchers to hypothesize that transient hypoglycemia accounts for some PMS symptoms.

Prostaglandins

Prostaglandins are associated with breast pain, fluid retention, abdominal cramping, headaches, irritability, and depression.[11] Physical premenstrual complaints and dysmenorrhea have been shown to respond to prostaglandin inhibitors.

Box **3-2**

Symptoms of premenstrual syndrome

More than 150 symptoms have been associated with PMS. The most common ones are listed.

Nervousness	Anxiety	Irritability
Fatigue	Lethargy	Depression
Mood swings	Water retention	Abdominal bloating
Breast tenderness	Headache	Changes in appetite
Back pain	Acne	Sugar/chocolate cravings
Diarrhea	Diminished libido	Constipation
Clumsiness	Dizziness	Low self-esteem
Social isolation	Insomnia	Joint pain

Psychosocial Theory

Emotional and physical stressors have been found to influence the levels of certain hormones and neurotransmitter substances. Travel, illness, stress, weather changes, and other environmental factors may affect ovulation, duration of the menstrual cycle, and the severity of PMS.[12] Cultural, societal, and personal attitudes toward menstruation also appear to play a role in the presence and severity of PMS. The dynamic interplay of environment, spirit, and physiology suggests that an integrated approach to treatment is most effective in many women (Box 3-2).

The American Psychiatric Association has defined diagnostic criteria for premenstrual dysphoric disorder (PMDD), considered by most physicians to be a more severe form of PMS. For this disorder to be diagnosed, a woman must have at least five of the following symptoms on a cyclical basis, and they must be serious enough to interfere with her normal activities:

- Feelings of sadness or hopelessness; possible suicidal thoughts
- Feelings of tension or anxiety
- Mood swings marked by periods of teariness
- Persistent irritability or anger
- Loss of interest in daily activities and relationships
- Trouble concentrating
- Fatigue or a low energy level
- Food cravings or eating binges
- Sleep disturbances
- Feelings of being out of control
- Physical symptoms, such as bloating, breast tenderness, headaches, and joint or muscle pain

CLASSIFICATION OF PREMENSTRUAL SYNDROME

Many women have a dominant set of symptoms, leading researchers to attempt to classify and categorize PMS symptoms. Guy Abraham developed one of the more popular classification schemes by breaking PMS symptoms into four distinct subgroups.[13] A summary of these categories follows:

- PMS-A (anxiety): Believed to be related to high levels of estrogen, deficiency of progesterone, or both. Affected women experience irritability, anxiety, and emotional lability.
- PMS-C (carbohydrate craving): Origin is unclear; may be due to enhanced intracellular binding of insulin. Affected individuals experience increased appetite, sugar and carbohydrate cravings, headache, and heart palpitations.
- PMS-D (depression): Thought to be a result of a low level of estrogen leading to an excessive breakdown of neurotransmitters, which results in depression.
- PMS-H (hyperhydration): Possibly due to increased water retention resulting from increased levels of aldosterone. Higher levels of aldosterone during the premenstrual period may be the result of excess estrogen, excessive salt intake, stress, or magnesium deficiency. Affected women report weight gain, breast tenderness and fullness, swelling of the hands and feet, and abdominal bloating.

Although categorizing the symptoms women experience may be of some value for identifying subgroups of PMS, many women experience considerable overlap of symptoms and do not fit neatly into this schema.

Again, since no single definite treatment adequately addresses all the symptoms women with PMS experience, this makes the condition quite amenable to an integrated, individual approach in which multiple treatment strategies are used.[4]

CLINICAL EVALUATION OF PREMENSTRUAL SYNDROME

A thorough evaluation should be performed before the diagnosis of premenstrual syndrome is made. This evaluation should include a careful history of the nature, timing, and severity of symptoms, as well as a detailed accounting of stress levels, diet, exercise, known medical problems, and alcohol and drug use. A complete physical and pelvic examination should be performed and laboratory tests conducted to rule out anemia and hypothyroidism. Some providers may check the prolactin level. Self-recording of a woman's symptoms on a daily basis for at least two complete menstrual cycles is useful to more accurately identify her symptoms and determine their relation to the menses.

Any other underlying medical conditions that may be misidentified as PMS should be addressed. The authors of one report found that 75% of women undergoing treatment for PMS at specialized clinics had another diagnosis that accounted for many of their symptoms, primarily major depression and other mood disorders.[14]

TREATMENT OPTIONS FOR PREMENSTRUAL SYNDROME

Practitioners will likely use a number of the following approaches to assist women with PMS. The multimodal strategy is probably best and would likely include at the very least exercise, dietary intervention, and the use of a multiple vitamin and possibly calcium/ magnesium.

Exercise

The few studies of exercise and PMS that have been conducted have clearly shown that women who engage in regular physical exercise have fewer symptoms than women who do not exercise.[15] The frequency, not the intensity, of exercise apparently relieves the negative mood and physical symptoms that occur during the premenstrual period.[16] It is postulated that exercise reduces symptoms by decreasing estrogen levels, decreasing circulating catecholamines, improving glucose tolerance, and increasing endorphin levels.[17] Given the many health benefits of exercise, practitioners should certainly consider regular exercise a part of the therapeutic approach to PMS.

Diet and Nutrition

A 1983 report found that women with PMS consumed 275% more refined sugar, 79% more dairy products, 78% more sodium, 62% more refined carbohydrates, 77% less manganese, and 53% less iron than women without PMS.[13] These dietary excesses and deficiencies may help explain some of the symptoms women experience during the premenstrual period. Refined sugars increase the urinary excretion of magnesium.[18] Heavy intake of sugar can increase sodium and water retention as a result of the rapid release of insulin. Dietary salt may exacerbate swelling. Although the data on caffeine and premenstrual breast tenderness are conflicting, many women obtain relief by eliminating or reducing consumption of caffeinated beverages and foods 2 weeks before the onset of menstruation. Consumption of caffeine-containing beverages has been associated with increases in both the prevalence and severity of PMS in college students.[19] A study of Chinese women found that increasing tea consumption was linked to an increasing prevalence of PMS.[20] Women experiencing irritability or difficulty sleeping during the premenstrual period should be encouraged to reduce or limit intake of caffeine (Table 3-1).

Dietary fat and premenstrual syndrome. Some practitioners advocate a high-fiber diet for women with PMS based on the premise that fiber helps reduce blood levels of estrogen. Estrogen is conjugated in the liver and is passed to the small intestine by way of bile for elimination in the feces. Intestinal bacteria deconjugate estrogen and allow it to be reabsorbed into the body. A fiber-rich, low-fat diet suppresses the ability of fecal bacteria to deconjugate estrogen, thereby enhancing fecal excretion. Several studies have shown

Table **3-1**

Caffeine in common foods and beverages

PRODUCT	CAFFEINE CONTENT (MG)
Coffee, instant (6-8 oz)	65-100
Coffee, percolated (6-8 oz)	80-135
Coffee, filtered (6-8 oz)	115-175
Coffee, decaffeinated (6-8 oz)	1-5
Tea, instant (6-8 oz)	1-5
Tea, brewed (6-8 oz)	28-150
Tea, iced (6-8 oz)	40-45
Tea, green (6-8 oz)	14-20
Chocolate, dark semisweet (1 oz)	3-35
Chocolate, milk (1 oz)	1-15
Cola beverage (8 oz)	25-30

that reducing fat (<20% in diet) and increasing fiber for only 3 months can reduce a woman's serum estrogen level.[21] This approach presupposes that an increased level of estrogen is the cause of PMS symptoms, a hypothesis not yet proven. In addition, many women would find it difficult to maintain such a low-fat diet. No rigorous studies are available with which to evaluate the effectiveness of this dietary intervention. However, a diet high in fruits, vegetables, and whole grains and low in saturated fat is still a wise recommendation for most women.

Calcium. Ovarian hormones influence calcium, magnesium, and vitamin D metabolism. Estrogen is involved in calcium metabolism, calcium absorption, and parathyroid gene expression and secretion. Clinical trials in women with PMS have found that calcium supplementation improves several mood and somatic symptoms.[22]

A randomized, double-blind, controlled clinical trial was conducted to evaluate the effectiveness of calcium carbonate in relieving PMS. Healthy premenopausal women were recruited nationally at 12 outpatient centers and screened for moderate to severe, cyclically recurring premenstrual symptoms. Symptoms were prospectively documented over the course of two menstrual cycles with the use of a daily rating scale that included 17 core symptoms and four symptom factors (negative affect, water retention, food cravings, and pain). Seven hundred twenty women were screened for the trial, 497 were enrolled, and 466 were valid for the efficacy analysis. Women were randomly assigned to receive 1200 mg of calcium carbonate or placebo daily for three menstrual cycles. Routine laboratory tests, complete blood cell counts, and urinalyses were performed in all participants. Each woman kept a daily diary to document symptoms, adverse effects, and compliance with therapy. The main outcome measure was a 17-parameter symptom-complex score. No difference was noted with regard to age, weight, height, use of oral contraceptives, or duration of menstrual cycle between the treatment and control groups. No differences were found between groups with regard to the mean screening symptom-complex score of the luteal ($P = 0.659$), menstrual ($P = 0.818$), or intermenstrual phase ($P = 0.726$) of the menstrual cycle. During the luteal phase of the treatment cycle, the mean symptom-complex score was significantly lower in the calcium-treated group by the third month of the study ($P < 0.001$). The authors concluded that calcium supplementation is a simple and effective treatment for PMS, resulting in a major reduction in overall luteal-phase symptoms.[23]

A review of studies focusing on calcium for the management of premenstrual symptoms was published in the *Annals of Pharmacotherapy*.[24] On the basis of data in the medical literature, the author concluded that "calcium supplementation of 1200 to 1600 mg/day, unless contraindicated, should be considered a sound treatment option in women who experience premenstrual syndrome." Although most experts believe that it is premature to consider calcium a "cure" for PMS, most would agree that calcium supplementation is a safe treatment recommendation for otherwise healthy women with PMS.

Magnesium. On the basis of research demonstrating that women with PMS have low red blood cell levels of magnesium compared with those of controls,[25] a randomized, double-blind, controlled crossover study was conducted to evaluate the effect of magnesium on PMS symptoms. A daily 200-mg magnesium oxide supplement or placebo was given to trial participants for two menstrual cycles. Evaluation consisted of a daily record of symptoms ranked on a 4-point scale for 22 symptoms grouped into 6 categories: PMS-A, PMS-C, PMS-D, PMS-H, PMS-O (other), and PMS-T (total overall symptoms). Twenty-four-hour urinary magnesium output was estimated from spot samples, with the magnesium/creatinine ratio used to assess compliance. No difference was observed between the two groups in any symptom category during the first month of supplementation. Reduction of PMS-H symptoms (weight gain, swelling of extremities, breast tenderness, abdominal bloating) was greater in the treatment group during the second month compared with women taking placebo ($P = 0.009$). Some would question the dose used in this study. Most practitioners of natural medicine recommend 400 to 800 mg/day of magnesium for addressing PMS complaints. More research on efficacy and optimal dose is needed.

Vitamin B$_6$. Pyridoxine is a water-soluble B vitamin that serves as a cofactor in more than 100 enzyme reactions, many of which are related to the metabolism of amino acids and proteins. Current thinking postulates that pyridoxine eases the symptoms of PMS by increasing the synthesis of serotonin, dopamine, norepinephrine, histamine, and taurine.[26] Serotonin is important in the regulation of sleep and appetite, and low levels of serotonin are associated with depressed mood. Low levels of serotonin and dopamine may play a role in premenstrual symptoms.[27] The use of pyridoxine to alleviate PMS symptoms has been studied in more than 25 trials since 1975.

A systematic review of pyridoxine for PMS was published in the *British Medical Journal*.[28] Nine randomized, controlled, double-blind, parallel, or crossover studies representing 940 patients with PMS were included. Studies of cyclical mastalgia and multivitamin preparations containing at least 50 mg of vitamin B$_6$ were also included in the review. Only one trial scored a 6 of a possible 8 points for classification as a high-quality trial according to the author's criteria, but it comprised too few subjects to achieve sufficient power.[29] Only one trial included a sufficient number of patients,[30] and the other trials were affected by low statistical power. None of the trials included power calculations. The author of the systematic review found the overall odds ratio in favor of pyridoxine to be 1.57 (95% confidence interval 1.40 to 1.77). When the effects on depressive symptoms in five trials were examined, the overall odds ratio in favor of pyridoxine was 2.12 (95% confidence interval 1.80 to 2.48). The authors of the systematic review caution that the "conclusions that can be drawn from our systematic review are limited. Although the results from the available data suggest that vitamin B$_6$ is more effective than placebo, there is insufficient evidence of high enough quality to give a confident recommendation for using vitamin B$_6$ in the treatment of premenstrual syndrome."

Clinical trials have involved pyridoxine doses ranging from 50 to 500 mg/day. For most women, it is prudent to limit single doses of B$_6$ to 50 mg and to not exceed 100 to 150 mg/day. Although pyridoxine is a water-soluble vitamin, it can be associated with toxicity when taken in large doses for prolonged periods. A few reports have noted toxicity occurring with prolonged ingestion of 150 mg/day.[31] Toxicity may result as large doses of pyridoxine overwhelm the liver's ability to form pyridoxal-5-phosphate, the active form of vitamin B$_6$. Research suggests that the liver cannot process more than 50 mg of pyridoxine at one time.[32] Conversion of pyridoxine to its active form depends on other nutrients such as magnesium and riboflavin. It may be prudent to take vitamin B$_6$ as part of a multivitamin/mineral supplement or to simply use pyridoxal-5-phosphate.

Given the low cost and relative safety of appropriate doses of pyridoxine, even in the face of incomplete information regarding efficacy, practitioners may wish to consider the use of a multivitamin containing 50 to 100 mg of vitamin B$_6$ for women with symptoms of PMS, especially when the diet is less than optimal.

Herbal Remedies

***Chaste or chastetree berry* (Vitex agnus-castus).** The Greek physician
Dioscorides described the medicinal uses for the dried ripe fruits of the chastetree (Fig. 3-1)
some 2000 years ago. The Latin designation *agnus castus* means "chaste lamb," in reference to the belief that the seeds reduce sexual desire; hence its other common name,
monk's pepper. The herb has been studied for more than five decades for its possible
benefit as a lactagogue and as an agent for the relief of PMS and infertility.

Several large, published drug-monitoring studies describe the use of Agnolyt (proprietary product of Dr. Madause GmbH, Cologne, Germany; a chasteberry-fruit tincture
containing 9 g of a 1:5 tincture for each 100 g of aqueous alcoholic solution) for numerous menstrual complaints, including PMS. Feldmann et al.[33] studied 1571 women with
menstrual disturbances related to "corpus luteum insufficiency or ovarian dysfunction."
The average duration of treatment was 135 days, with an average daily dose of 40 drops
of Agnolyt taken on an empty stomach. The response rate was roughly 90%, with assessments being provided by both physicians and participants. Adverse effects were seen in
fewer than 2% of the women: 12 cases of malaise, gastrointestinal complaints, nausea, or

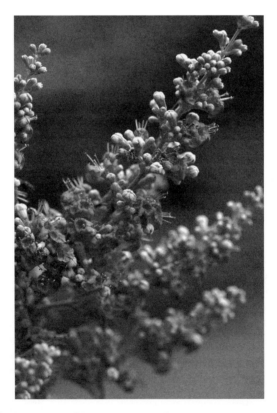

Figure **3-1 Chastetree** *(Vitex agnus-castus)*. *(Courtesy Martin Wall Botanical
Services.)*

diarrhea. Single cases of hypermenorrhea, dizziness, weight gain, allergy, and pyrosis were reported; no explanation was given for the other 13 cases.

Dittmar et al.[34] published another focused drug monitoring study using Agnolyt in 1542 women with PMS (age range 13 to 62 years). The average dose was 42 drops/day (range 20 to 120 drops/day). Symptom improvement was seen after a mean of 25.3 days (range 1 to 365 days); 33% of patients reported total relief of symptoms, 57% reported partial relief, and treatment was discontinued in fewer than 4% of cases because the effects were inadequate. Adverse effects were reported in 32 women, but only 17 (2%) discontinued treatment. The most common complaint was nausea. Treatment was rated as good or very good in 92% of cases by both participants and physicians.

Complete assessment of these drug monitoring studies is not possible because of the vague inclusion and exclusion criteria, lack of definable end points, large dosage range, lack of randomization, lack of a control group, no intention-to-treat analysis, and no power analysis. It is also unclear whether women from one drug monitoring study were included in the other. Although limited meaningful information can be extracted from these reports, the lack of significant adverse events is reassuring.

The studies described in Table 3-2 are randomized, double-blind trials as of January 2002 using chastetree berry as the sole agent for the alleviation of PMS.

The mechanism by which *Vitex* alleviates PMS symptoms is uncertain. One theory suggests that the symptoms of PMS are improved by way of its inhibitory action on prolactin.[35] Ethanol extracts of *Vitex* fruit have been shown to bind directly to dopamine (D_2) receptors, inhibiting prolactin in rat pituitary cells.[35]

Women with hyperprolactinemia often experience irregularities of the menstrual cycle. Some authors suggest that as many as 62% of women with menstrual disorders have some degree of increased prolactin.[4] The correction of hyperprolactinemia is believed to cause a reversal of LH suppression, resulting in full development of the corpus luteum during the luteal phase of the cycle, thereby regulating the menses.[4] Researchers have reported that *Vitex* restores progesterone concentration and prolongs the hyperthermic phase in the basal body-temperature curve when 40 drops/day of Agnolyt tincture is taken for 3 months.[36]

Preliminary evidence suggests that *Vitex* is beneficial in the relief of PMS symptoms in some women and that it may be of value in women with irregular menses. Given the relatively good safety profile of *Vitex*, the use of a high-quality product for a 3-month trial in women with PMS may be considered. The German health authorities have approved the use of *Vitex* fruit for irregularities of the menstrual cycle, premenstrual complaints, and mastodynia.[37] The chastetree berry products that were studied in Europe are not currently available in the United States. The average daily dose of crude herb is 500 to 1000 mg/day, which is the equivalent of 3 to 5 mL of a 1:5 strength hydroethanolic tincture.

Evening primrose oil. Some researchers have reported that women with PMS have impaired conversion of linoleic acid to γ-linolenic acid (GLA).[38] This finding has led to the investigation of GLA supplementation for the alleviation of PMS symptoms. A systematic review identified seven placebo-controlled trials of evening primrose oil and concluded that all had methodological flaws. The two highest-quality studies of evening primrose oil showed no beneficial effects in PMS, although sample size was small in both.[39] The following is a brief review of those two trials.

The authors of a randomized, double-blind crossover trial studied 27 women with PMS for 10 menstrual cycles. All 27 women were given placebo during the second cycle and

Table 3-2

Randomized clinical trials of Vitex for premenstrual syndrome

STUDY	METHODS	PARTICIPANTS	OUTCOME
Lauritzen et al.[58]	*Study design:* Randomized, double-blind, comparative trial lasting 3 months. *Dose/preparation:* Participants received 1 Agnolyt capsule containing 3.5-4.2 mg *Vitex* fruit, dry native extract plus placebo per day or 1 placebo BID on days 1-5 and then 100 mg pyridoxine BID on days 16-35. *Evaluation:* CGIC and PMTS last 7 days of each menstrual cycle	*Inclusion criteria:* Patients 18-45 years with PMS symptoms consistently correlated with the luteal phase and severe enough to interfere with quality of life. Participants had to be symptom-free at least 1 week per month. *Exclusion criteria:* Subjects who had taken herbs, medications, vitamins, or minerals in the preceding 3 months; women with significant depression, premenopausal symptoms, corpus luteum irregularities, drug/alcohol abuse, or physical disease and women who were pregnant or nursing. *Study size:* 85 treatment, 90 control. *Dropouts:* 39 in treatment group (4 because of adverse effects), 31 in control group (5 because of adverse effects).	*Authors' major conclusions:* CGIC scale showed overall efficacy at 77.1% for *Vitex* and 60.6% for pyridoxine. Investigators rated efficacy of *Vitex* as 24.6% and that of pyridoxine as 12.1%. In *Vitex* group, 36.1% of participants were free of symptoms; 21.1% were free of symptoms in pyridoxine group. Authors note that although not statistically valid, these findings support the view that Agnolyt is superior to pyridoxine with regard to these parameters. *Flaws/comments:* No placebo arm (10 published randomized controlled trials of pyridoxine for PMS); no intention-to-treat analysis.

Turner and Mills[59]	*Type of study:* RCT lasting 3 months *Dose/preparation:* 600 mg of dried *Vitex* fruit in capsule form, 3 times daily, or soya-based placebo.	*Inclusion criteria:* Women with physiologic symptoms of PMS as assessed with a form of the Moos Menstrual Distress Questionnaire. Average age 32 years. *Study size:* Total population, 600; total evaluated at end of trial, 217 (105 from *Vitex* group, 112 from control group). Statistical analysis revealed no difference between those who completed the trial and those who withdrew with regard to age, marital status, cycle length, or employment.	*Authors' major conclusions:* No statistical difference was found between the treatment and control groups with regard to symptoms of impaired concentration, fluid retention, or pain. *Vitex* conferred statistically significant relief of "feeling jittery or restless" that was sustained throughout the trial. *Flaws/comments:* This trial involved a high dosage of *Vitex* (1800 mg/day) compared with the dosages used in other studies (3.5-175 mg/day). The number of withdrawals from the study was significant.
Schellenberg[60]	*Type of study:* RCT lasting 3 months *Dose/preparation:* Fruit extract ZE 440: 60% ethanol extract ratio 6-12:1, standardized for casticin; one 20-mg tablet daily or placebo	*Inclusion criteria:* Women aged ≥18 years with PMS diagnosed in accordance with the DSM-III-R. *Exclusion criteria:* Participation in other trials, concomitant psychotherapy, pregnancy, breastfeeding, inadequate contraception, dementia, alcohol/drug dependence, serious concomitant medical condition, hypersensitivity to *Vitex agnus-castus*, fever, pituitary disease,	*Author's major conclusions:* "*Agnus castus* is well tolerated and effective for the treatment of premenstrual syndrome, the effects being confirmed by physicians and patients alike. The effects are detected in most main symptoms of the syndrome." Five of the six self-assessment items indicated significant superiority of *Vitex agnus-castus* (irritability, mood

Continued

Table 3-2

Randomized clinical trials of Vitex for premenstrual syndrome—cont'd

STUDY	METHODS	PARTICIPANTS	OUTCOME
		concomitant use of sex hormones (except oral contraceptives, whose dosages were left unchanged) *Study size:* 178 women were initially screened and randomized; 170 were evaluated at the end of the trial.	alteration, anger; headache, breast fullness); other symptoms, including bloating, were unaffected by treatment. *Flaws/comments:* Well-done study; statistically significant improvement in multiple parameters; no significant adverse effects. All patients accounted for.

CGIC, Clinical global impression of change; *DSM-III-R,* Diagnostic and Statistical Manual of Mental Disorders, ed 3, revised; *PMTS,* premenstrual tension syndrome; *RCT,* randomized controlled trial.

then were randomly assigned to four cycles of active treatment with essential fatty acids or four cycles of placebo, with a crossover after completion of the fourth cycle. Daily symptom records were kept. No difference was found between the placebo and essential fatty acids in the relief of premenstrual symptoms. The authors did note that "time had a significant effect on a number of symptoms, indicating either a placebo effect or an effect from participation in the study." They concluded that essential fatty acids are ineffective in the treatment of PMS.[40]

A randomized, double-blind, placebo-controlled crossover trial was conducted in 38 women with PMS. Women were randomly assigned to receive placebo or evening primrose oil for 3 months and then were crossed over to the other treatment for an additional 3 months. The beneficial effect on all symptoms (psychological symptoms, fluid retention, breast tenderness) was rapid; the scores decreased during the first menstrual cycle but increased slightly during the changeover period after the third month, regardless of whether the active agent or placebo was the next medication received. The authors concluded, "These finding indicate that the improvement experienced by these women with moderate PMS was solely a placebo effect."[41]

The problem with simply dismissing (or accepting) the use of evening primrose oil for the relief of PMS is that even the best studies have lacked sufficient power, making them vulnerable to false-negative results. A high-quality randomized, placebo-controlled trial with a sample size based on a power analysis is needed to answer the question of whether evening primrose oil is effective in the treatment of PMS. The trial must also be of adequate duration because treatment effects may be slower to appear with any dietary intervention. The dose generally recommended by practitioners of natural medicine is 3 g/day of evening primrose oil.

Black cohosh (Cimicifuga racemosa). Early American physicians used black cohosh for a variety of menstrual complaints, including nervousness, breast pain, and headaches.[42] Although most research has been focused on black cohosh for the alleviation of menopausal complaints, one study of 135 women with PMS revealed that a standardized extract of black cohosh was effective in reducing symptoms of anxiety, tension, and depression.[34] Preliminary research on an Asian species of *Cimicifuga* suggests that the rhizome acts as a mild serotonin reuptake inhibitor.[43] If this effect occurs with *C. racemosa*, it could partially explain the positive benefits reported by women with PMS (and those in menopause). German health authorities have endorsed the use of black cohosh for premenstrual discomfort, dysmenorrhea, and menopausal complaints.[44] The dose for extracts standardized to triterpene glycosides (marker compound) is generally 20 to 80 mg bid. The dose for crude herb is 250 to 500 mg/day.

Ginkgo (Ginkgo biloba). Although gingko is associated primarily with the treatment of mild dementia, cerebrovascular insufficiency, and intermittent claudication, preliminary data suggest that it may also have some value in relieving certain PMS symptoms. A double-blind, placebo-controlled trial was conducted with 165 women (ages 18 to 45 years) who experienced congestive premenstrual symptoms for at least 7 days per cycle for at least 3 cycles. The diagnosis of PMS was confirmed during the first month, after which the women were randomly assigned to receive placebo or 80 mg of standardized extract of ginkgo (Egb761, product standardized to contain 24% ginkgoflavones and 6% terpenes) twice daily from day 16 of the menstrual cycle through day 5 of the next cycle for 2 cycles. Evaluation of 143 patients at the end of the trial revealed a statistically significant difference in favor of ginkgo for the alleviation of breast pain and tenderness, as well as reduction of fluid retention.[45]

St. John's wort **(Hypericum perforatum).** Several trials have been conducted with selective serotonin reuptake–inhibiting medications for the alleviation of severe premenstrual symptoms, with approximately 60% of women obtaining significant relief. A number of herbalists recommend St. John's wort for women who complain of depression and irritability during the premenstrual phase.

One clinical trial addressing the question of whether St. John's wort is effective in treating PMS is a prospective, open, uncontrolled, observational study. Nineteen physically and mentally healthy women with PMS completed a daily symptom-rating diary for one cycle and attended a medical screening interview before being given the diagnosis of PMS. Participants were then given 300 mg/day of St. John's wort extract standardized to 0.3% hypericin. Symptoms were rated daily with the use of validated measures. The Hospital Anxiety and Depression Scale and Social Adjustment Scale were administered at baseline and after one and two menstrual cycles. The authors reported a reduction of greater than 50% in PMS-symptom scores between baseline and the end of the trial. More than two thirds of the participants noted a 50% decrease in symptom severity. The authors conclude, "The results of this pilot study suggest that there is scope for conducting a randomized, placebo-controlled, double-blind trial to investigate the value of *Hypericum* as a treatment for premenstrual syndrome."[46]

The dose of St. John's wort recommended in the clinical trials for depression is 300 mg standardized to contain 0.3% hypericin (products may also be standardized to 4% to 5% hyperforin) three times per day. The pilot study mentioned previously involved a much lower dose (300 mg/day). A well-designed trial is necessary to assess the efficacy and most appropriate dose for the treatment of PMS.

AUTHORS' NOTE: People taking medications that increase photosensitivity, protease inhibitors (for human immunodeficiency virus infection), cyclosporine, digoxin, or other medications metabolized by the P450 CYP3A4 enzyme system should avoid St. John's wort.

Kava **(Piper methysticum).** Physicians occasionally prescribe alprazolam, a benzodiazepine, for the treatment of PMS. Because this drug has some potential for habituation and abuse, other anxiolytic agents should be considered. Kava, an herb that has been used as a beverage and medicinal agent in the South Pacific for centuries, is the most extensively studied botanical for the treatment of anxiety. A meta-analysis concluded that kava is an effective treatment for anxiety compared with placebo. The trials were found to have methodological flaws, but none was considered "fatal."[47] No studies of kava in the treatment of PMS are available for review.

Concerns over the safety of kava have been raised. Approximately 30 cases of liver toxicity that may have been related to the use of kava products have been reported in the literature. Germany, Switzerland, Ireland, Canada, Australia, and the United Kingdom have banned the sale of kava. The U.S. Food and Drug Administration is evaluating the safety data, and, at the time of this writing, the herb is still being sold in the United States. While a recent survey of traditional healers and biomedical practitioners in Samoa showed a lack of evidence of kava-related hepatotoxicity,[48] practitioners should be cautious about the use of the herb until the issue of safety has been more clearly elucidated. This caution is especially true for those with underlying liver disease or those taking hepatotoxic substances.

Other Treatment Options

Natural progesterone. Katherina Dalton first postulated that PMS symptoms could be alleviated by administration of progesterone during the 1950s. Dalton administered natural progesterone in the form of injection, suppository, or subcutaneous pellets, and 83% of her subjects reported complete relief of PMS symptoms.[49] Since the early days of Dalton's work, several studies have been conducted to determine the effectiveness of natural progesterone in the treatment of PMS. Trials have varied in quality, providing inconsistent results.

A prospective, double-blind multicenter study randomly assigned 141 women with the diagnosis of PMS to receive progesterone pessaries (400 mg twice a day) or matching placebo, vaginally or rectally, starting 14 days before the expected onset of menstruation and continuing until the onset of vaginal bleeding, for 4 cycles. Efficacy was evaluated in 93 patients. Reduction of symptoms was superior for progesterone compared with placebo in all four cycles. Adverse events were reported by 51% of women in the progesterone group and by 43% of those using the placebo. The subjects using progesterone pessaries reported menstrual irregularities, headache, and vaginal pruritus more often than did those receiving the placebo.[50]

Another study failed to demonstrate any benefit for oral micronized progesterone over placebo for treatment of PMS. One hundred eighty-five women with the diagnosis of PMS were randomly assigned to a double blind, placebo-controlled 3-month trial. Women took 300 mg of oral micronized progesterone, 0.25 mg of alprazolam, or placebo four times a day from days 18 of the menstrual cycle through day 2 of the next cycle. Participants were assigned to either 20- or 50-minute clinic visits. One third of the alprazolam group experienced a 50% reduction in total daily symptom report scores and this treatment was superior to both placebo and progesterone for symptoms of mood, pain, and mental function. Oral micronized progesterone was no more effective than placebo. The duration of clinic visits did not affect treatment outcome. The authors reported no clinically significant withdrawal symptoms associated with alprazolam. The authors concluded, "Alprazolam has a role in PMS treatment and offers a therapy limited to the luteal phase. Oral micronized progesterone is ineffective for PMS."

Numerous uncontrolled trials of varying quality have assessed the use of varying doses of progesterone in oral micronized form or pessary for the relief of PMS symptoms. The data are conflicting. Currently the evidence is insufficient to recommend use of progesterone for the relief of PMS.

Selective serotonin reuptake inhibitors. Several controlled studies have shown that selective serotonin reuptake inhibitors (SSRIs) are effective in the treatment of PMDD. In one double-blind, randomized, controlled study, a group of 120 women was divided into 4 groups of 30 patients each. Participants received 3 months of placebo followed by 3 months of active treatment. Active treatments included pyridoxine (300 mg/day), alprazolam (0.75 mg/day), fluoxetine (10 mg/day), and propanolol (20 mg/day and 40 mg/day during the menstrual period). The fluoxetine group had a mean 65% reduction of symptoms, propanolol 59%, alprazolam 56%, pyridoxine 45%, and placebo 46%. The authors concluded that fluoxetine in a dosage of 10 mg yielded the best results in the treatment of PMS.[51]

The question of intermittent dosing of fluoxetine was addressed in a trial comparing 20 mg/day continuous treatment with fluoxetine 20 mg/day for 14 days of premenstrual treatment only. The authors concluded that "intermittent dosing of fluoxetine appears to be effective and mostly free of side effects in women with PMDD and, therefore, may offer an attractive treatment option for a disorder that is itself intermittent."[52]

The authors of a recent review concluded that fluoxetine 20 mg/day is an effective and well-tolerated treatment for women with PMDD, a severe variant of PMS.[53] Sertraline and paroxetine appear to be equally effective. The SSRIs have been shown to be superior to and better tolerated than tricyclic antidepressants for treatment of PMS symptoms.[54]

Acupuncture. The data are limited with regard to the efficacy of acupuncture in alleviating PMS symptoms. The findings of preliminary studies do suggest that acupuncture is useful for some women, either alone or in combination with other treatment therapies such as SSRIs.[55]

MIND/BODY

Mind/body therapies (MBTs) are those therapies grounded in the emerging scientific understanding that thoughts and feelings affect physiology and physical health. MBTs for PMS vary widely in their approach and include interventions such as progressive muscle relaxation, biofeedback, stress management, cognitive-behavioral ("talk") therapy, massage, hypnotherapy, biofeedback, guided imagery, and yoga. Research is growing in this field but is still scant. However, practitioners should use a common sense approach when considering recommendations for "mind/body" approaches. Little harm, and possibly much good, can be found in patients taking a yoga class, getting a monthly massage, or doing 10 minutes of relaxation in the evening while listening to soothing music.

Relaxation Therapy

A randomized clinical trial of 46 women with PMS found that subjects assigned to the relaxation response group (progressive muscle relaxation combined with slow, deep breathing) reported significantly greater reduction of mood symptoms compared with controls assigned either charting of symptoms or reading over a 5-month period.[56]

Yoga

A 10-month empirical study of 40 women was undertaken to investigate the effectiveness of certain yogic practices in relieving menstrual-related stress. Women assigned to the study group underwent yoga training (regular practice of specific yoga postures and transcendental meditation); the control group had no training. The authors found significantly lower scores on the subscales of the menstrual distress questionnaire for subjects in the yoga-trained group compared with the control group in both the premenstrual and menstrual periods.[57]

Summary

Premenstrual syndrome is likely a combination of environmental, biological, and societal factors. Many treatment options have been presented in this chapter: oral micronized progesterone, SSRIs, vitamin B_6, calcium, magnesium, dietary changes, exercise, evening primrose oil, *Vitex*, black cohosh, St. John's wort, kava, and other botanicals. Although some have shown varying degrees of success, none is universally effective and none can be represented as a cure for PMS. Obviously the first approach should be lifestyle recommendations, including nutritious diet, regular exercise, and stress-management strategies. If these measures are not sufficient, multivitamin and calcium dietary supplementation, and *Vitex* should be considered. Subsequently, practitioners should make recommendations on the basis of patient preferences and evidence of safety/efficacy as to which further interventions should be administered.

References

1. American College of Obstetrics and Gynecology: Committee opinion: premenstrual syndrome, *Int J Gynaecol Obstet* 50:80-84, 1995.
2. Rubinow DR, Hoban HC, Groven GN, et al: Changes in plasma hormones across the menstrual cycle in patients with menstrually related mood disorder and in control subjects, *Am J Obstet Gynecol* 158:5-11, 1988.
3. Kellner R, Buckman MT, Fava GA, et al: Hyperprolactinemia, distress, and hostility, *Am J Psychiatry* 141:759-763, 1984.
4. Bohnert KJ: Clinical study on chaste tree for menstrual disorders, *Q Rev Nat Med* Spring:19-21, 1997.
5. Munday MR, Brush MG, Taylor RW: Correlations between progesterone, oestradiol, and aldosterone levels in the premenstrual syndrome, *Clin Endocrinol* 14:1-9, 1981.
6. Chuong CJ, Coulam CB, Kao PC, et al: Neuropeptide levels in the premenstrual syndrome, *Fertil Steril* 44:760-765, 1985.
7. Chuong CJ, His BP, Gibbons WE: Periovulatory beta-endorphin levels in premenstrual syndrome, *Obstet Gynecol* 83:755-760, 1994.
8. Bloch M, Schmidt PJ, Su TP, et al: Pituitary-adrenal hormones and testosterone across the menstrual cycle in women with premenstrual syndrome and controls, *Biol Psychiatyr* 43:897-903, 1998.
9. Clare AW: Premenstrual syndrome: single or multiple causes? *Can J Psychiatry* 30:474-482, 1985.
10. Sherwood RA, Rocks BF, Steward A, et al: Magnesium and premenstrual syndrome, *Ann Clin Biochem* 23:667-670, 1986.
11. Budoff PW: The use of prostaglandin inhibitors for the premenstrual syndrome, *J Reprod Med* 28:465-468, 1983.
12. Hamilton JA, Parry B, Alagna S, et al: Premenstrual mood changes: a guide to evaluation and treatment, *Psychiatr Ann* 14:426-435, 1984.
13. Abraham GE: Nutritional factors in the etiology of premenstrual tension syndromes, *J Reprod Med* 28:446-464, 1983.
14. DeJong R, Rubinow DR, Roy-Byrne P, et al: Premenstrual mood disorder and psychiatric illness, *Am J Psychiatry* 142:1359-1361, 1985.
15. Aganoff J, Boyle G: Aerobic exercise, mood states and menstrual cycle symptoms, *J Psychosom Res* 38:183-192, 1994.
16. Johnson W, Carr-Nangle R, Bergeron K: Macronutrient intake, eating habits, and exercise as moderators of menstrual distress in healthy women, *Psychosom Med* 57:324-330, 1995.
17. Gannon L: The potential role of exercise in the alleviation of menstrual disorders and menopausal symptoms: a theoretical synthesis of current research, *Women Health* 4:105-127, 1988.
18. Abraham G: Magnesium deficiency in premenstrual tension, *Magnes Bull* 4:68, 1982.
19. Rossignol AM: Caffeine-containing beverages and premenstrual syndrome in young women, *Am J Publ Health* 75:1335-1337, 1985.
20. Rossignol AM, Zhang J, Chen Y, et al: Tea and premenstrual syndrome in the People's Republic of China. *Am J Publ Health* 79:66-67, 1989.
21. Rose D: Diet, hormones, and cancer, *Annu Rev Publ Health* 14:1-7, 1993.
22. Thys-Jacobs S: Micronutrients and the premenstrual syndrome: the case for calcium, *J Am Coll Nutr* 19:220-227, 2000.

23. Thys-Jacobs S, Starkey P, Bernstein D, et al: Calcium carbonate and the premenstrual syndrome: effects on premenstrual and menstrual symptoms. Premenstrual Syndrome Study Group, *Am J Obstet Gynecol* 179:444-452, 1998.

24. Ward MW, Holimon TD: Calcium treatment for premenstrual syndrome, *Ann Pharmacother* 33:1356-1358, 1999.

25. Rosenstein DL, Elin RJ, Hosseini JM, et al: Magnesium measures across the menstrual cycle in premenstrual syndrome, *Biol Psychiatry* 35:557-561, 1994.

26. Ebadi M, Govitrapong P: Pyridoxal phosphate and neurotransmitters in the brain. In Tryfiates G, editor: *Vitamin B6: metabolism and role in growth*, Westport, Ct, 1980, Food and Nutrition Press, p 223.

27. Taylor D, Mathew RJ, Ho BT, et al: Serotonin levels and platelet uptake during premenstrual tension, *Neuropsychobiology* 12:16-18, 1984.

28. Wyatt KM, Dimmock PW, Jones PW, et al: Efficacy of vitamin B-6 in the treatment of premenstrual syndrome: a systematic review, *BMJ* 318:1375-1381, 1999.

29. Kendall KE, Schnurr PP: The effects of vitamin B6 supplementation on premenstrual symptoms, *Obstet Gynecol* 70:145-149, 1987.

30. Williams MJ, Harris RI, Dean BC: Controlled trial of pyridoxine in the premenstrual syndrome, *J Int Med Res* 13:174-179, 1985.

31. Cohen M, Bendich A: Safety of pyridoxine: a review of human and animal studies, *Toxicol Lett* 34:129-139, 1986.

32. Zempleni J: Pharmacokinetics of vitamin B6 supplements in humans, *J Am Coll Nutr* 14:579-586, 1995.

33. Feldmann HU, Albrecht M, Lamertz M, et al: The treatment of corpus luteum insufficiency and premenstrual syndrome. Experience in a multicenter study under clinical practice conditions [in German], *Gyne* 12:422-425, 1990.

34. Dittmar FW, Bohnert KJ, Peeters M, et al: Premenstrual syndrome treatment with a phytophar maceutical [in German], *T W Gynakologie* 5:60-68, 1992.

35. Sliutz G, Speiser P, Schultz AM, et al: *Agnus castus* extracts inhibit prolactin secretion of rat pituitary cells, *Horm Metab Res* 25:253-255, 1993.

36. Newall CA, Anderson LA, Phillipson JD: *Herbal medicines: a guide for health-care professionals*, London, 1996, Pharmaceutical Press, pp 19-20.

37. Blumenthal M, Gruenwald J, Hall T, Rister RS, editors: *The complete German Commission E monographs: therapeutic guide to herbal medicine*, Boston, 1998, Integrative Medicine Communications, p 108.

38. Horrobin DF, Manku MS, Brush M, et al: Abnormalities in plasma essential fatty acid levels in women with premenstrual syndrome and nonmalignant breast disease, *J Nutr Med* 2:259-264, 1991.

39. Budeiri D, Li Wan Po A, Dornan JC: Is evening primrose oil of value in the treatment of premenstrual syndrome? *Cont Clin Trial* 17:60-68, 1996.

40. Collins A, Cerin A, Coleman G, et al: Essential fatty acids in the treatment of premenstrual syndrome, *Obstet Gynecol* 81:93-98, 1993.

41. Khoo SK, Munro C, Battistutta D: Evening primrose oil and treatment of premenstrual syndrome, *Med J Aust* 153:189-192, 1990.

42. Felter HW: *The eclectic Materia Medica: pharmacology and therapeutics*. Cincinnati, 1922, John K. Scudder.

43. Liao JF, Jan YM, Huang SY, et al: Evaluation with receptor binding assay on the water extracts of ten CNS-active Chinese herbal drugs. Proceedings of the National Science Council, Republic of China, *Life Sci* 19:151-158, 1995.

44. Blumenthal M, Gruenwald J, Hall T, et al, editors: *The Complete German Commission E monographs: therapeutic guide to herbal medicine*. Boston, 1998, Integrative Medicine Communications, p 90.

45. Tamborini A, Taurelle R: Value of a standardized *Ginkgo biloba* extract in the management of congestive symptoms of premenstrual syndrome, *Rev Fr Gynecol Obstet* 88:447-457, 1993.

46. Stevinson C, Ernst E: A pilot study of *Hypericum perforatum* for the treatment of premenstrual syndrome, *Br J Obstet Gynaecol* 107:870-876, 2000.

47. Pittler MH, Ernst E: Efficacy of kava extract for treating anxiety: systematic review and meta-analysis, *J Clin Psychopharmacol* 20:84-90, 2000.

48. Tavana G, Stewart P, Snyder S, et al: Lack of evidence of kava-related hepatotoxicity in native populations in Savaii, Samoa, *HerbalGram* 59:28-32, 2003.

49. Keye W: Medical treatment of premenstrual syndrome, *Can J Psychiatry* 30:483-487, 1985.

50. Magill PJ: Investigation of the efficacy of progesterone pessaries in the relief of symptoms of premenstrual syndrome. Progesterone Study Group, *Br J Gen Pract* 45:589-593, 1995.

51. Diegoli MS, daFonseca AM, Diegoli CA, et al: A double-blind trial of four medications to treat severe premenstrual syndrome, *Int J Gynaecol Obstet* 62:63-67, 1998.

52. Steiner M, Korzekwa M, Lamont J, et al: Intermittent fluoxetine dosing in the treatment of women with premenstrual dysphoria, *Psychopharm Bull* 33:771-774, 1997.

53. Romano S, Judge R, Dillon J, et al: The role of fluoxetine in the treatment of premenstrual dysphoric disorder, *Clin Ther* 21:615-633, 1999.

54. Freeman EW, Rickels K, Sondheimer SJ, et al: Differential response to antidepressants in women with premenstrual syndrome/premenstrual dysphoric disorder: a randomized controlled trial, *Arch Gen Psychiatr* 56:932-939, 1999.

55. Habek D, Habek JC, Barbir A: Using acupuncture to treat premenstrual syndrome, *Arch Gynecol Obstet* 267:23-26, 2002.

56. Goodale IL, Domar AD, Benson H: Alleviation of premenstrual syndrome symptoms with the relaxation response, *Obstet Gynecol* 75:649-655, 1990.

57. Sridevi K, Krishna Rao PV: Yoga practice and menstrual distress, *J Indian Acad Applied Psychol* 22:47-54, 1996.

58. Lauritzen CH, Reuter HD, Repges R, et al: Treatment of premenstrual tension syndrome with *Vitex agnus-castus*. Controlled, double-blind study versus pyridoxine, *Phytomedicine* 4:183-189, 1997.

59. Turner S, Mills S: A double-blind clinical trial on a herbal remedy for premenstrual syndrome: a case study, *Compl Ther Med* 1:73-77, 1993.

60. Schellenberg R: Treatment for the premenstrual syndrome with agnus castus fruit extract: prospective, randomized, placebo controlled study, *BMJ* 322:134-137, 2001.

Menstrual Cramps

Dysmenorrhea, commonly referred to as menstrual cramps, affects more than 50% of menstruating women. Women between the ages of 20 and 24 years typically experience the most severe pain. Dysmenorrhea is generally divided into two subcategories. When the menstrual cramps are associated with an identifiable pathology, such as endometriosis (see Chapter 5), it is referred to as secondary dysmenorrhea. When no organic pathologic condition exists, it is classified as primary dysmenorrhea.[1] The pain of primary dysmenorrhea usually begins with the onset of menstrual flow and lasts 8 to 72 hours, whereas cramping often occurs before, as well as during menstruation with secondary dysmenorrhea.

Menstrual cramps are believed to be the result of excessive prostaglandin production in the secretory endometrium, which leads to painful uterine contractions. Other symptoms—such as headache, nausea, diarrhea, and back pain—can also be explained by the entry of prostaglandins into the systemic circulation.[2] Prostaglandin release is greatest during the first 48 hours of menstruation, which is the period during which most women state their symptoms are worst. Prostaglandin $F_{2\alpha}$ ($PGF_{2\alpha}$) appears to be the primary cause. $PGF_{2\alpha}$ stimulates the nonpregnant uterus, whereas prostaglandins of the E series induce uterine relaxation. Overproduction of vasopressin, a hormone that stimulates muscle contraction, may be another cause.[3] Pain is also partly mediated by ischemia, which is induced by the contraction of the myometrium itself.

TREATMENT
Nonsteroidal Antiinflammatory Drugs

Nonsteroidal antiinflammatory drugs (NSAIDs) are often used to suppress the production of prostaglandins from the arachidonic acid chemical precursor by the enzyme prostaglandin synthetase. Of more than 50 clinical trials conducted on prostaglandin synthetase inhibitors, the fenamates have been shown to be the most effective in relieving menstrual pain.[4] These agents not only inhibit prostaglandin production but also compete for prostaglandin-binding sites. Treatment should begin at the first sign of menstrual cramping. Most women only need to use these medications for 2 or 3 days. Side effects may include gastrointestinal upset, blurred vision, headache, and dizziness. Contraindications to the use of NSAIDs include gastrointestinal bleeding, peptic-ulcer disease, and sensitivity to aspirin.

Oral Contraceptives

Oral contraceptives are effective in the treatment of dysmenorrhea. They create an atrophic decidualized endometrium that produces fewer prostaglandins. However, oral contraceptives are not a viable treatment in women who smoke, those with clotting disorders or liver disease, or those who wish to become pregnant.

Omega-3 Fatty Acids

Preliminary data suggest that women with low dietary intake of omega-3 fatty acids (essential fatty acids) experience greater menstrual pain.[5] In a small randomized, placebo-controlled crossover study, 42 adolescent girls with primary dysmenorrhea were administered fish oil (1080 mg eicosapentaenoic acid [EPA] and 720 mg docosahexaenoic [DHA] per day) and 1.5 mg of vitamin E per day for 2 months, followed by placebo; or placebo for 2 months followed by the fish oil and vitamin E for 2 months. On a 7-point scale with a score of 4 indicating moderate effectiveness, 73% of the girls rated the treatment a 4 or better.[6] The authors of a double-blind, randomized, controlled trial found that a low-temperature extract of the Antarctic krill *(Euphausia superba)* effectively reduced the amount of analgesics required by women with dysmenorrhea after 45 and 90 days of treatment compared with baseline and compared with women receiving omega-3 fish oil.[7]

SOUND FISHY?

Eskimos consume more fat than just about any other people on the planet and yet they have a much lower incidence of heart disease. The secret may lie in the amount of fish consumed in their diet. Omega-3 fatty acids are polyunsaturated fatty acids found in all seafood, including shellfish, oysters, and shrimp, although the richest sources are salmon, tuna, mackerel, herring, sea bass, and trout. The American Heart Association now recommends eating fish two times a week to prevent heart disease. Other research suggests that fish may also reduce the risk of stroke and improve mood. Although fish are healthy, low in fat, and protein rich, swordfish, shark, tilefish, king mackerel, and tuna steak can contain high levels of mercury. Women should limit consumption of these fish and avoid them altogether during pregnancy and early childhood.

Although the research is preliminary, given the relative safety of fish and fish oil, women with dysmenorrhea may want to eat oily, cold-water fish two or three times per week or consider taking fish-oil supplements. Concerns have been raised with regard to the presence of heavy metals in some sources of fish oil. However, an evaluation of 20 varieties of commercially available fish oil capsules by Consumer Labs showed that none of them contained any detectable level of mercury (<1.5 parts per billion [ppb]).[8] By comparison, mercury levels in fish generally range from 10 to 1000 ppb, depending on the fish. Researchers note several possible explanations for the lack of mercury in these supplements, including the use of species of fish that are less likely to accumulate mercury, the fact that most mercury is found in fish meat and not fish oil, and distillation processes that remove contaminants. Flax and pumpkin seeds also contain omega-3 fatty acids and may be used instead of, or in addition to, fish.

Thiamine (Vitamin B₁)

A randomized, double blind, placebo-controlled study was conducted in 556 girls ages 12 to 21 years experiencing moderate to very severe primary spasmodic dysmenorrhea. Thiamine hydrochloride (vitamin B_1) at a dose of 100 mg/day was found to completely alleviate pain in 87% of participants; 8% experienced some pain relief, and 5% showed no effect.[9] This study was conducted in India, where thiamine deficiency is more common than it is in the United States or Europe. At this time, no other trials are available for evaluation. In addition to supplementation, thiamine is present in many foods; it is most abundant in pork, dried fortified cereals, oatmeal, and sunflower seeds.

Vitamin E

In a double-blind clinical study of 100 girls ages 16 to 18 years with primary dysmenorrhea, the participants were randomly assigned to receive 500 IU/day vitamin E or placebo for 2 months. The treatment began 2 days before the onset of menstruation and continued through the first 3 days of bleeding. The severity of pain in the two groups was reduced after treatment, but the reduction was modestly superior in the group treated with vitamin E.[10] At the start of the study, the median pain scores on a scale of 0 to 10 were similar: 5.5 in the vitamin E group and 5.4 in the control group. Two months later the girls in the vitamin E group reported an average pain score of 3.5, whereas those receiving placebo reported a pain score of 4.3.

Magnesium

Three small trials have evaluated the efficacy of magnesium for the relief of dysmenorrhea. Overall, magnesium was more effective than placebo for pain relief, and the need for additional medication was less. The investigators noted no significant difference in the number of adverse effects experienced.[11] A reduction in inflammatory prostaglandins may be responsible. One study included data on levels of prostaglandin $F_{2\alpha}$. Women taking magnesium therapy had substantially lower levels of prostaglandin $F_{2\alpha}$ in their menstrual blood than those on the placebo ($P < 0.05$); these lower levels correlated with a decrease in pain by the participants. Dosage recommendations vary, but the range is generally 300 to 600 mg/day for 3 to 5 days, starting the day before the onset of menses.

Botanical Remedies

Pelvic pain and menstrual cramps are discussed in many classic herbal texts. Various herbal treatments are primarily directed at easing pain and trying to restore a "balanced" constitution. In traditional Chinese medicine, the problem is seen as one of blood stagnation, and herbs and acupuncture are used to correct the underlying imbalance. A practitioner of *ayurveda* would attempt to restore balance by making recommendations regarding all aspects of life, including diet, exercise, and botanicals, to ultimately help rebalance the constitution. Western-trained herbalists have traditionally relied on botanicals with antispasmodic and anti-inflammatory activity. Bitter herbs that enhance digestion and act on the liver are also included in some formulations.

Much of what has been done over the history of herbalism to relieve pelvic pain and menstrual cramps continues to be relied on by contemporary herbalists. Most practitioners of these systems of medicine still take a "holistic" approach to treatment. The following text presents some of the dietary measures and botanicals that are currently being recommended for menstrual cramps or show some promise of efficacy. Readers should be aware that very few randomized studies have been conducted to support the use of these approaches, although many are well founded in a biologically plausible approach.

Black haw **(Viburnum prunifolium).** Black haw was valued in early American medicine for its effectiveness in easing uterine cramping, be it spasmodic dysmenorrhea or threatened miscarriage. *King's American Dispensatory* states that black haw "acts promptly in spasmodic dysmenorrhea, especially with excessive flow."[12] The herb was highly valued for its ability to prevent miscarriage. A dark part of U.S. history is reflected in another passage: "It was for a long time customary for planters to compel their female slaves to drink an infusion of black haw daily whilst pregnant to prevent abortion."[12] Black haw was officially entered into the United States Pharmacopoeia in 1882 and remained in the National Formulary until 1960.

An article published in 1939 described the uterine-relaxant effects of a preparation of *V. prunifolium* in a woman whose uterus was subsequently removed for therapeutic reasons. Strips of uterine tissue were tested with the same extract. Uterine relaxation was found to occur in a dose-dependent manner.[13] An active glycoside from *V. prunifolium* was later shown to bring about relaxation in both animal and human uteri.[14]

Scopoletin and esculetin, substances found in the bark of black haw, exert antispasmodic effects on uterine muscle. Scopoletin has an antispasmodic activity approximately one twentieth of that of papaverine; esculetin exerts approximately one eighth of the activity.[15] The potency of the whole root is 0.05% that of papaverine.[16]

As in test tube studies, animal research has demonstrated complete relaxation of uterine tissue in rats with the administration of extracts from black haw, cramp bark (*V. opulus*), *V. carlcephalum*, and *V. chenaulti*. *V. chenaulti* was found to have twice the uterine-relaxant activity of the other species. Constituents have been identified in black haw and cramp bark that exert uterine-relaxant properties.[17]

Herbalists practicing in the United States and United Kingdom commonly recommend black haw, cramp bark, or both for painful menstrual cramps, threatened miscarriage, leg cramps, tension headaches, afterbirth pains, and muscle spasm. However, despite the praise from physicians of old and contemporary practitioners of botanical medicine, sadly no clinical trials have been conducted to evaluate the antispasmodic effects of either herb. Black haw appears to be relatively safe but has been given a restriction by the American Herbal Products Association (AHPA)—"Individuals with a history of kidney stones should use this herb cautiously"[18]—because of the presence of oxalates. (Cramp bark does not contain oxalates.) The AHPA does not say that the use of black haw or cramp bark is contraindicated during pregnancy or lactation.[18]

Dose and administration. To prepare an infusion, or tea, simmer 2 or 3 teaspoons of bark in 8 oz of water for 10 minutes. Strain and drink 1 cup two or three times a day as needed. The dose for fluid extract (1:1) is 4 to 8 mL, taken three or four times a day.[19]

Wild yam (Dioscorea villosa). Eclectic physicians of the 19th century considered wild yam a useful antispasmodic for dysmenorrhea and ovarian neuralgia. Older in vitro studies of *Dioscorea villosa* extracts failed to demonstrate any antispasmodic effects on the uterus.[20] It is interesting to note that the old name for wild yam was "colic root," from the extensive use of this herb in easing gastrointestinal pain and griping. A study published in 1997 found that dietary diosgenin, a key component of wild yam, reduced intestinal inflammation induced by indomethacin.[21] No current research is available with which to validate or dispute the historical use of wild yam as a remedy for dysmenorrhea.

Pulsatilla (Anemone pulsatilla). Pulsatilla, also known as pasque flower, has been shown to reduce uterine contractions in vitro,[22] and the extract is said to exert sedative and analgesic activity. The *British Herbal Compendium* lists the following indications for pulsatilla: "Painful spasmodic conditions of the male and female reproductive systems; dysmenorrhea."[23] No randomized, controlled studies of this plant are available. Members of the buttercup family, to which pulsatilla belongs, contain the glycoside ranunculin. When converted by plant enzymes to protoanemonin, it becomes a strong irritant,[24] causing blistering of the skin and irritation of the oral and gut mucosa.[25] Protoanemonin is rapidly polymerized to anemonin on drying. Anemonin is nontoxic. Therefore only dried pulsatilla should be used in herbal remedies. The use of pulsatilla is contraindicated during pregnancy and lactation.

Dose and administration. The dose recommended in the *British Herbal Compendium* is 0.1 to 0.3 g in infusion three times a day or 0.5 to 3 mL of tincture (1:10, 25% ethanol) three times a day.[23] Mild overdose acts as a strong gastric irritant; larger doses can lead to coma and convulsions. It is important to stay within the appropriate dosage range.

Black cohosh (Cimicifuga racemosa). Older literature reports claim that black cohosh was used to treat breast pain and menstrual cramps and that it was favored for "melancholia" around the time of menses. The presence of aromatic acids accounts for much of the plant's antiinflammatory, analgesic, and antipyretic activity.[26] This may be the result of prostaglandin inhibition, which could partially explain the historical use of black cohosh in the treatment of menstrual cramps. German health authorities have endorsed the use of black cohosh for the treatment of premenstrual discomfort and dysmenorrhea.[27]

Dose and administration. The herb is typically blended with other herbs for the treatment of dysmenorrhea. The dose for tincture (1:5) is generally in the range of 2 or 3 mL, twice a day. The crude herb is taken at a dosage of 500 to 1000 mg/day.

Dong quai (Angelica sinensis). *Dong quai* has been used in traditional medicine of China for at least 20 centuries and is found in Lei Gong's *Treatise on Preparation of Materia Medica* (588 AD): "The root is used medicinally as a strengthener of the heart, lung, and liver meridians; it is a tonic of the blood and promotes blood circulation; it regulates the menstrual cycle and stops menstrual pain."[28] Although it is used to treat a variety of ailments, *dong quai* is regarded as a tonic for women with fatigue or low vitality and those who are recovering from illness.

A volatile-oil component has been found to inhibit spontaneous uterine contractions in isolated uteri through antagonism of the effects of histamine and epinephrine, and a nonvolatile oil, water/alcohol-soluble component, appears to exert uterine stimulant activity in vivo. These contrasting effects were noted in animal studies involving both pregnant and nonpregnant cats, dogs, and rabbits.[29] Ferulic acid, an organic acid found in *dong quai* root, has demonstrated uterine-relaxant activity in rat uteri.[30] The fact that certain constituents of *dong quai* stimulate and others relax the uterus is often used by herbalists to explain the "tonic" effect of the herb.

A 1992 article by Ozaki noted that high doses of ferulic acid (300 mg/kg) inhibited edema induced by carrageenan in rats. It was hypothesized that the effect is a result of inhibition of prostaglandins.[31] Given the antiinflammatory and possible analgesic activity of *dong quai*, this herb has a plausible role in easing menstrual cramping.

Traditional Chinese practitioners caution that because *dong quai* is a "heating" herb, it may cause symptoms such as hot flashes, red face, sweating, insomnia, and irritability. Use during the first trimester of pregnancy cannot be recommended because of the uncertain effects of the herb on the uterus. The AHPA states that *A. sinensis* should not be taken during pregnancy, although the association notes that most Chinese herbal references do not list pregnancy as a contraindication to its use.[32]

Dose and administration. The dose is generally 3.5 to 4.0 g/day of the dried root, or 200 mg three times a day of an extract standardized to contain 1% ligustilide. The dose for tincture (1:5) is generally in the range of 5 to 8 mL, three times a day.

Fennel seed (Foeniculum vulgare). Preliminary research has demonstrated that fennel essential oil inhibits prostaglandin- and oxytocin-induced uterine contractions.[33] Anethole and other terpenoids present in the volatile oil fraction of fennel seed inhibit spasms in smooth muscle, likely accounting for fennel seed's long history of use as a remedy for colic and intestinal spasm. A small 3-month study was conducted in 30 women ages 15 to 24 years with moderate to severe primary dysmenorrhea to compare the efficacy of mefenamic acid (250 mg every 6 hours) and a 2% concentration of fennel seed essence (25 drops every 4 hours, taken orally). No medication was given in the first (control) cycle; in the second cycle women were treated with mefenamic acid, and in the third cycle essence of fennel fruit at a 2% concentration was prescribed at the beginning of the cycle. These cycles were compared day by day for their effect, potency, time of initiation of action, and complications through the use of a self-scoring system. Both treatments effectively relieved menstrual pain compared with that during the control cycles ($P < 0.001$). Mefenamic acid had a more potent effect than did fennel on the second and third menstrual days ($P < 0.05$); however, the difference on the other days was not significant. No complications were reported for mefenamic acid treatment cycles, but five participants (16.6%) withdrew from the study because of the odor of the fennel and one woman (3.11%) reported a mild increase in the amount of menstrual flow.[34]

Dose and administration. Many women have difficulty locating the fennel seed essence used in the previously mentioned clinical trial. Tincture of fennel seed would likely yield better results than tea, given the superior extraction of the volatile/essential-oil fraction by ethanol. Fennel is generally well tolerated by most, although the licorice-like taste and smell can be off-putting to some. The dosage for tincture is 1 to 3 mL, taken every 4 hours as needed.

Partridgeberry (Mitchella repens). Partridgeberry is an indigenous North American plant that found its way into Western herbal medicine by way of colonial interactions with Eastern Native American tribes. Its colloquial name, squaw vine, was coined by early settlers who observed its use by Native American women. However, we find the term *squaw* inappropriate and use the plant's other common name, partridgeberry. The partridgeberry fruits were eaten raw or dried and used in jams and breads. Early practitioners praised the herb for its ability to ease the pain associated with childbirth and menstruation. It was also used as a mild diuretic. No contemporary research has been conducted with the herb, but it contains a variety of potentially active tannins, glycosides, and saponins. Studies conducted in the early 1900s failed to note any significant action on isolated uterine muscle tissue.[22]

Despite the lack of contemporary research, partridgeberry remains popular among herbalists in the United States and is often found in combination with other herbs such as black haw, wild yam, *donq quai*, and raspberry leaf.

Dose and administration. To prepare a partridgeberry infusion, pour a cup of boiling water over 1 teaspoon of the herb and let it infuse for 10 to 15 minutes. The resulting infusion should be taken three times a day. The dosage for tincture (1:5) is generally 2 to 3 mL, three times a day. The crude herb is taken in a dosage of 1000 to 1500 mg/day.

Acupuncture

The National Institutes of Health Consensus Review Panel recommended acupuncture as either a supplemental or alternative treatment for dysmenorrhea. This recommendation appears to be supported by one small but methodologically sound trial of 43 women with dysmenorrhea. Researchers reported 91% efficacy with acupuncture, compared with 36% for women administered sham acupuncture and 18% of subjects in an untreated control group.[35] Open trials have also shown beneficial effects.[36,37] A study of 216 girls ages 14 to 18 years with primary dysmenorrhea found acupressure to be equivalent in efficacy to ibuprofen and superior to sham acupressure.[38]

Cochrane reviewers found that high-frequency transcutaneous electrical nerve stimulation (TENS) was effective in the treatment of primary dysmenorrhea. They found insufficient evidence to determine the effectiveness of low-frequency TENS or acupuncture in reducing dysmenorrhea.[39] The conclusion was drawn because of the lack of any large clinical trials addressing the efficacy of acupuncture and dysmenorrhea.

Chiropractic Manipulation (Spinal Manual Therapy)

Some women turn to spinal manual therapy (chiropractic care) for the treatment of their menstrual pain. Several hypotheses have been suggested to explain why it may be an effective intervention. The parasympathetic and sympathetic pelvic-nerve pathways are closely associated with the spinal vertebrae. One hypothesis is that mechanical dysfunction in these vertebrae causes decreased spinal mobility. This dysfunction could affect sympathetic-nerve distribution to the blood vessels supplying the pelvic viscera, leading to dysmenorrhea as a result of vasoconstriction.[40] Another theory holds that dysmenorrhea is the result of referred pain from musculoskeletal structures in the pelvis. Cochrane reviewers found that the results from four clinical trials of high-velocity, low-amplitude spinal manipulation suggest that the technique was no more effective than sham manipulation in the treatment of dysmenorrhea, although it was possibly more effective than no treatment at all. The reviewers concluded, "Overall there is no evidence to suggest that spinal manipulation is effective in the treatment of primary or secondary dysmenorrhea. There is no greater risk of adverse effects with spinal manipulation than there is with sham manipulation."[40]

Summary

Conventional medicine offers NSAIDS and oral contraceptives for the management of mild to moderate dysmenorrhea. Surgical interruption of the pelvic-nerve pathways is sometimes used as a last resort for severe, intractable cases of dysmenorrhea. Although NSAIDs and oral contraceptives are effective for many women, these treatments are not without side effects, leaving women to seek alternatives for the management of menstrual cramps. Dietary interventions, vitamin supplementation, botanical remedies, and acupuncture all appear to offer some benefit to women with dysmenorrhea. Some of these interventions have both a long history of use and a strong contemporary following for their alleviation of menstrual pain. The virtually empty pool of clinical trials with which to assess their efficacy presents limitations.

References

1. Lichten EM, Bombard J: Surgical treatment of primary dysmenorrhea with laparoscopic uterine nerve ablation, *J Reprod Med* 32:37-41, 1987.
2. Speroff L, Glass RH, Kase NG: Clinical gynecologic endocrinology and infertility, ed 4, Baltimore, 1989, Williams & Wilkins, pp 133-134.
3. Stromberg P, Akerlund M, Forsling ML, et al: Vasopressin and prostaglandins in premenstrual pain and primary dysmenorrhea, *Acta Obstet Gynecol Scand* 63:533-538, 1984.
4. Owens PR: Prostaglandin synthetase inhibitors in the treatment of primary dysmenorrhea: outcome trials reviewed, *Am J Obstet Gynecol* 148:96, 1984.
5. Deutch B: Menstrual pain in Danish women correlated with low omega-3 polyunsaturated fatty acid intake, *Eur J Clin Nutr* 49:508-516, 1995.
6. Harel Z, Biro FM, Kottenhan RK, et al: Supplementation with omega-3 polyunsaturated fatty acids in the management of dysmenorrhea in adolescents, *Am J Obstet Gynecol* 174:1335-1338, 1996.
7. Sampalis F, Bunea R, Pelland MF, et al: Evaluation of the effects of Neptune Krill Oil on the management of premenstrual syndrome and dysmenorrhea, *Altern Med Rev* 8:171-179, 2003.
8. Product review: Omega-3 fatty acids (EPA and DHA) from fish/marine oils. Available at: www.consumerlabs.com. Accessed September 2003.
9. Gokhale LB: Curative treatment of primary (spasmodic) dysmenorrhoea, *Ind J Med Res* 103:227-231, 1996.
10. Ziaei S, Faghihzadeh S, Sohrabvand F, et al: A randomised placebo-controlled trial to determine the effect of vitamin E in treatment of primary dysmenorrhoea, *Br J Obstet Gynaecol* 108:1181-1183, 2001.
11. Wilson ML, Murphy PA: Herbal and dietary therapies for primary and secondary dysmenorrhoea, The Cochrane Library, Issue 2, 2002, Oxford: Update Software.
12. Felter HW, Lloyd JU: *King's American Dispensatory*, ed 18, rev 3, vol II, Portland, Oregon, 1983, Eclectic Medical Publications, pp 2059-2062.
13. Munch JC: *Viburnum* studies. V. Uterine sedative action, *J Am Pharm Assoc* 28:886-887, 1939.
14. Evans WE, Harne WG, Krantz JC: A uterine principle from *Viburnum prunifolium*, *J Pharmacol Exp Ther* 75:174-177, 1942.
15. Hoerhammer L, Wagner H, Reinhardt H: On new constituents from the barks of *Viburnum prunifolium* L. (American snowball) and *Viburnum opulus* (common snowball), *Z Naturforschg* 22b:768-776, 1967.
16. Sloane AB, Latven AR, Munch JC: *Viburnum* studies. XVI. Rate of extraction of uterine sedative potency, *J Am Pharm Assoc* 38:457-459, 1949.

17. Nicholson JA, Darby TD, Jarboe CH: Viopudial, a hypotensive and smooth muscle antispasmodic from *Viburnum opulus, Proc Soc Exp Biol Med* 140:457-461, 1972.

18. McGuffin M, Hobbs C, Upton R, et al, editors: *American Herbal Products Association's Botanical Safety Handbook*, Boca Raton, Fla, 1997, CRC Press, p 122.

19. Council of the Pharmaceutical Society of Great Britain: *The British Pharmaceutical Codex,* London, 1934, Pharmaceutical Press, pp 1108-1109.

20. Pilcher JD: The action of certain drugs on the excised uterus of the guinea-pig, *J Pharmacol Exp Ther* 8:110-111, 1916.

21. Yamada T, Hoshino M, Hayakawa T, et al: Dietary diosgenin attenuates subacute intestinal inflammation associated with indomethacin in rats, *Am J Physiol* 273 (2 Pt 1):G355-G364, 1997.

22. Pilcher JD, Burman GE, Delzell WR: The action of the so-called female remedies on the excised uterus of the guinea pig, *Arch Intern Med* 18:557-583, 1916.

23. Bradley PR: *British Herbal Compendium: A handbook of scientific information on widely used plant drugs*, vol 1, Dorset, England, 1992, British Herbal Medicine Association, pp 179-180.

24. Nachman NJ, Olsen JD: Ranunculin: a toxic constituent of the poisonous range plant bur buttercup (*Ceratocephalus testiculatus*), *J Am Agric Food Chem* 31:1358-1560, 1983.

25. Winters JB: Severe urticarial reaction in a dog following ingestion of tall field buttercup, *Vet Med Small Anim Clin* 71:307, 1976.

26. Liske E: Therapeutic efficacy and safety of *Cimicifuga racemosa* for gynecologic disorders, *Adv Ther* 15:45-53, 1998.

27. Blumenthal M, Gruenwald J, Hall T, Rister RS, editors: *The Complete German Commission E Monographs: therapeutic guide to herbal medicine*, Boston, 1998, Integrative Medicine Communications, p 90.

28. Zhu DP: Dong quai, *Am J Chin Med* 15:117-125, 1987.

29. Mei QB, Tao JY, Cui B: Advances in the pharmacological studies of radix *Angelica sinensis* (Oliv) Diels (Chinese dang gui), *Chin Med J* 104:776-781, 1991.

30. Ozaki Y, Ma JP: Inhibitory effects of tetramethylpyrazine and ferulic acid on spontaneous movement of rat uterus in situ, *Chem Pharm Bull* 38:1620-1623, 1990.

31. Ozaki Y: Anti-inflammatory effect of tetramethylpyrazine and ferulic acid, *Chem Pharm Bull* 40:954-956, 1992.

32. McGuffin M, Hobbs C, Upton R, et al: A: *American Herbal Products Association's botanical safety handbook*, Boca Raton, Fla, 1997, CRC Press, p 11.

33. Ostad SN, Soodi M, Shariffzadeh M, et al: The effect of fennel essential oil on uterine contraction as a model for dysmenorrhea: pharmacology and toxicology study, *J Ethnopharmacol* 76:299-304, August 2001.

34. Namavar Jahromi B, Tartifizadeh A, Khabnadideh S: Comparison of fennel and mefenamic acid for the treatment of primary dysmenorrhea, *Int J Gynaecol Obstet* 80:153-157, 2003.

35. Helms JM: Acupuncture for the management of primary dysmenorrhea, *Obstet Gynecol* 69:51-56, 1987.

36. Xiaoma W: Observations of the therapeutic effects of acupuncture and moxibustion in 100 cases of dysmenorrhea, *J Trad Chin Med* 7:15-17, 1987.

37. Chuang Z: Treatment of 32 cases of dysmenorrhea by puncturing hegu and sanyinjiao acupoints, *J Trad Chin Med* 10:33-35, 1990.

38. Pouresmail Z, Ibrahimzadeh R: Effects of acupressure and ibuprofen on the severity of primary dysmenorrhea, *J Trad Chin Med* 22:205-210, 2002.

39. Proctor ML, Smith CA, Farquhar CM, et al: Transcutaneous electrical nerve stimulation and acupuncture for primary dysmenorrhoea, *Cochrane Database Syst Rev* (1):CD002123, 2002.

40. Proctor ML, Hing W, Johnson TC, et al: Spinal manipulation for primary and secondary dysmenorrhoea, *Cochrane Database Syst Rev* (4):CD002119, 2001.

CHAPTER

5

Endometriosis

Endometriosis is a condition in which endometrial tissue implants in sites outside the uterus, most commonly in the ovaries, fallopian tubes, and peritoneum. It is estimated to affect as many as 15% of all women.[1] Endometriosis is the third leading cause of hospitalization for gynecologic problems in the United States and a major reason for hysterectomy.

The implants of endometrial tissue in endometriosis are derived from the glandular and stromal tissues of the endometrium, the lining of the uterus. These hormone-responsive tissues maintain their response to hormonal stimulation even outside the uterus. During the normal shedding of the endometrial lining at the end of each menstrual cycle, the endometriotic tissue bleeds into the surrounding tissue, causing local inflammation. This peritoneal inflammation leads to the formation of adhesions and ovarian cysts, resulting in pain[2] and sometimes infertility.[3] Symptoms typically include dysmenorrhea, dyspareunia, and abdominal pain. The risk of ectopic (tubal) pregnancy is increased if the fallopian tube becomes narrowed as a result of the formation of adhesions. Infertility occurs in many women with endometriosis.

The origin of endometriosis is not completely understood, but retrograde menstruation, which occurs in roughly 90% of women may play a role.[4] When a woman menstruates, some menstrual blood, containing endometrial tissue, flows into the fallopian tubes instead of through the cervix and into the vagina. This tissue can then implant and grow on surrounding organs. But if so many women experience retrograde flow, why does endometriosis develop in so few? Researchers hypothesize that the immune system fails to seek out and eliminate this aberrant tissue. It is thought that these endometrial cells implant in women with deficient cell-mediated immunity.[5]

Endometriosis also appears to involve the humoral immune system; the formation of autoantibodies to endometrial tissue has been noted.[6]

Environmental factors may play a role in the development of endometriosis. A team of investigators has linked the environmental toxin dioxin (2,7,8-tetra-chloro-dibenzo-*p*-dioxin) to endometriosis in primates.[7] It is speculated that endometriosis develops after excessive dietary exposure to dioxin and related pesticides. Chemotoxins such as dioxin are known to disrupt the reproductive and immune systems[8] and have also been found to increase the risk of breast and prostate cancer.

Genetics may be a contributing factor in endometriosis; first-degree relatives of women with the condition are at approximately 10 times greater risk of having it themselves.[9] The reality is that the cause of endometriosis is likely multifactorial and that it comprises a combination of physiologic, immunologic, genetic, and environmental factors.

EVALUATION

Health care providers should be alert to the triad of menstrual pain, painful intercourse, and infertility that signals the presence of endometriosis. Dysmenorrhea that develops after years of pain-free menstrual cycles should raise suspicions of endometriosis. Some women experience painful or difficult bowel movements when the intestines are involved. The differential diagnosis includes irritable bowel syndrome, dysmenorrhea, peptic ulcer disease, appendicitis, pelvic inflammatory disease, urinary-tract infection, ovarian cysts or torsion, ectopic pregnancy, and inflammatory bowel disease. Physical examination may be helpful if the clinician is able to palpate pelvic nodules or tender nodules on the fallopian tubes or if painful discolored areas are visible on the back wall of the vagina. Depending on the patient's presentation, a complete blood cell count, urinalysis, cervical culture, and assessment of the patient's level of β-human chorionic gonadotropin may be ordered.

The definitive diagnosis of endometriosis requires laparoscopic confirmation of the presence of one or more endometriotic implants on the peritoneum or ovaries. In laparoscopy, several small incisions are made in the abdomen and a telescope-like instrument is inserted into the pelvis to permit visualization of the endometriotic lesions. Lesions generally appear as black, dark-brown, or bluish nodules or small cysts containing old hemorrhage, surrounded by a variable degree of fibrosis. Samples of the tissue are taken for laboratory analysis and pathologic diagnosis.

TREATMENT

Endometriosis is a chronic disorder that varies in severity. Treatment must be tailored to the needs of each woman. Is the primary goal pain relief? Fertility? What are the risks and benefits of each treatment? With these considerations in mind, a woman might consider some of the following options for the treatment of endometriosis.

Nonsteroidal Antiinflammatory Drugs

For mild to moderate pain associated with endometriosis, nonsteroidal antiinflammatory agents can offer effective, temporary relief. Ibuprofen, naproxen, and mefenamic acid, among others, are effective and safe when used appropriately for short periods. As many as 80% of all women experience some relief with these agents; however, complete alleviation of pain does not always occur. Something more than just prostaglandins is probably responsible for the pain associated with the disorder. Acetaminophen has not been as effective, probably because of its lack of antiinflammatory activity.[10] Women with a history of peptic ulcer disease or renal failure should check with a health care provider before using nonsteroidal antiinflammatory drugs.

Hormonal Therapies

Endometrial tissue contains receptors for estrogen, progesterone, and androgens, and so hormonal manipulation may be a relatively effective method of treating this disorder.

Oral contraceptives. For women who are not attempting pregnancy, oral contraceptives (OCs) can be used to control pelvic pain. Cyclic therapy (3 weeks on, 1 week off) may be used; however, continuous therapy is most often recommended. Combination OCs that contain both estrogen and progesterone are taken every day. This places the woman in a state of "pseudopregnancy" and prevents the endometrial implants from enlarging, bleeding, and causing pain. In clinical trials, as many as 90% of women with endometriosis have achieved improvement with this therapy.[11] Symptoms often recur when treatment is discontinued; thus use of OCs offers a long-term treatment strategy. Common adverse effects associated with OCs include nausea, breakthrough bleeding, breast tenderness, headache, and weight gain. This therapy works best for women who do not currently desire pregnancy, who do not smoke, and who do not have a history of blood clots. Some practitioners recommend OCs for patients at high risk for endometriosis.

Progestins. Prolonged administration of progestin induces endometrial atrophy, which limits the growth of endometrial implants. The progestin medroxyprogesterone acetate (MPA), administered orally or as a long-acting depot injection, is commonly prescribed for endometriosis, although it is no longer approved by the U.S. Food and Drug Administration (FDA) for this indication. When given by injection, MPA suppresses ovulation and provides pain relief for many women.[12] The most common adverse effects of MPA are weight gain, depression, breast tenderness, and reduced libido.

Gonadotropin-releasing hormone agonists. When continuous therapy with OCs does not effectively control endometriosis-related pain, gonadotropin-releasing hormone (GnRH) agonists are usually tried. Initially these agents increase circulating levels of luteinizing hormone (LH) and follicle-stimulating hormone (FSH), resulting in a worsening of symptoms during the first month of therapy. However, long-term administration leads to a decline in LH and FSH secretion, followed by inhibition of ovulation and menstruation. These drugs place the body in a state of "pseudomenopause." The pituitary gland decreases production of LH and FSH, which in turn causes a reduction in ovarian secretion of estrogen. Menstrual cycles become irregular or cease, and implants of endometrial tissue shrink as hormone levels decrease.[13] At the time of this writing, three GnRH agonists have been approved by the FDA for the treatment of endometriosis: goserelin, leuprolide, and nafarelin.

Although these drugs are often effective, their side effects must be considered. The patient who takes such an agent is placed in a menopausal state (reversible with discontinuation of the drug) and may accordingly experience hot flashes, vaginal dryness, depression, weight gain, insomnia, and bone loss. Because of the loss of bone density and because long-term effects of therapy are uncertain, treatment with GnRH agonists has been limited to 6 months. However, this practice may change; newer research has shown that "add-back" hormone replacement therapy (HRT) can maintain bone mineral density (BMD) and reduce both the incidence and severity of hot flashes.[14] The authors of one prospective, randomized, placebo-controlled trial found that goserelin plus HRT is as effective as goserelin alone in alleviating the pain and symptoms of endometriosis while reducing the loss of BMD and the physiologic side effects of hot flashes and vaginal dryness.[15] When a GnRH agonist is the treatment of choice, HRT should be used in combination.[16]

Danazol. The first drug approved for the treatment of endometriosis was danazol, a synthetic male hormone. The antiestrogenic activity of danazol causes regression and shrinkage of both the uterine lining (endometrium) and endometrial implants. Evidence also suggests that it helps reduce the extent of endometriosis associated with autoimmune abnormalities.[17] Relief of pain is obtained while the drug is being used but returns once the woman stops taking it. Practitioners should note that this drug is pregnancy category X and advise patients to use appropriate barrier methods, even though danazol inhibits ovulation. Side effects include hot flashes, weight gain, acne, male pattern hair growth, muscle cramps, reduction of breast size, and increased cholesterol levels. The androgenic effects may be irreversible, so patients must be instructed to watch closely for signs of virilization.

Surgery

Surgical treatment may offer some women long-lasting pain relief, the opportunity to become pregnant, and the avoidance of side effects associated with drug therapies. However, not all surgeons have the same experience with laparoscopy, and careful inquiry should be made with regard to a surgeon's qualifications. The goal of surgery is to remove or destroy as much abnormal tissue as possible. Surgical techniques currently include laser surgery, electrocautery (burning), knife excision, and curettage (scraping). Sometimes a surgeon cuts specific nerves in the lower back to reduce the transmission of pain impulses to the brain. Recovery time from laparoscopic surgery is usually quite short. Many women are able to achieve pregnancy after surgery.

Laparotomy may be necessary if scar tissue is excessive or if the endometrial implants are very large (endometriomas). This surgery is more extensive and the recovery time is longer, but laparotomy is often necessary for those with extensive implants and adhesions. The results of surgical treatment are not permanent in all women. Recurrence rates range from 5% to 20% per year, with a rate of 40% after 5 years.[18] The rate of recurrence depends on the severity and extent of endometriosis, the surgical method used, and the skill of the surgeon.[19] Some practitioners recommend hormone therapy to prevent the reappearance of endometriotic implants in women who do not desire pregnancy.

Integrative Approaches

Our forebears likely did not understand the complex interaction of physiology, immunology, and genetics that accompanies endometriosis. The extent to which this condition existed in the distant past is also unclear. Pelvic pain and menstrual cramps are frequently discussed in ancient medical texts, but treatments were aimed mainly at easing pain and trying to restore a "balanced" constitution. In traditional Chinese medicine, the problem is regarded as being one of blood stagnation, and herbs and acupuncture are used to correct the underlying imbalance. In the ancient Indian system of *ayurveda*, recommendations are made with regard to all aspects of life, including diet, exercise, and botanical remedies to ultimately rebalance the constitution. Herbalists rely on herbs: bitter herbs that enhance digestion and act on the liver, herbs that reduce inflammation, ease spasms, and "purify" the body.

Many of the measures taken in the past to relieve pelvic pain and menstrual cramps are still used by herbalists. Most contemporary practitioners of these systems of medicine rely on a holistic approach to treatment. The following is a review of some of the dietary approaches and botanical remedies that are either being recommended for the treatment endometriosis or show some promise of efficacy. Few randomized studies have been conducted to support the use of these recommendations, although many are well founded in a biologically plausible approach.

Dietary considerations. Common sense indicates that a woman living with endometriosis should focus on a diet rich in vegetables and fiber, as this type of diet has been shown to reduce the level of active estrogens in the bloodstream.[20] A high-fiber diet can reduce the amount of estrogen that is reabsorbed and increase the amount that is excreted in the feces. Because estrogen has been shown to support the growth of endometriotic implants, a decrease in the circulating level of this hormone might be beneficial.

Some women choose to eat organically grown foods, when possible, to reduce their dietary intake of chemotoxins. The Environmental Protection Agency estimates that 90% of human dioxin exposure comes through food, and dioxin levels are highest in sources such as meat and dairy products.[21] Increased consumption of plant-based foods and fish paired with a reduced intake of other animal products may be beneficial to health in general and specifically helpful for women with endometriosis and those at high risk for the condition because of the presence of established risk factors (discussed previously). In many traditional systems of medicine, reduced intake of animal products is recommended for patients with inflammatory conditions. Such recommendations are biochemically plausible. For example, arachidonic acid (AA) is found preformed in animal fats and dairy products. When AA is liberated from the cell membrane, it is converted to the inflammatory prostaglandin-2 series and thromboxanes by the enzyme cyclooxygenase or to the inflammatory leukotrienes by way of the lipoxygenase pathway. All roads lead to inflammation.

Essential fatty acids. Essential fatty acids (EFAs) help reduce the production of harmful prostaglandins (hormone-like chemicals) that are associated with swelling and inflammation. Beneficial omega-3 fatty acids are found mainly in cold-water fish (cod, salmon, mackerel), whereas oils from the black currant seed, borage seed, and evening primrose are rich sources of gamma-linolenic acid. Vegetarians can use flaxseed instead of fish oil. Theoretically, the addition of EFAs to the diet helps reduce inflammation and consequently helps control the development of adhesions, as well as tissue destruction.

Several articles addressing the association of low omega-3 intake and dysmenorrhea have been published. Danish researchers found that a higher intake of marine omega-3 fatty acids was associated with less menstrual pain.[22] In one small randomized crossover study of 42 adolescent girls with primary dysmenorrhea, participants took fish oil (1,080 mg of eicosapentaenoic acid and 720 mg of docosahexaenoic acid) and 1.5 mg of vitamin E each day for 2 months and then took placebo or took placebo for 2 months and followed it with the active treatment. On a 7-point scale (4 representing "moderately effective"), 73% of the girls rated the treatment a 4 or higher.[23] Although this study focused on primary dysmenorrhea in adolescents, not endometriosis, the biochemical rationale remains the same. The purpose of reducing AA and increasing omega-3 fatty acids in the diet is to increase the levels of the antiinflammatory prostaglandin-1 and -3 series while decreasing the presence of the proinflammatory prostaglandin-2 series.

Although virtually no randomized double-blind studies have been conducted to evaluate the effect of dietary manipulation on endometriosis, this should not preclude practitioners from guiding women toward a diet that is primarily plant-based, with an emphasis on fiber and vegetables and some consumption of red meat shifted to cold-water fish.

Botanical remedies. Herbal therapies are primarily focused on the reduction of pain and inflammation. Many herbalists prescribe herbs traditionally used to benefit the liver, believing they will improve the metabolism of steroid hormones, thereby reducing serum estrogen levels through enhanced breakdown and excretion. Herbs that reduce levels of circulating autoantibodies may also play a beneficial role in the treatment of endometriosis, although this application has not been extensively investigated. Herbs that enhance the immune response also are found in a number of herbal formulations.

Herbs commonly used in the treatment of endometriosis include chastetree berry (*Vitex agnus castus*), black cohosh (*Cimicifuga racemosa*), black haw (*Viburnum prunifolium*), dong quai (*Angelica sinensis*), kava (*Piper methysticum*), pulsatilla (*Anemone pulsatilla*), and ginger (*Zingiber officinale*). Herbs that are believed to enhance liver function include bitters such as dandelion, milk thistle, and gentian. Cotton root bark (*Gossypium* spp.) has been shown to induce endometrial atrophy; however, its therapeutic use is limited by side effects. Yellow vine (*Tripterygium wilfordii*) has primarily been studied in rheumatoid arthritis (RA) but also shows promise in the treatment of endometriosis. Herbs such as echinacea (*Echinacea purpurea, E. angustifolia*) and astragalus (*Astragalus membranaceus*) are often included in herbal formulations to enhance immune surveillance for wayward endometrial tissue. Licorice (*Glycyrrhiza uralensis*) is frequently used for its antiinflammatory action. *Shakuyaku-kanzo-to,* an herbal medicine containing peony (*Paeonia* spp) and licorice, has been found to inhibit prostaglandin production in human uterine myometrium in vitro through its inhibition of phospholipase A_2 activity. These herbs are generally not given as single agents but are instead combined in herbal formulations.

Chastetree berry (Vitex agnus castus). Herbalists and naturopathic physicians frequently recommend chastetree berry as part of a treatment protocol for endometriosis,[24] probably because of the widely held belief that chastetree "balances" ovarian hormones. This herbal remedy is commonly used to treat premenstrual syndrome and is thought to work by normalizing the estrogen/progesterone ratio. Research does indicate that chastetree enhances the production and binding of progesterone. In vitro research has shown that chastetree stimulates progesterone-receptor expression in endometrial cells.[25] The authors of an open study in women with infertility noted that chastetree berry restores progesterone levels and prolongs the hyperthermic phase of the basal body temperature curve when used daily for at least 3 months.[26]

Chastetree is also recommended for the infertility that accompanies endometriosis. The herb inhibits prolactin production as a result of its dopamine-agonist properties. In vitro animal and human studies have demonstrated prolactin inhibition with higher doses of chastetree. Some researchers postulate that occult hyperprolactinemia is one cause of infertility in women with endometriosis.[27] If hyperprolactinemia is indeed present, chastetree may be of some benefit with regard to infertility. Practitioners in the United States, United Kingdom, and Germany commonly recommend chastetree for female infertility; however, the clinical data are difficult to interpret, given the design limitations of most studies.

Chastetree appears to be relatively safe when used appropriately. The German Commission E (German health authorities) states that there is "no application during pregnancy."[28] However, it is occasionally used to treat corpus luteum insufficiency during early pregnancy in women subject to frequent miscarriage. The offspring of women treated for infertility with chastetree preparations were not noted to have an increased incidence of malformations.[24] Some authors recommend that women taking OCs, HRT, or other hormonal agents avoid the concomitant use of chastetree.[29] The dose commonly used in Germany is equivalent to roughly 200 mg/day of dried fruit, whereas a dose of 500 to 1000 mg/day is typically used in the United States and United Kingdom. Most clinical trials using botanicals do not include dose escalation, making "optimal" dosing difficult.

Black cohosh (Cimicifuga racemosa). Although black cohosh is thought of mainly as an herb for women going through menopause, the rhizome and roots of this North American plant have a long history of use for numerous reproductive and rheumatic complaints. The antispasmodic and antiinflammatory properties of black cohosh are believed to be a result of the aromatic acids in the root. German health authorities recognize the use of black cohosh in the treatment of premenstrual discomfort, dysmenorrhea, and menopausal complaints.[28]

Black cohosh appears to be relatively safe when used appropriately. The use of black cohosh during pregnancy and lactation is contraindicated by most authorities. In vitro research indicates that black cohosh does not increase the proliferation of breast cancer cells,[30] although some authors recommend caution in women with a history of breast cancer. The German Commission E limits the use of black cohosh to 6 months because of the scarcity of long-term studies. Most studies have been based on standardized extracts equivalent to 40 to 80 mg/day of dried root and rhizome. Traditional doses have ranged from 0.5 to 1.0 g/day of dried root and rhizome.[31]

Black haw (Viburnum prunifolium). Perhaps one of the most commonly used herbs for the treatment of dysmenorrhea is black haw. Extracts of black haw, cramp bark (*V. opulus*), and two other *Viburnum* species were observed to bring about complete uterine relaxation in early animal studies.[32] Later investigation found at least four constituents in black haw and cramp bark that possess uterine-relaxant properties.[33] The bark of the root and stem were used by indigenous North American women to relieve menstrual pain, slow uterine bleeding, and prevent miscarriage. Black haw was once listed officially in the *United States Pharmacopoeia* and remained in the National Formulary until 1960. Black haw is often combined with black cohosh or kava to treat endometrial pain. It was historically used to relieve uterine and pelvic inflammation and was considered to be of specific benefit to those with intermittent painful spasms associated with menses.[34]

Although black haw is considered relatively safe, it should not be used by women with a history of oxalate-containing kidney stones. In such cases, cramp bark, which does not contain oxalate, is generally recommended.[29] Black haw and cramp bark are considered by herbalists to be the herbs of choice for the treatment of menstrual pain. However, no human clinical trials are available for review. The usual dose is 5 to 10 mL of tincture (1:5 strength) taken three or four times daily.

Dong quai (Angelica sinensis). *Dong quai* (Figure 5-1) has been used in the traditional medicine of China for at least 20 centuries and can be found in Lei Gong's *Treatise on Preparation of Materia Medica* (588 AD): "The root is used medicinally as a strengthener of the heart, lung, and liver meridians; it is a tonic of the blood and promotes blood circulation; it regulates the menstrual cycle and stops menstrual pain."[35] Researchers have found substances in the root that relax[36] the uterus and others that cause uterine stimulation.[37] Herbalists often cite this dual action to explain the "tonic" effect of the herb.

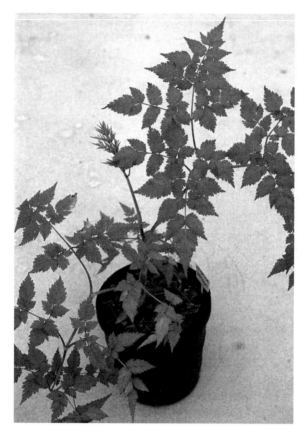

Figure 5-1 Dong quai *(Angelica sinensis)*. *(Courtesy Martin Wall Botanical Services.)*

Antiinflammatory and analgesic activities have also been demonstrated for constituents of *dong quai*.[38]

Given *dong quai's* antiinflammatory and analgesic effects, this herb may prove beneficial for women with endometriosis. The use of *dong quai* is contraindicated during pregnancy.[29] Doses of 2 g/kg were found to increase prothrombin time in rabbits given warfarin.[39] Patients taking warfarin should be monitored if *dong quai* therapy is initiated.

Ginger (Zingiber officinale). Ginger rhizome, widely used as both a spice and a medicinal agent, has been used on the Asian continent for more than 2500 years. Human trials have demonstrated benefit in the treatment of motion sickness, pregnancy-related nausea and vomiting, arthritis, and indigestion. An effective antispasmodic agent, ginger is valued in traditional Chinese medicine for its purported relief of menstrual cramps. Ginger is commonly found in herbal formulas for dysmenorrhea and endometriosis. Although no clinical trials are available for evaluation, the pharmacologic activity of the herb (antiinflammatory) would be expected to be of benefit in the treatment of mild symptoms.

Ginger is relatively safe when used appropriately. Pregnant women should limit their daily intake of dried ginger to 1 g/day.[40] Caution should be exercised by patients with active gallstone disease.[41] Patients who are taking anticoagulants or large doses of antiplatelet agents should not exceed 4 g/day of dried ginger.[42] The usual dose is 1 or 2 g/day of dried ginger.

Kava (Piper methysticum). Kava root is used in the preparation of a social beverage and as a medicinal agent throughout the South Pacific. Traditionally the rhizome is used to treat conditions including chronic cystitis, menstrual cramping, and migraines. Among the constituents of kava, four pyrones of the kawain-methysticin type have been found to act centrally as muscle relaxants. These substances have also been shown to reduce the excitability of the limbic system, an effect analogous to that of benzodiazepines.[43] Herbalists often make use of the antispasmodic, analgesic, and mild tranquilizing effects of kava for the treatment of premenstrual syndrome, menopause, dysmenorrhea and endometriosis.

The German Commission E lists pregnancy, lactation, and endogenous depression[28] as contraindications to the use of kava because of a lack of data. Kava may act synergistically with central nervous system agents such as alcohol and barbiturates. It may also act as a dopamine antagonist[44]; practitioners should be aware of this interaction in patients taking psychiatric medications and in those with Parkinson's disease. Large doses (>9 g/day) are associated with a dermopathy that is reversible on discontinuation of the herb.[45] More than 30 reports of suspected kava-induced hepatotoxicity have been reported in the literature. A causal relationship has not been scientifically determined at the time of this writing; however, practitioners may wish to avoid prescribing this herb until the issue has been further clarified. Most clinical studies have involved a product standardized to provide 100 to 200 mg/d of kavalactones taken in divided doses.

Pulsatilla (Anemone pulsatilla). Pulsatilla, also known as pasque flower, has been shown to reduce the amplitude of uterine contractions in vitro; historically the extract has been said to exert sedative and analgesic activity. The *British Herbal Compendium* lists the following indications for pulsatilla, which is popular among British herbalists: "Painful spasmodic conditions of the male and female reproductive systems; dysmenorrhea."[46] No randomized controlled studies are available for review.

The fresh plant contains protoanemonin, a strong local irritant, but this compound is not present in the dried plant. The use of pulsatilla is contraindicated during pregnancy and lactation. The dose recommended in the *British Herbal Compendium* is 0.1 to 0.3 g in infusion three times per day or tincture (1:10, 25% ethanol), 0.5 to 3 mL three times a day.

Cotton root bark (Gossypium *spp.*). Gossypol is a polyphenolic bisesquiterpene present in the subepidermal glands found throughout the cotton plant and in its seed. Gossypol has been shown to exert antifertility activity in both men and women. In China it was tested as a contraceptive in 12,000 men.[47] Antifertility activity exceeding 99% efficacy has been noted. Research to discover improved systems of delivery and methods of reducing adverse effects is ongoing. The primary serious side effect is hypokalemia that is not readily reversed with potassium supplementation.

In addition to the contraceptive effects of gossypol in women, evidence suggests that it may be useful in the treatment of endometriosis and uterine fibroids.[48] This usefulness probably stems from the induction of amenorrhea and endometrial changes that result in infertility. One report in the literature states that endometrial atrophy occurred in all 67 women administered gossypol in one study and that complete recovery of the endometrium occurred within 6 months of cessation of gossypol treatment.[47] Atrophy of endometrial tissue is the primary treatment goal for endometriosis. This herb should be further investigated for possible use in the treatment of this debilitating disorder.

Toxicity during pregnancy is likely. Gossypol's antiprogesterone effect and subsequent reduction of corpus luteum activity can cause abortion. Animal studies have shown that fetal implantation is impaired by gossypol.[49] Given the risk of hypokalemia and the possibility of unintended use by pregnant women, cotton root bark is not recommended for the treatment of endometriosis until more data are available.

Yellow vine (Tripterygium wilfordii). Yellow vine has been shown to exert antiinflammatory and immunosuppressive activity. A study of 70 patients with RA who were given 60 mg/day of a glycoside extract of yellow vine revealed significant improvement in symptoms; however, approximately one third of the women experienced cessation of the menstrual cycle within 12 weeks. Another study comprising 144 patients with RA revealed an overall effective rate of 90%, but almost a quarter of the women experienced menstrual irregularities or amenorrhea. This side effect has limited the use of this herb in RA. In light of this activity, the potential role in endometriosis is interesting. However, it is premature to recommend the use of this herb for the treatment of endometriosis.

Turska's formula. Many naturopathic physicians recommend an old remedy known as Turska's formula for the treatment of endometriosis.[50] The formula contains monkshood (*Aconitum napellus*), yellow jessamine (*Gelsemium sempervirens*), bryony (*Bryonia alba*), and poke root (*Phytolacca americana*). The recommended dose is 5 to 10 drops three times daily. Aconite poisoning still occurs, albeit more frequently in Asia, where the herb is used in several traditional remedies.[51] The alkaloids present in the monkshood plant manifest powerful actions upon the heart through interference with voltage-dependent sodium channels.[52] Even small doses of monkshood can be quite toxic. *Bryonia* has traditionally been used to relieve cough in pleurisy but is also considered toxic.[31] *Gelsemium* has been used to treat neuralgia and migraines, but "it should be used with care, since untoward symptoms sometimes result from comparatively low doses. Excessive doses cause giddiness, double vision, and loss of power, with slowing and subsequent cessation of respiration."[31] Poke root is frequently recommended by herbalists for its effects on the immune system, yet it contains potent lectins with hemagglutinating and mitotic activity.[29] Turska's formula may indeed prove beneficial to women with endometriosis but should be subjected to rigorous scientific inquiry before it is recommended, given its content of potentially toxic herbs.

Other Therapies

Some women with primary dysmenorrhea report improvement with the use of acupuncture. Acupuncture has been shown to produce analgesia in several medical conditions; however, no clinical trials have been conducted to assess its effectiveness in the treatment of endometriosis. Doctors of Oriental medicine often use a combination of herbs and acupuncture to treat endometriosis.

Women who experience lower back pain associated with endometriosis may benefit from chiropractic and osteopathic manipulation. Massage may be therapeutic and relaxing for women with pelvic and low back pain.

Yoga, tai chi, stretching, and other forms of exercise may relieve discomfort. Stress management and relaxation techniques may also be of benefit; stress can disrupt hormonal balance and diminish a woman's ability to cope with pain.

Summary

A number of strategies are available for women living with endometriosis. An integrated approach that comprises diet, movement, stress management, pharmacologic treatment (herbal or pharmaceutical), or surgical intervention—or any number of these approaches—will likely yield the most effective treatment, as well as the most satisfied patient. Individualization of therapy and honoring a woman's complaint of pain are important. The authors of one study reported that as many as 70% of women with endometriosis have been wrongly told that their symptoms were psychogenic in origin. Although much remains to be learned about the management of this disorder, with an accurate diagnosis and thoughtful consideration of the needs of each woman, much can be done to improve quality of life.

References

1. Houston DE, Noller KL, Melton LJ, et al: Incidence of pelvic endometriosis in Rochester, Minnesota, 1970-79, *Am J Epidemiol* 125:959-969, 1987.
2. Barlow DH, Glynn CJ: Endometriosis and pelvic pain, *Clin Obstet Gynecol* 7:775-789, 1993.
3. Prentice A, Ingamells S: Endometriosis and infertility, *J Br Fertil Soc* 1:51-55, 1996.
4. McLaren J, Prentice A: New aspects of pathogenesis of endometriosis, *Curr Obstet Gynecol* 6:85-91, 1996.
5. Giudice LC, Tazuke SI, Swiersz L: Status of current research on endometriosis, *J Reprod Med* 43:252-262, 1998.
6. Stratseva NV: Clinical-immunological aspects of genital endometriosis. *Akush Ginekol* 3:23-26, 1980.
7. Rier S, Martin D, Bowman RE, et al: Immunoresponsiveness in endometriosis: implications of estrogenic toxicants, *Envir Health Perspect* 103:151-156, 1995.
8. Osteen KG, Sierra-Rivera E: Does disruption of immune and endocrine systems by environmental toxins contribute to the development of endometriosis? *Semin Reprod Endocrinol* 15:301-308, 1997.
9. Dmowski WP, Lesniewicz R, Rana N, et al: Changing trends in the diagnosis of endometriosis: a comparative study of women with pelvic endometriosis presenting with chronic pelvic pain or infertility, *Fertil Steril* 67:238-243, 1997.
10. Milsom I, Andersch B: Effect of ibuprofen, naproxen sodium and paracetamol on intrauterine pressure and menstrual pain in dysmenorrhea, *Br J Obstet Gynaecol* 91:1129-1135, 1984.
11. Schmidt CL: Endometriosis: a reappraisal of pathogenesis and treatment. *Fertil Steril* 44:157-173, 1985.
12. Malinak R: Endometriosis, *ACOG Technical Bull* 184:1-5, 1993.
13. Cahill M, editor: *Physician's drug handbook*, ed 7, Springhouse, Pa, Springhouse, 1997, pp 554-555.
14. Schlaff WD: Extending the treatment boundaries: Zoladex and add-back, *Int J Gynaecol Obstet* 64(suppl 1):S25-S31, 1999.
15. Moghissi KS, Schlaff WD, Olive DL, et al: Goserelin acetate (Zoladex) with or without hormone replacement therapy for the treatment of endometriosis, *Fertil Steril* 69:1056-1062, 1998.
16. Edmonds DK: Add-back therapy in the treatment of endometriosis: the European experience, *Br J Obstet Gynaecol* 103(suppl 14):10-13, 1996.
17. el-Roeiy A, Dmowski W, Gleicher N, et al: Danazol but not gonadotropin-releasing hormone agonists suppresses autoantibodies in endometriosis, *Fertil Steril* 70:115-119, 1987.
18. Fedele L, Bianchi S, DiNola G, et al: The recurrence of endometriosis, *Ann N Y Acad Sci* 734:358-364, 1994.

19. Redwine D: Conservative laparoscopic excision of endometriosis by sharp dissection: life table analysis of re-operation and persistent or recurrent disease, *Fertil Steril* 56:628-634, 1991.
20. Goldin B, Adlercreutz H, Dwyer JT, et al: Effect of diet on excretion of estrogens in pre- and postmenopausal women, *Cancer Res* 41:3771-3773, 1981.
21. Tremblay L: Reproductive Toxins Conference—Pollution Prevention Network, *Endomet Assoc News* 17(5-6):13-15, 1996.
22. Deutch B: Menstrual pain in Danish women correlated with low omega-3 polyunsaturated fatty acid intake. *Eur J Clin Nutr* 49:508-516, 1995.
23. Harel Z, Biro FM, Kottenhahn RK, et al: Supplementation with omega-3 polyunsaturated fatty acids in the management of dysmenorrhea in adolescents. *Am J Obstet Gynecol* 174:1335-1338, 1996.
24. Newall CA, Andersen LA, Phillipson JD: *Herbal medicines: a guide for health care professionals*, London, 1996, Pharmaceutical Press.
25. Liu J, Burdette JE, Xu H, et al: Evaluation of estrogenic activity of plant extracts for the potential treatment of menopausal symptoms, *J Agric Food Chem* 49:2472-2479, 2001.
26. Propping D, Katzorke T, Belkien L: Diagnosis and therapy of corpus luteum deficiency in general practice, *Therapiewoche* 38:2992-3001, 1988.
27. Gregoriou G, Bakas P, Vitoratos N, et al: Evaluation of serum prolactin levels in patients with endometriosis and infertility. *Gynecol Obstet Invest* 48:48-51, 1999.
28. Blumenthal M, Busse W, Goldberg A, et al, editors: *The complete German Commission E Monographs: therapeutic guide to herbal medicines*, Boston, 1998, Integrative Medicine Communications.
29. McGuffin M, Hobbs C, Upton R, et al: *American Herbal Products Association's botanical safety handbook*, Boca Raton, Fla, 1997, CRC Press.
30. Zava DT, Dollbaum CM, Bien M: Estrogen and progestin bioactivity of foods, herbs, and spices. *Proc Soc Exp Biol Med* 217:369-378, 1998.
31. Pharmaceutical Society of Great Britain. *British Pharmaceutical Codex*, London, 1934, Pharmaceutical Press.
32. Jarboe CH, Schmidt CM, Nicholson JA, et al: Uterine relaxant properties of *Viburnum*, *Nature* 212:837, 1966.
33. Jarboe CH: One-methyl 2,3-dibutyl hemimellitate: a novel component of *Viburnum prunifolium*, *J Org Chem* 34:4202-4203, 1969.
34. Felter HW, Lloyd JU: *King's American Dispensatory*, ed 18, revision 3, vol II [originally rewritten and enlarged in 1898 and reprinted in 1983 by Eclectic Medical Publications, Portland, Ore, pp 2060-2061].
35. Zhu DP: Dong quai, *Am J Chin Med* 15:117-125, 1987.
36. Ozaki Y, Ma JP: Inhibitory effects of tetramethylpyrazine and ferulic acid on spontaneous movement of rat uterus in situ. *Chem Pharm Bull* 38:1620-1623, 1990.
37. Shi M, Chang L, He G: Stimulating action of *Carthamus tinctorius* L., *Angelica sinensis* (Oliv.) Diels and *Leonurus sibiricus* L. on the uterus, *Zhongguo Zhong Yao Za Zhi* 20:173-175, 1995 [originally in Chinese].
38. Ozaki Y: Anti-inflammatory effect of tetramethylpyrazine and ferulic acid. *Chem Pharm Bull* 40:954-956, 1992.
39. Lo AC, Chan K, Yeung JH, et al: Dang gui (*Angelica sinensis*) affects the pharmacodynamics but not the pharmacokinetics of warfarin in rabbits, *Eur J Drug Metab Pharmacokinet* 20:55-60, 1995.
40. Muller JL, Clauson KA: Pharmaceutical considerations of common herbal medicine. *Am J Managed Care* 3:1753-1770, 1997.
41. Bissett NG, editor: *Herbal drugs and phytopharmaceuticals*, Stuttgart, Germany, 1994, Medpharm GmBH Scientific Publishers.
42. Lumb AB: Effect of dried ginger on human platelet function, *Thromb Haemost* 71:110-111, 1994.
43. Schulz V, Hansel R, Tyler V: *Rational phytotherapy: a physician's guide to herbal medicine*, New York, 1998, Springer-Verlag, pp 65-73.
44. Schelosky L, Raffauf C, Jendroska K, et al: Kava and dopamine antagonism, *J Neurol Neurosurg Psychol* 58:639-640, 1995.

45. Norton SA, Ruze P, Kava dermopathy, *J Am Acad Dermatol* 31:89-97, 1994.
46. Bradley PR, editor: *British herbal compendium: a handbook of scientific information on widely used plant drugs*, vol 1, Dorset, UK, 1992, British Herbal Medicine Association, pp 179-180.
47. Evans WC: *Trease and Evans' pharmacognosy*, ed 14, London, 1996, Saunders, p 326.
48. Wu DF: An overview of the clinical pharmacology and therapeutic potential of gossypol as a male contraceptive agent and in gynaecological disease, *Drugs* 38:333-341, 1989.
49. Gossypol. In De Smet PAGM, Keller K, editors: *Adverse effects of herbal drugs*, vol 2, Berlin, 1993, Springer-Verlag, pp 195-207.
50. Hudson T: *Women's encyclopedia of natural medicine*, Lincolnwood, Ill, 1999, Keats Publishing, pp 85-86.
51. Chan TY: Aconite poisoning: a global perspective, *Vet Hum Toxicol* 36:326-328, 1994.
52. Ameri A: The effects of Aconitum alkaloids on the central nervous system, *Prog Neurobiol* 56:211-235, 1998.

CHAPTER

6

Menopause

The word *menopause* comes from the words *meno* (monthly menses) and *pausis* (pause), meaning a pause in menstruation, or, more correctly, the cessation of menstrual cycles. Menopause is a natural and normal part of aging, except when brought about through surgery or as the result of medication or illness. The average age of menopause is 52 years, and it commonly occurs between the ages of 42 and 56 years. The signs and symptoms generally ascribed to menopause include hot flashes, mood swings, depression, vaginal dryness, sleep disturbances, heart palpitations, headaches, urinary tract infections, and decreased libido. As women lose the support of estrogen, they are at increased risk for developing osteoporosis and heart disease. Some women pass through menopause with few physical or emotional complaints, whereas others become debilitated by the physical and emotional manifestations of the "change." By the year 2015, nearly 50% of American women will be in menopause.

The recent flood of often-conflicting information about the risks and benefits of hormone replacement therapy (HRT) has raised interest among many women and health care providers about the efficacy and safety of complementary and alternative medicinal approaches to managing menopausal effects in lieu of conventional HRT. The following is an overview of conventional and alternative therapies currently being offered to women in menopause. The abbreviation HRT is used in this chapter because of its wide recognition in the field. However, I believe that the term "hormone therapy" would be more accurate to describe the use of estrogen and progestin/progesterone because these hormones are not truly "replacement" in nature.

MENOPAUSAL SYMPTOMS AND THERAPIES

The primary symptoms of menopause for many women are hot flashes and night sweats. However, a great deal of variation exists among individual women and cultures. Approximately 70% of American women have at least one hot flash during their menopausal years, Greek women report a higher rate of hot flashes, Japanese women report fewer hot flashes, and Mayan women report no symptoms at all. A number of cultures do not even have a word for hot flash even though all women go through menopause. Variance in symptoms could be the result of diet, lifestyle, environment, or societal perception.

Hormone Therapy

HRT has been successfully used for decades to treat the symptoms of menopause. Minor side effects associated with HRT include bloating, breast tenderness, cramping, irritability, depression, breakthrough bleeding, or a return of monthly periods. Many women find these side effects unpleasant, and even before the release of the Women's Health Initiative (WHI) findings that put the safety of HRT in doubt, approximately two in three women who started either estrogen replacement therapy or HRT discontinued therapy within a year, regardless of hysterectomy status.[1] But these minor side effects did not compare to the concerns for more severe adverse events that were generated with the release of the findings of the WHI in July 2002.

The WHI is a large-scale, randomized, controlled clinical trial of 16,608 menopausal women aged 50 to 79 years with an intact uterus at the time of enrollment who were randomly assigned to receive either HRT in the form of 0.625 mg of conjugated equine estrogens and 2.5 mg of medroxyprogesterone acetate (Prempro) or placebo. The study was halted after 5.2 years on the recommendation of an independent review board because of an unacceptably higher risk of breast cancer in women receiving HRT.[2] When compared with those receiving placebo, women assigned to the combination HRT group also had more strokes, heart attacks, and blood clots. Although the HRT users also had a reduced risk of colorectal cancer and fractures (including hip fractures), overall the observed risks outweighed these benefits.[3] Patients and practitioners then waited for the results of the estrogen-only arm of the WHI, which was to finish in 2005. However, on March 1, 2004, the National Institutes of Health (NIH) informed study participants that they should stop study medications in the trial of conjugated equine estrogens (Premarin, Estrogen-alone) versus placebo in the WHI. Participant follow-up will continue for several more years, including ascertainment of outcomes and mammogram reports. Almost 11,000 women with a prior hysterectomy aged 50-79 at baseline participated in the WHI estrogen-alone trial, which was designed to determine whether estrogen prevents heart disease in healthy older women. Hip fractures were the major secondary outcome, and breast cancer the major possible risk. When the study was stopped by the NIH, women, who now have an average age of almost 70 years and have been followed for approximately 7 years, were told that the current results show that estrogen alone does not appear to affect (either decrease or increase) coronary heart disease and appears to increase the risk of stroke. Other findings included a decreased risk of hip fracture and no increase in the risk of breast cancer during the time period of this study.[4]

The WHI Memory Study (WHIMS), an ancillary study of the WHI, found that estrogen plus progestin did not improve cognitive function when compared with placebo in postmenopausal women aged 65 years or older. This study also found a small increased risk of clinically meaningful cognitive decline in the estrogen plus progestin group.[5] On the basis of these collective findings, the U.S. Preventive Services Task Force has recommended against the routine use of HRT for the prevention of chronic conditions in postmenopausal women.[6]

Women and health care providers are understandably concerned with the results from the WHI study. Statistics can be confusing to interpret, and practitioners should clarify the difference between relative and absolute risks when talking to women about the results of the WHI, which include the following:

- A 26% increase in breast cancer risk means that if 10,000 women were taking HRT for 1 year, 8 more women would develop breast cancer when compared with 10,000 women not taking HRT.
- A 29% increase in heart attack risk means if 10,000 women were taking HRT for 1 year, 7 more women would have a heart attack when compared with 10,000 women not taking HRT.
- A 41% increase in stroke risk means that if 10,000 women were taking HRT for 1 year, 8 more women would have a stroke when compared with 10,000 women not taking HRT.
- A 37% decrease in colorectal cancer risk means that if 10,000 women were taking HRT for 1 year, 6 fewer cases of colorectal cancer would be seen in this group when compared with 10,000 women not taking HRT.
- A 34% decrease in hip fracture risk means that if 10,000 women were taking HRT for 1 year, 5 fewer hip fractures would be seen in this group compared with 10,000 women not taking HRT.

As demonstrated, the absolute risk of an adverse outcome for an individual woman is very small; however, these findings should not be minimized. When considering the millions of women taking HRT for reasons other than simply the relief from vasomotor symptoms of menopause, the number of cases of breast cancer, strokes, and heart attacks becomes unacceptable, especially because this therapy does not provide the protection against cardiovascular disease and cognitive decline as originally thought.

For many American women, one of the major concerns of the study was the increased risk of breast cancer. The WHI found that relatively short-term combined estrogen plus progestin use increases incident breast cancers, which are diagnosed at a more advanced stage, compared with placebo and also substantially increases the percentage of women with abnormal mammograms.[7] However, it must be asked whether the addition of progestin to estrogen increased the risk of breast cancer in this trial population, especially since the estrogen-only arm, at least at the time of this writing, did not appear to be associated with increased risk. Although the data on progestin and breast cancer risk are limited, some observational studies do suggest a relation. In a cohort of 46,355 postmenopausal women, after 4 years of use, combined estrogen and progestin therapy was associated with a higher incidence of breast cancer than therapy with estrogen alone (relative risk, 1.4 and 1.2, respectively; 95% confidence interval [CI], 1.1-1.8 and 1.0-1.4, respectively).[8] The relative risk increased by 8% (95% CI, 2%-16%) per year of use of estrogen plus progestin compared with 1% (95% CI, 2%-3%) per year of estrogen use alone. This finding is consistent with a recent report from Sweden that found longer use of HRT containing progestins significantly elevated breast carcinoma risk, whereas estradiol use alone did not. Continued use of progestins rendered the highest risks.[9] Other questions that remain to be answered include whether natural progesterone is safer than progestin, and whether it is safer to administer progestin every 3 months to induce withdrawal bleeding than to use it cyclically every month or continuously.

Prempro is only one of many formulations of hormone therapy available in the marketplace. This must be considered when confronted with the WHI report of increased risk of adverse events. Premarin is a mixture of sodium estrone sulfate and sodium equilin sulfate.[10] Equilin occurs naturally in horses but is not found in human beings. A number of researchers and health care practitioners question what the results would have been if a low-dose 17β-estradiol had been used. Or what about the use of a transdermal estrogen that is less likely to stimulate the production of oncogenic metabolites? While researchers and practitioners speculate, the Food and Drug Administration (FDA) has stated that though combinations of other estrogens and progestins were not studied in the WHI, in the absence of comparable data, the risks should be assumed to be similar. More research is obviously needed before definitive answers are available.

Individually Compounded Hormone Replacement Therapy

A growing trend among complementary medicine practitioners is the use of individually compounded HRT (ICHRT) containing "natural" or "bioidentical" hormones made from soy or yams. Proponents of this type of therapy claim that hormones that are bioidentical to those produced by the human body are safer than other forms, such as conjugated equine estrogen. Jonathan Wright, MD, a strong proponent of using ICHRT, has proposed that hormone replacement should mimic the ratios of estrogen that naturally occur in a woman's body, which he purports to be 90% estriol, 3% estrone, and 7% estradiol.[11]

Based on this ratio, a popular preparation of ICHRT is Tri-Est 2.5 mg, or triple-estrogen therapy. This blend of estriol (1 mg), estrone (0.125 mg), and estradiol (0.125 mg) is taken twice a day. Tri-Est 2.5 mg is said to be roughly equal to 0.625 mg Premarin.[12] Bi-Est is another popular compounded blend composed of estriol (80%) and estradiol (20%).

Complementary practitioners often claim that higher estriol levels protect against the more potent effects of estrone and estradiol, making the development of estrogen-driven cancers less likely. Diet and environment may play a role in the relative amounts of these hormones in a woman's body. Premenopausal Asian women have a lower breast cancer risk than white women and have a higher rate of urinary estriol excretion. When Asian women migrate to the United States, urinary excretion of estriol decreases and the risk for breast cancer increases.[13] Estriol has been shown to protect rats against breast cancer induced by various chemical carcinogens.[14] Estriol may prove to have a protective effect against the development of breast cancer, but it is premature to make this claim.

Estriol is sometimes prescribed without progesterone because some proponents claim that it does not stimulate endometrial proliferation. However, a population-based, case-control study in Sweden found that 5 years of oral use of estriol, 1 to 2 mg/day, increased the relative risk of endometrial cancer compared with women who had never used estriol. The odds ratio was 8.3 for atypical endometrial hyperplasia and 3.0 for endometrial cancer.[15] Women using estriol, or a compounded formulation, should be instructed to use progesterone either cyclically or every 3 months to protect the endometrium.

Consumers are often confused over the terms *natural, synthetic,* and *artificial* when it comes to hormones. In reality, estrogens used in hormone therapy, with a few exceptions such as ethinyl estrogen, are from natural sources. Cost can be an issue. A month's supply of Tri-Est at the local compounding pharmacy in Albuquerque, New Mexico, is five times the price of most other estrogens. It remains unclear if there is any benefit from these compounded blends compared with 17β-estradiol, an inexpensive and readily available bioidentical hormone.

Table **6-1**

Estrogen replacement compounds containing estradiol derived from natural sources			
NAME	**COMPANY**	**SOURCE**	**EQUIVALENT DOSE**
Estrace	Mead-Johnson	Soybeans	1.0 mg = 0.625 mg Premarin
Ortho-Est	Ortho	Wild yam, soybean	0.75 mg = 0.625 mg Premarin
Climara (patch changed once per week; can be cut in half)	Berlex Lab	Soybeans	0.05 mg = 0.625 mg Premarin
Estraderm (patch that can be changed twice per week but cannot be cut in half)	Ciba-Geigy	Wild yam, soybean	0.5 mg = 0.625 mg Premarin

Table 6-1 lists a few estrogen replacement compounds containing estradiol derived from natural sources that can be taken orally or as a transdermal patch. Table 6-2 lists a few examples of estrogen creams derived from natural sources.

The route of administration should be based on the patient's history, risks, and personal preferences. When estrogen is given orally, it must pass through the liver, where it is

Table **6-2**

Examples of estrogen creams derived from natural sources			
NAME	**COMPANY**	**SOURCE**	**DOSE**
Estrace	Mead-Johnson	Soybeans	0.1 mg estradiol per gram (2 g per night for 2 weeks and then 1 g three times per week)
Ogen	Upjohn	Wild yam, soybean	1.5 mg per gram (2 g per day for 3 weeks and then 1 week off)
Estriol	Compounding pharmacies	Soybean	Usually 0.5 mg/g (apply 2 g per night for 2 weeks and then 1 g three times per week)

converted to a less active form of estrogen before it reaches the bloodstream. When the hormone is given in the form of a patch, it is directly absorbed into the bloodstream before it passes through the liver. Oral estrogens elevate C-reactive protein[16] and triglycerides, whereas the patch does not.[17]

Options for Progesterone Replacement

Women who have a uterus must take a progestational agent if they are using estrogen replacement therapy to prevent endometrial cancer. For the past 20 years, the most commonly prescribed progestin in the United States has been medroxyprogesterone acetate (MPA).[18] Oral progesterone administration has always been problematic because of poor absorption and short biologic half-life. Natural progesterone in powder form is destroyed by stomach acid. This has been overcome by decreasing the size of progesterone particles through the process of "micronization"[19] followed by dissolution in oils consisting primarily of long-chain fatty acids. Micronized progesterone (MP) is identical in chemical structure to endogenous progesterone and manufactured from the wild yam or soybean precursor diosgenin.[20] It is available as Prometrium or through compounding pharmacists as oral MP. Side effects include bloating, breast tenderness, and drowsiness. Drowsiness can be minimized by taking it before bed. Bloating and breast tenderness are dose related. The Food and Drug Administration recognizes a dose of 200 mg for 12 sequential days per 28-day cycle for prevention of endometrial hyperplasia in women who are taking estrogen replacement therapy. Now that a bioavailable form of natural progesterone has entered the U.S. marketplace, the question arises of which progestogen to use.

Few studies have compared MP with MPA. The Postmenopausal Estrogen/Progestin Interventions (PEPI) study is the largest study addressing the question of therapeutic differences between progestogens. A total of 875 postmenopausal women (aged 45 to 64 years) without known contraindications to HRT were randomly assigned to this placebo-controlled, double-blinded study with 3 years of follow-up. The study had 5 treatment regimens: (1) placebo, (2) conjugated equine estrogen (CEE) 0.625 mg daily, (3) CEE plus MPA 10 mg on days 1 through 12, (4) CEE plus MPA 2.5 mg daily, and (5) CEE plus MP 200 mg on days 1 through 12. Primary end points were high-density lipoprotein (HDL) cholesterol, systolic blood pressure, fibrinogen, and 2-hour insulin level after glucose tolerance test. A secondary end point was weight gain. One third of the women had a previous hysterectomy. Exclusion criteria included hyperlipidemia, obesity, hypertension, diabetes, hypothyroidism, history of breast or endometrial cancer, abnormal mammograms during screening, myocardial infarction within the previous 6 months, history of transient ischemic attack or stroke, and severe menopausal symptoms.

All treatment groups had higher HDL levels (CEE only and CEE plus MP regimens more than CEE plus MPA regimens), lower low-density lipoprotein (LDL) levels, and higher triglyceride levels compared with the placebo group. Both systolic and diastolic blood pressure readings increased over time in all groups, including the placebo group. Fibrinogen levels increased in the placebo group but remained at baseline in all treatment groups. Glucose levels were higher in all treatment groups. The placebo group had the most weight gain, whereas the CEE-only group had the least.[21] The authors concluded "in women with a uterus, CEE with cyclic MP has the most favorable effect on HDL-C and no excess risk of endometrial hyperplasia."

A 1985 Swedish study included 58 postmenopausal women who received 2 mg oral estradiol daily for 3 months followed by an additional 3-month course of 2 mg of estradiol daily plus 10 mg of MPA, 200 mg of MP, or 20 μg of levonorgestrel given for 20 days of each menstrual cycle. There was a significant decrease in HDL cholesterol in the groups receiving estradiol plus MPA or levonorgestrel. No change in HDL cholesterol was noted in the group receiving estradiol with MP.[22] Two other small trials by Hargrove et al.[23] and Jensen et al.[24] have shown similar results.

However, a 1998 study of 123 postmenopausal Asian women receiving CEE alone, CEE plus MPA, or CEE plus MP did not show the same favorable effect on lipids. At the end of the 6-month trial, the groups receiving CEE alone and CEE plus MPA had a significant decrease in LDL levels that was not observed in the CEE plus MP group. An increase in HDL cholesterol was only noted in the group receiving CEE alone. A confounding factor in this study could be diet because many Asian diets are rich in phytoestrogens. Japanese women consuming a traditional diet were found to have 100 to 1000 times higher levels of urinary phytoestrogens than American and Finnish women eating an omnivorous diet.[25] Because diets high in phytoestrogens have a favorable effect on cholesterol, there may have been little room for improvement in the lipid profiles of the Asian women in this study.

No comparative trials had been conducted between MPA and MP for their effects on bone density. When MPA is given alone, no beneficial effect results on bone density in postmenopausal women. When combined with estrogen therapy, studies demonstrate a neutral[26] or additional beneficial effect[27] on bone density. A Danish study found that MP did not affect the bone-preserving effects of estrogen.[28] Although some authors suggest that MP is safer,[29] there are no comparative studies addressing the question of breast cancer risk and the use of MP versus MPA.

Wild Yam and Progesterone Creams

Wild yam (*Dioscorea villosa*) has been promoted as an herb that, when either taken internally or applied topically, can be converted in vivo into progesterone. Despite such claims, wild yam is not converted to progesterone in the body, and a double-blind, randomized, placebo-controlled study failed to show any statistical difference between a topically applied cream containing wild yam extract and placebo in alleviating menopausal symptoms or altering serum and salivary hormone levels.[30] Although these products are prevalent in the marketplace and claim to "balance" women's hormones, no historic or contemporary evidence validates this use.

John Lee, MD, has been a major force behind the use of progesterone cream for menopausal symptoms and for the treatment of osteoporosis. Lee describes an unselected case series of 100 postmenopausal women (aged 38 to 83 years) who received a 3% progesterone cream that was applied 12 consecutive nights per month or during the last 2 weeks of estrogen use. Total dose was one half to one third of an ounce of cream per month. The cream was applied to the neck, face, or under the arms, rotating sites. Women were given strict dietary instructions that included increasing green vegetables, avoiding all carbonated sodas, limiting alcohol intake, and reducing red meat consumption to three or fewer times per week. The following were also given: 400 IU of vitamin D, 2000 mg of vitamin C, 25,000 IU of beta carotene, and calcium, 800 to 1000 mg/day. Conjugated estrogens (0.3 or 0.625 mg/day) were taken 3 weeks per month unless contraindicated. Women were prescribed exercise for 20 minutes per day or 30 minutes three times per week. Serial bone densities were performed at 6- to 12-month intervals. Sixty-three of the 100 women underwent dual-photon absorptiometry. The author reported an overall increase of more than 15% in bone mineral density (BMD) over a 3-year period. The development of endometrial carcinoma in one 74-year-old woman is concerning and not surprising, given that estrogen was administered without an oral progestational agent.[31]

The obvious problems with this study include lack of a placebo arm and double-blinding, as well as the fact that some women were given dietary supplements, some exercised, some made dietary changes, and some were taking estrogen. No breakdown of patients by menopausal status, age, risk factors, or diagnosis of osteoporosis is provided in any of the bone density reports. No attempt to record compliance with dietary instructions, smoking cessation, or exercise prescriptions was made. Little can be made from this study of the relation between progesterone cream and increased bone density.

In a randomized, placebo-controlled trial of 102 healthy menopausal women who had not taken HRT for 1 year, a cream containing 20 mg/dose of progesterone or a placebo was applied once daily for 12 months. All women were given a multivitamin and 1200 mg of calcium daily and were evaluated for symptoms every 4 months for a 1-year period. Evaluation of BMD by dual-energy x-ray absorptiometry and lipid profiles were done at baseline and repeated after 12 months. The study found no significant difference between the progesterone and placebo groups regarding BMD of the spine and hip or lipids; however, women in the progesterone group showed a reduction in the frequency of hot flashes. Among women with vasomotor symptoms at the onset of the study, 25 of 30 in the topical progesterone group reported an improvement compared with 5 of 26 in the control group.[32]

However, other researchers have failed to note any beneficial effect of progesterone cream on menopausal symptoms. A parallel, double-blind, randomized, placebo-controlled trial comparing the effect of a transdermal cream containing a progesterone (32 mg daily) with a placebo cream in 80 postmenopausal women failed to note any detectable change in vasomotor symptoms, mood characteristics, sexual feelings, blood lipid levels, or bone metabolic markers despite a slight elevation of blood progesterone levels.[33]

On the basis of evidence to date, topical progesterone cream should not be relied on to maintain bone density or protect the uterine endometrium from exogenous estrogen. It is concerning that some practitioners are prescribing oral estrogen and using topical progesterone creams to protect the endometrium. A crossover study enrolled 20 surgically menopausal women not receiving HRT who were randomly assigned to apply 1 tsp of Progest cream or placebo cream two times daily for 10 days, followed by a 4-day washout before participants switched creams. Participants were then given oral MP (100 mg every morning and 200 every evening) for 5 days. Plasma progesterone, 17-hydroxyprogesterone (17-OHP), and pregnanediol-3α-glucuronide (P3G) levels were used for evaluation purposes. Median plasma levels were 2.9 nmol/L after 10 days of Progest cream compared with 9.5 nmol/L after oral progesterone. Urine P3G levels were 4.2 μmol after Progest administration and 291 μmol with oral progesterone. Serum levels of 17-OHP were similar for Progest cream (1.1) and oral progesterone (1.2). The authors stated that 3 nmol/L is not enough to protect the endometrium from estrogen stimulation.[34]

These findings are consistent with a recent study of 27 women who were given a combined regimen of transdermal estrogen on a continuous basis throughout the 28 days of an average menstrual cycle in addition to sequential use of a cream containing 16, 32, or 64 mg of progesterone on a daily basis from days 15 to 28 of the cycle for three cycles. The study failed to show any secretory change in the subjects' proliferative endometrium.[35] Levels of salivary progesterone in the study were so variable as to be considered completely unreliable in determining the potential influence of the regimen on biologic progesterone activity. This finding is in accord with other research questioning the value of salivary progesterone testing.[36]

Topical progesterone is available as a 3% transdermal gel from compounding pharmacies and it is also available over the counter either alone or in combination with other herbs and vitamins.

Herbs And Other Therapies

Black Cohosh Root (*Cimicifuga racemosa*)

Cohosh is an Algonquian word meaning "rough," in reference to the root. Black cohosh is an indigenous herb that was used by Native Americans to treat musculoskeletal pain, aid in childbirth, and treat respiratory complaints (Figure 6-1). A popular remedy among physicians and the general public, use of the root spread to England where it was used as a treatment for rheumatic symptoms and chorea. Black cohosh was also used for the treatment of depression during the nineteenth century.[37] The sedative effects of the herb were not overlooked by the physicians of the day. The American Medical Association stated in 1849 that they "uniformly found *Cimicifuga* to lessen the frequency and force of the pulse, to soothe pain and allay irritability."[38] A survey of physicians in 1912 found that at the time it was one of the most popularly prescribed herbs in the United States.[39] Black cohosh was referred to as *black snakeroot (Cimicifuga, black cohosh, black snakeroot,* and *Macrotys)* in the United States Pharmacopoeia from 1820 until 1890, when it was referred to as Black cohosh remained an official drug until 1926. A very popular female remedy of the nineteenth century was Lydia E. Pinkham's Vegetable Compound, of which black cohosh was a prominent component. This remedy can still be found, but it no longer contains black cohosh.

A wide variety of black cohosh products are available in the United States, including combination formulae, designed for a wide variety of female complaints. The German health authorities approve the use of *C. racemosa* extract as a nonprescription drug for premenstrual discomfort, dysmenorrhea, and menopause. Clinical trials have almost been exclusively conducted on a proprietary isopropanolic extract called Remifemin (Schaper & Brummer GmbH & Co. KG, Salzgitter, Germany). Eleven clinical trials for black cohosh have been published according to MEDLINE, EMBASE, Cochrane Library, and Napralert. Table 6-3 is a summary of six controlled clinical trials. The other five trials[40-44] were not included because they were open, uncontrolled trials.

Although the majority of studies show a beneficial effect of black cohosh for the alleviation of menopausal symptoms, most have methodologic flaws that limit their findings. A large, long-term study with rigorous methods is needed to more accurately determine the size and mechanism of treatment effect before formal recommendations can be made. However, a recent safety review found the extract to be well tolerated and adverse events rare when taken for up to 6 months.[48]

The precise mechanism of action is not currently understood. Early research suggested an estrogen-like activity. On injection of black cohosh extract, animal studies demonstrated

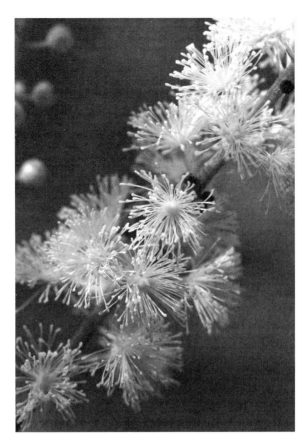

Figure 6-1 Black cohosh *(Cimicifuga racemosa). (Courtesy Martin Wall Botanical Services.)*

an increase in the weight of the uterus and enhanced circulation in the genital region, thought to be caused by the presence of formononetin. In vitro studies show that the isoflavone formononetin binds to estrogen receptors in rat uteri.[49] Recent studies, however, have found that *Cimicifuga* extracts (aqueous isopropanolic and aqueous ethanolic extracts) do not contain formononetin.[50,51]

Although older studies showed a reduction of luteinizing hormone (LH), newer studies have failed to show any effect on LH, follicle-stimulating hormone (FSH), prolactin, or serum hormone-binding globulin.[52] New data dispute the estrogenic theory and indicate that extracts of black cohosh do not bind to the estrogen receptor, upregulate estrogen-dependent genes, or stimulate the growth of estrogen-dependent tumors in animal models.[53] Studies using estrogen-positive or progesterone-positive breast cancer cell lines MCF-7, MDA-MB-435S, T-47D,[54-57] and various in vitro assays[58] demonstrate that *Cimicifuga* extracts do not induce estrogenic effects on breast tissue or mammary tumors. A study by Jacobson et al. found that *Cimicifuga* treatment did not significantly alter LH and FSH levels in breast cancer survivors compared with placebo-treated breast cancer patients, and

Table 6-3

Comparison of six clinical trials of black cohosh

Reference	Date	Design	Product and Dose	Evaluation Criteria and Duration	Results
45	1985	Open, randomized, controlled, comparative; 60 patients initially, 55 evaluated	Remefemin 40 drops bid; conjugated estrogens 0.6 mg/day; diazepam 2 mg/day	SDS, CGI, HAM-A, vaginal cytology; 12 weeks	*Author's conclusions:* All three groups showed significant decrease in neurovegetative and psychologic symptoms. Black cohosh and estrogen group experienced proliferation of vaginal epithelium. No significant adverse effects noted. *Comments:* Study did not discuss randomization process, no placebo control, no *P* values.
46	1987	Randomized, double-blind, comparative, placebo-controlled; 80 patients initially, 16 dropouts from groups; 12 estrogen, three placebo, one black cohosh; five patients unable to be evaluated	Remefemin extract 80 mg bid; conjugated estrogens 0.625 mg/day; placebo	Kupperman Menopause Index, HAM-A, vaginal cytology; 12 weeks	*Author's conclusions:* Remefemin group had most pronounced reduction in Kupperman and HAM-A scores compared with estrogen and placebo groups (*P* < 0.001). Remefemin group had most significant change in proliferation of vaginal epithelium (*P* < 0.01). *Comments:* Randomization process not described. Attrition bias likely (12 of 30 women in estrogen group discontinued medication between weeks 5 and 8 because of perceived lack of efficacy).
47	1998	Randomized, comparative	Remefemin 40 mg bid;	Kupperman Index	*Authors' conclusions:* No statistically significant differences between the

#	Year	Study design	Intervention/dose	Outcomes/duration	Comments
		study in women with "surgical menopause"; 60 patients	estriol 1 mg/day; conjugated estrogens 1.25 mg/day; estradiol 2 mg/day + norethisterone 1 mg/day	(modified), serum LH and FSH; 6 months	groups. Decrease in Kupperman Index scores, no change in LH and FSH levels. *Comments:* Hormone therapies achieved slightly better scores in modified Kupperman Index compared with black cohosh. No placebo control. No description of randomization process. Not double blinded. No clear inclusion/exclusion criteria.
34	1991	Single-blind, placebo-controlled	Remefemin 40 mg bid; placebo	LH and FSH; 8 weeks	*Authors' conclusions: Cimicifuga racemosa* suppresses LH secretion in menopausal women compared with placebo ($P < 0.05$), pointing to an estrogenic effect. FSH levels were not affected. *Comments:* No description is given for randomization process. The graph and text do not include baseline FSH and LH levels for either group. Method for evaluating compliance not included. No exclusion criteria provided.
30	1992	Double-blind, randomized, controlled, parallel-group study; 149 patients evaluated for first 12 weeks; 116 for	Remefemin 40 mg/day; Remefemin 127 mg/day	Kupperman Index, SDS, CGI vaginal cytology serum LH, FSH, prolactin, SHBG estradiol;	*Authors' conclusions:* Both doses showed similar results in efficacy and safety. By the end of the trial Kupperman Index reduced from 31 to 15 in 90% of patients. No changes noted in LH, FSH, SHBG, prolactin, estradiol, or vaginal

continued

Table 6-3

Comparison of six clinical trials of black cohosh—cont'd

Reference	Date	Design	Product and Dose	Evaluation Criteria and Duration	Results
		full 24 weeks		6 months	cytology parameters during study, "thus clearly indicating a non-hormone-like (estrogen) effect for the *C. racemosa* preparation." *Comments:* No placebo group.
59	2001	Double-blind, placebo-controlled, randomized study in breast cancer patients; 85 initially, 69 completed study	Remefemin 20 mg bid	Hot flash diary; FSH and LH drawn at baseline and conclusion of study; 59 patients taking tamoxifen and 26 not	*Authors' conclusions:* Black cohosh was not significantly more efficacious than placebo against most menopause symptoms, including number and intensity of hot flashes. Sweating-only symptom showed significantly greater improvement over placebo. Changes in FSH and LH were not different between the two groups. *Comments:* Majority of patients taking tamoxifen in study; a drug known to induce significant menopausal symptoms. The group of patients not taking tamoxifen was too small for any significant statistical information regarding treatment effect. The dose of 20 mg bid may not be high enough in this treatment group.

bid, Twice per day; *FSH,* follicle-stimulating hormone; *LH,* luteinizing hormone; *SHBG,* sex hormone–binding globulin; *SDS,* Self-Assessment Depression Scale; *CGI,* Clinical Global Impression.

the extract did not induce cancerous regrowth of breast tissue.[59] Likewise, a study of 50 women, including 5 breast cancer survivors, treated with 20 mg/day of a *Cimicifuga* extract for relief of hot flashes and night sweats found that mammography, Papanicolaou smear, and vaginal ultrasound results were comparable to baseline over a 24-week period.[60] In contradiction to the aforementioned data, a recently presented abstract suggested that black cohosh at doses equivalent to 40 mg/day may be unsafe for women with breast cancer. Although this study did not find any increased incidence of breast cancer, lung metastases were greater in those mice that developed breast cancer than in mice that served as controls.[61] Although it is important not to overinterpret one study in transgenic mice, it does raise the question about other mechanisms by which herbs and other medications may increase the rate of metastases without affecting the incidence or latency of breast tumors.

Current thinking is that *Cimicifuga* extracts may work by serotonergic or dopaminergic mechanisms. Research on an Asian species of *Cimicifuga* has indicated a possible central nervous system effect. In vitro studies have demonstrated binding of serotonin (5-HT$_{1A}$) receptors,[62] while animal research shows serotonin blocking activity.[63] Dopaminergic activity of *Cimicifuga* extract has been demonstrated with the D(2)-receptor assay.[64]

Very preliminary data suggest that *Cimicifuga* species may have a beneficial effect on bone. Hydrophilic and lipophilic extracts of *C. heracleifolia* and *C. foetida* have demonstrated inhibition of parathyroid-induced bone resorption in vitro and in ovariectomized rats.[65] The mechanism is unknown. A recent study of *C. racemosa* extract found it to be equipotent to conjugated equine estrogen in reducing climacteric complaints and showed positive effects on bone metabolism in a double-blind, randomized, placebo-controlled study of 62 postmenopausal women.[66] Bone metabolism was monitored by following levels of crosslaps (marker of bone degradation), as determined by the ELECSYS system and bone-specific alkaline phosphatase (marker of bone formation) by enzymatic assay.

Black cohosh is the most widely studied botanical therapy for alleviation of menopausal complaints. Although newer research suggests a nonhormonal mechanism of action, long-term effects on the uterine endometrium have not been well documented. Research is currently under way at Columbia University to assess the long-term effects of black cohosh on the endometrium. A three-arm, 12-month study (beginning June 2003) at the University of Illinois at Chicago will compare the effects of black cohosh, red clover, or conjugated equine estrogen/MPA on menopause symptoms. It is hoped that these larger long-term studies will provide more definitive answers about efficacy and long-term safety for both practitioners and patients.

More data are needed to assess genotoxicity. Studies on other *Cimicifuga* species failed to show teratogenicity in female rats at doses up to 2000 mg/kg per day[67]; however, similar studies in *C. racemosa* have not been published. The American Herbal Products Association states that black cohosh should not be used during pregnancy.[68]

The dose of standardized extract is 20 to 80 mg twice daily. The extract is generally an isopropanolic extract standardized to 2.5% triterpene glycosides; some researchers, however, question the rationale of standardizing to these compounds because it is uncertain that they are the key "actives" in the herb. *The British Herbal Compendium* recommends a daily dose of 40 to 200 mg of dried root and rhizome or its equivalent, a tincture (1:10) of 60% ethanol 0.4 to 2 mL. Black cohosh is often found in combination with other dietary supplements, including soy, dong quai, licorice, chastetree berry, and ginseng.

Interestingly, a combination of soy, black cohosh, and dong quai was found to be more effective than placebo for the prevention of menstrual migraine when taken for 6 months.[69] Although these combinations may have an additive/synergistic effect, they have not been subjected to clinical evaluation for effectiveness in menopause.

Dong Quai Root (*Angelica sinensis*)

Dong quai has been used in traditional Chinese medicine for at least 20 centuries and can be found in Lei Gong's *Treatise on Preparation of Materia Medica* (588 AD): "The root is used medicinally as a strengthener of the heart, lung, and liver meridians; it is a tonic of the blood and promotes blood circulation; it regulates the menstrual cycle and stops menstrual pain."[70] Merck introduced the herb to the Western world in 1899 under the trade name Eumenol, a product that was said to positively affect menstrual disorders.[71]

Today, dong quai can be found in many Western herbals and is considered to be a valuable female tonic by herbalists around the world. *Angelica* species native to Europe and North America are primarily used for digestive disorders (*A. archangelica* and *A. atropurpurea*); the distilled essential oils are used for flavoring gin and vermouth. Comparative chemical studies between Western and Asian species are only now being rigorously conducted.

The question of estrogenic activity has been hotly debated over the years. It appears that if dong quai is estrogenic, it is only weakly so. A Chinese study failed to note any change in vaginal smears or increased uterine weight in rodents who were fed dong quai as 5% of their diet.[70] A 1998 study found that dong quai does not bind to estrogen receptors in vitro and does not stimulate estrogen receptor–positive human breast cancer cell lines.[55] A 2001 study demonstrated that dong quai and licorice (*Glycyrrhiza glabra* L.) exhibited only weak estrogen receptor binding and progesterone receptor and pS2 (presenelin-2, an inducible breast cancer gene) messenger RNA induction.[58] A 2002 in vitro study reported that dong quai significantly induced the growth of MCF-7 cells by 16-fold over that of untreated control cells by an estrogen-independent mechanism.[72] More research is needed to clarify the safety of dong quai in women who have had a history of breast cancer.

Although dong quai may be beneficial for a variety of "female" complaints, a study casts doubt on the effectiveness of dong quai for menopause. Seventy-one women with hot flashes entered a randomized, double-blind, placebo-controlled trial and were given 1500 mg of dong quai or placebo three times per day for 12 weeks. At the end of the 3 months no difference was observed between the groups in blood hormone levels or relief of menopausal symptoms, including hot flashes and vaginal dryness. No signs of estrogen-like stimulation of the uterine lining were noted.[73]

Dong quai is not usually administered as a single herb in traditional Chinese medicine but is combined with other herbs in a formula designed specifically for the individual. Traditional Chinese medicine practitioners caution that because dong quai is a "heating" herb it may cause symptoms such as hot flashes, red face, sweating, insomnia, and irritability. Clearly, this herb is prescribed to only a subset of menopausal women who meet specific diagnostic criteria in accordance with traditional Chinese medicine. Practitioners of this discipline argue that the clinical study failed because herbs were not given in accordance with traditional diagnostic and prescribing methods. However, even if traditional Chinese diagnostic and prescribing methods were not used, if much benefit existed for menopausal vasomotor symptoms, this trial should have showed it.

The dong quai dose is generally 3.5 to 4.0 g/day of the dried root, or 200 mg three times daily of an extract standardized to contain 1% ligustilide. The dose for tincture (1:5) is 5 to 8 mL three times daily. Numerous authors mention a risk of increased vaginal bleeding during menstruation and possible risk of uterine stimulation during pregnancy. For these reasons, dong quai is best avoided during pregnancy. Animals receiving warfarin for several days were found to have an increased prothrombin time when given 2 g/kg twice daily of dong quai.[74] This dose is much higher than what is normally used, yet it is probably wise to closely monitor patients taking anticoagulants and using this herb.

Chastetree Berries (*Vitex agnus-castus*)

Vitex is often recommended for women who are in early menopause and having irregular menstrual cycles. The overall action of the herb appears to be a relative increase in progesterone. This progesterogenic effect has been verified by endometrial biopsy, analysis of blood hormone levels, and examination of vaginal secretions.[75] Progesterone has a stabilizing effect on the uterine lining and may help prevent heavy bleeding and reduce spotting between cycles. Clinical trials are lacking for efficacy in menopausal flooding and irregular cycles, although I have successfully used the herb for these conditions for many years. Several large drug-monitoring studies have been conducted looking at the use of *Vitex* for a variety of menstrual and menopausal symptoms. Unfortunately, the data from these studies are difficult to evaluate (poor inclusion criteria, inadequate reporting of other therapies, ill-defined end points, etc.). No randomized trials have looked specifically at *Vitex* for the treatment of menopausal symptoms. It is endorsed by the German health authorities for the treatment of premenstrual syndrome, irregular menses, and mastalgia.[76] The herb is generally well tolerated. A small number of women have reported nausea, diarrhea, gastrointestinal symptoms, mild skin rash, and increased acne. The herb is commonly found in combination with other dietary supplements and botanicals such as soy, black cohosh, and licorice.

Soy

Phytoestrogens (i.e., isoflavones, phytosterols, and lignans) are compounds present within plants that exert mild estrogenic effects within the human body. Isoflavones are found in legumes such as soy, chickpeas, pinto beans, lima beans, and alfalfa. Lignans and lignins are present in seeds, fruits, vegetables, and whole grains. Gut bacteria break down lignin precursors in food to enterolactone and enterodiol to form the active isoflavones genistein, daidzein, and equol. The high intake of soy and other dietary phytoestrogens is believed to partially explain why hot flashes and other menopausal symptoms do not occur with the same frequency in cultures that eat a primarily plant-based diet.[77]

Phytoestrogens are only weakly estrogenic, but high concentrations can be achieved in the body with diet. A study comparing American and Finnish women noted that the highest levels of urinary phytoestrogens are in women who consume a macrobiotic diet and lowest in those with an omnivorous diet.[78] Japanese women consuming a traditional diet were found to have 100 to 1000 times higher levels of urinary phytoestrogens than American and Finnish women eating an omnivorous diet.[25] This could partially account for why Japanese women are reported to have fewer hot flashes than American women during menopause.

Twelve clinical trials have been published evaluating the effects of soy on menopausal symptoms. Soy seems to have modest benefit for hot flashes, but studies are not conclusive. Isoflavone preparations seem to be less effective than soy foods.

Soy does appear to have a modest role in modulating endocrine function in the body. A small but well-conducted crossover study of fourteen premenopausal women was performed to determine the effects of soy on hormone levels. Women were given high isoflavone soy powder (2 mg/kg per day), low isoflavone soy powder (1 mg/kg per day), or isoflavone-free soy powder for three periods of 3 months with a 3-week washout period in between. Participants consumed their regular diet but were given careful instructions about avoiding vitamins, alcohol, and phytoestrogens. Hormone levels were collected every other day during the last 6 weeks of each cycle. At the end of the study the high-isoflavone group was noted to have decreased free triiodothyronine (T_3) and dehydroepiandrosterone sulfate (DHEA-S) levels during the follicular phase and decreased estrone in the mid-follicular phase. The low isoflavone group had lower LH and FSH levels in the periovulatory phase. Other than those noted, no significant changes occurred in hormone levels (thyroxine, prolactin, progesterone, testosterone, androstenedione, cortisol, insulin, or thyroid-stimulating hormone) or length of menstrual cycles.[79]

The availability of more data may enhance understanding of the role of dietary phytoestrogens in health. Phytoestrogens vary greatly in complexity and diversity, making these compounds a challenge for researchers because in vitro and in vivo studies often provide conflicting results. Specific cellular response depends on the type of phytoestrogen, the level of estrogen receptor beta and alpha, co-activators, co-repressors, and duration of exposure. As one author states, "overall, it is naive to assume that exposure to these compounds is always good; inappropriate or excessive exposure may be detrimental."[80] Although the benefit for women with hot flashes appears to be small, the addition of soy foods to the diet can have a beneficial effect on cholesterol and possibly a beneficial effect on the bone density of the spine. Recommending large doses of isolated isoflavones is premature.

Red Clover (*Trifolium pratense*)

Red clover has been used since antiquity as a treatment for skin disorders and minor respiratory ailments. The National Formulary listed red clover as a skin remedy until the mid-1900s. In the 1940s the flower heads found their way into Harry Hoxsey's controversial anticancer formula. Red clover contains formononetin, biochanin A, daidzein, genistein, and coumestrol, substances that act as weak estrogens in the body.[81] Constituents within red clover have been shown to alter vaginal cytology, increase FSH, and reduce LH in animal models.[55] Sheep grazing on a related clover (*T. subterraneum*) in Australia developed "clover disease," a condition associated with abnormal lactation, infertility, and prolapsed uterus. These adverse effects were thought to be the result of estrogenic substances in the clover.[82] Consumption of large amounts of red clover is associated with infertility in livestock.[83] Because of these "estrogenic" activities in animals some researchers and herbal manufacturers began to explore and promote the use of red clover for relief of menopausal symptoms.

Human trials have been small and conflicting. The largest and most recent randomized, double-blind, placebo-controlled trial of 252 menopausal women failed to find any significant benefit for two different strengths of red clover leaf extract. Women who were recently postmenopausal (mean [SD], 3.3 [4.5] years since menopause) experiencing 8.1 hot flashes per day were included in the trial. Exclusion criteria included vegetarianism, consumption of soy products more than once per week, or ingestion of medications that would affect isoflavone absorption. After a 2-week placebo run-in period, participants were randomly assigned to Promensil (82 mg of total isoflavones per day), Rimostil (57 mg of total isoflavones per day), or an identical placebo and followed up for 12 weeks. A total of 246 women (98%) completed the 12-week protocol. The reductions in mean daily hot flash count at 12 weeks were similar for the Promensil (5.1), Rimostil (5.4), and placebo (5.0) groups; however, women in the Promensil group (41%; 95% CI, 29%-51%; $P = 0.03$), but not in the Rimostil group (34%; 95% CI, 22%-46%; $P = 0.74$) had faster relief of hot flashes than women in the placebo group. Quality of life improvements and adverse events were comparable among the three groups.[84]

A 1999 double-blind, placebo-controlled, crossover trial was conducted with 51 menopausal women who had been at least 6 months without menses and were having at least three hot flashes per day. They received placebo or red clover extract (Promensil; 40 mg of total isoflavones; genistein, 4 mg; daidzein, 3.5 mg; biochanin, 24.5 mg; formononetin, 8 mg). The first phase lasted 3 months and was followed by a 4-week washout period. The second phase lasted 14 weeks. The Greene Climacteric Scale Score was used to evaluate symptoms in a diary kept by participants. At the beginning and conclusion of each phase of the trial, participants were evaluated by blood work that included a complete blood cell count, liver function tests, FSH, estradiol, and sex hormone–binding globulin; a 24-hour urine to test for isoflavone levels; vaginal cytology; and transvaginal ultrasound to evaluate endometrial thickness. Forty-three women completed the study. No significant differences were observed between groups in Greene scores, blood studies, vaginal cytology, endometrial thickness, or body weight. Hot flashes were reduced in the placebo group by 18% and in the treatment group by 20%.[85]

Another randomized, placebo-controlled study enrolled 37 postmenopausal women who were having at least three hot flashes per day. Participants received placebo, Promensil (40 mg total isoflavones), or Promensil (160 mg total isoflavones) per day for 12 weeks. Evaluation was similar to the previous trial. No significant differences were observed among the three groups in blood work or vaginal cytology. Urinary isoflavone levels rose in both of the groups taking Promensil. A small but insignificant rise in urinary isoflavones was noted in the placebo group. Although not adequately confirmed, this small rise may have been caused by the consumption of alfalfa (a phytoestrogen) by one participant.[86]

These three studies are in contrast to a small randomized, double-blind, placebo-controlled trial of 30 women with more than 12 months of amenorrhea and having more than five hot flashes per day that showed a beneficial effect with 80 mg/day isoflavones (Promensil).[87] After a single-blind placebo run-in period of 4 weeks, the women were randomly assigned to receive either 80 mg of isoflavones or placebo for 12 weeks. Efficacy was measured by the decrease in number of hot flashes per day and changes in Greene score. During the first 4 weeks of placebo the frequency of hot flashes decreased by 16%. During the subsequent double-blind phase, a further, statistically significant decrease of 44% was seen in the isoflavones group ($P < 0.01$), whereas no further reduction occurred within the placebo group. The Greene score decreased in the active group by 13% and remained unchanged in the placebo group. The small sample size and low placebo response challenge the results of this study.

Safety for women who have had an estrogen receptor–positive cancer is unclear. Although red clover is a prominent ingredient in the Hoxsey cancer formula, an in vitro study found that the herb was equipotent to estradiol in its ability to stimulate cell proliferation in estrogen receptor–positive breast cancer cells.[55] Other researchers found that methanol extracts of red clover showed significant competitive binding to estrogen receptors alpha and beta and exhibited estrogenic activity in cultured Ishikawa (endometrial) cells.[58] Until further research is available, avoidance of prolonged use of red clover leaf extract in women with a history of breast cancer seems prudent. This is especially true given the fact that three of four trials, including the largest and best done study, fail to show any clinically significant benefit for relieving menopausal symptoms. (NOTE: Red clover flowers are much lower in isoflavones than are the leaves.)

Ginseng (*Panax ginseng*)

Ginseng has been revered in Asian medicine for thousands of years. In the first Chinese *Materia Medica,* believed to be written more than 2000 years ago, Shen Nung said "ginseng is a tonic to the five viscera, quieting the animal spirit, revitalizing the soul, preventing fear, expelling the vicious energies, brightening the eye and improving vision, opening the heart benefiting the understanding, if taken for some time will invigorate the body and prolong life." The tonic effects of ginseng have been the focal point of research for more than 50 years. Many of the studies are plagued with methodologic flaws and results are contradictory, making it difficult to assess the true efficacy of the herb. The best evidence suggests that ginseng does improve sleep, appetite, and emotional lability and may enhance physical and mental performance in certain populations.[88] Ginseng remains one of the most popular herbal supplements sold on the American market. Two species dominate the trade: Asian ginseng (*Panax ginseng*) and American ginseng (*P. quinquefolius*).

Researchers have debated the estrogenicity of ginseng and questioned a potential role for the herb in relieving menopausal symptoms. Three incidents of hormone-like effects in older women have been reported.[89] A randomized, double-blind, placebo-controlled study of ginseng (*P. ginseng*) in 384 women with menopausal symptoms failed to note a reduction in vasomotor symptoms; however, using a validated instrument for evaluating mood and well-being, the study reported P values less than 0.05 for depression, well-being, and health subscales in favor of ginseng compared with placebo.[90] This is consistent with a small, open study that found 30 days of treatment with 6 g/day Korean red ginseng improved symptoms of fatigue, insomnia, and depression in women with menopausal symptoms.[91] These studies are intriguing given the fact that these women were still having hot flashes and night sweats and yet felt better. Could this be from a "tonic" effect?

Is ginseng estrogenic? Does it affect the uterine endometrium or stimulate the growth of breast cancer? Ginseng has been found to induce the growth of MCF-7 cells by 27-fold over that of untreated control cells[92] and to upregulate pS2 in S30 breast cancer cells but failed to demonstrate significant estrogen-binding affinity or alkaline phosphatase induction.[58] Other researchers report that concurrent use of American ginseng and breast cancer therapeutic agents resulted in a significant ($P < 0.005$) suppression of cell growth for most drugs evaluated, indicating an additive or synergistic inhibitory effect.[93] At this time, long-term safety of ginseng in menopausal women is simply not known and the question of estrogen activity not fully answered.

Given the problem with adulteration of ginseng, it is probably wisest to use whole root or purchase a standardized extract. The dose used in most studies is 100 to 200 mg/day standardized extract of ginseng or 3 to 6 g/day of crude root.

Shepard's Purse (*Capsella bursa-pastoris*)

Shepard's purse derives its name from the plant's heart-shaped delicate seed pods that look like little purses. The herb has been used for more than 2000 years to staunch the flow of blood. As late as World War I, soldiers used this humble plant to stop bleeding when other remedies were unavailable. Studies have verified that shepard's purse has hemostatic properties, and the German authorities endorse the internal use of the herb for the symptomatic treatment of mild menorrhagia and metrorrhagia and externally for superficial injuries to the skin.[94] After appropriate medical evaluation, shepard's purse may be helpful in reducing heavy menstrual flow. Tincture should not be older than 1 year and the dose for tincture (1:5) is 3 mL four to six times per day. There are no recent studies in the literature on the hemostatic properties of shepard's purse.

St. John's Wort (*Hypericum perforatum*)

St. John's wort is the most heavily studied of the botanical remedies for depression. Its use as a mood-elevating substance may date back at least 2000 years. *Hypericum perforatum* is the botanical name given by the ancient physician Dioscorides (70 CE), meaning "over an apparition." The name was apparently chosen because the plant was believed to protect one from evil or wandering spirits. Early users of St. John's wort may have found that the herb "lifted" the spirits, or eased depression.

The most recent Cochrane review found 27 trials with a total of 2291 patients who met inclusion criteria for a meta-analysis. Seventeen trials with 1168 patients were placebo controlled (16 were on monopreparations, one with St. John's wort plus four other herbs), and 10 trials (eight single preparations, two combinations of St. John's wort and valerian) with 1123 patients compared *Hypericum* with other antidepressant or sedative drugs. The duration of most trials was 4 to 6 weeks and the participants usually had a diagnosis of "neurotic depression" or "mild to moderate severe depressive disorders." The authors concluded "There is evidence that extracts of *Hypericum* are more effective than placebo for the short-term treatment of mild to moderately severe depressive disorders. The current evidence is inadequate to establish whether *Hypericum* is as effective as other antidepressants. Further studies comparing St. John's wort with standard antidepressants in well-defined groups of patients over longer observations periods, investigating long-term side effects, and comparing different extracts and doses are needed."[95]

A number of women have menopausal mood swings, although it remains unclear how much of this is caused by hormonal flux versus other social or environmental factors. A number of herbal formulae designed for menopausal symptoms contain St. John's wort. A 1997 survey of premenopausal, perimenopausal, and postmenopausal women with psychovegetative disorders reported a "synergistic" effect for a combination of black cohosh and St. John's wort.[96] There are no controlled trials of St. John's wort alone, or in combination with black cohosh, for the alleviation of menopausal symptoms.

The antidepressant dose used in most clinical trials is 900 to 1800 mg/day standardized extract (3% to 5% hyperforin and/or 0.3% hypericin). St. John's wort has shown to be relatively safe, but it does interact with P450 CYP3A4 and p-2 glycoprotein, contraindicating its use by those taking indinavir, cyclosporine, digoxin, oral contraceptives, warfarin, and other medications metabolized by these systems.

Kava (*Piper methysticum*)

Kava is an herb that has been used as a social beverage and medicinal agent in the South Pacific for many years. Although generally not thought of as an herb for menopause, kava has been shown to be an effective anxiolytic.[97] Some of the symptoms women mention with menopause include irritability, heart palpitations, nervousness, and difficulty sleeping. Warnecke[98] has published two placebo-controlled trials on the effectiveness of kava for menopausal symptoms. A 1991 study compared 210 mg/day standardized extract of kava (70% kavapyrones) with placebo in 40 menopausal women for 8 weeks. The Hamilton Anxiety Scale (HAM-A), Depression Status Inventory, and Kupperman Menopause Index were used to evaluate effectiveness. A statistically significant reduction in the HAM-A total score was apparent by week 8 in the kava group ($P < 0.01$). HAM-A scores fell from an average of 30 to 6 in the treatment group compared with an average score of 22 in the placebo group. Improvement was noted in the group receiving kava by the end of week 1 and reached a plateau by week 4.[99]

Approximately 30 cases of hepatotoxicity have been reported with the use of kava, leading Canada, Australia, and many European countries to ban its sale. At the time of this writing, kava is still available for sale in the United States but the FDA has cautioned consumers and health care providers to be alert and report any adverse events. Until this issue is further clarified, it is probably wise to avoid the use of kava or limit its use to 4 to 6 weeks. Gruenwald and Skrabal[100] uncovered reasons other than kava for the reported cases of liver toxicity.

Vitamin E

Many women report that taking 800 IU of vitamin E helps reduce their hot flashes; however, the scientific evidence is not convincing. Older studies had numerous methodologic flaws and more recent trials show only minimal benefit. A 1998 randomized, placebo-controlled crossover study enrolled 125 women with a history of breast cancer who were having at least 14 hot flashes per week. Exclusion criteria included women who were receiving treatment for hot flashes and women who took more than two multivitamins or 60 IU of vitamin E per day. Participants were given either placebo or 400 IU vitamin E for 4 weeks, and then the other treatment in a crossover fashion. Participants kept a daily diary to assess hot flash frequency and severity. One hundred four women finished the study (120 were available to assess toxicity). Hot flash frequency decreased by 25% with vitamin E compared with 22% with placebo. The hot flash score (frequency times average severity) fell 20% with placebo compared with 28% with vitamin E. Participants were asked which therapy they preferred; 38% had no preference, 29% preferred placebo, and 32% preferred vitamin E.[99] The clinical significance of this trial is important because 67% of women either had no preference or preferred placebo. Some practitioners argue that the dose was too low and that 800 IU vitamin E would have been a better test for efficacy.

Acupuncture

As acupuncture becomes more readily available to consumers across the United States, many women claim that treatments help to alleviate their menopausal symptoms. One study of 24 menopausal women found that acupuncture significantly reduced the number of hot flashes when receiving one to two 30-minute treatments per week over an 8-week period.[101] Several other small studies have also demonstrated some benefits for vasomotor symptoms; however, a trial with more rigorous methodology and sufficient size is needed to adequately assess efficacy.

Menopause is a time of change. Many women consider it a time to reflect on who they are and question where they are going. Every woman should be encouraged to take an active role in the decision-making process for addressing her menopause and post-menopausal years. The media and medical profession often provide conflicting information that confuses and sometimes frightens women. Health care professionals must be aware of the evidence that exists regarding a variety of available treatments and be open to discussing alternative options with women seeking guidance.

At present, estrogen therapy, with or without an accompanying progestin or progesterone, appears to be the most effective means for relieving the acute vasomotor symptoms of menopause; however, concerns over long-term use and adverse effects have led women to seek alternative treatments. Soy offers some minor benefits and has the advantage of being a safe food that can be added to the diet. Among the botanicals currently being used for menopause, black cohosh extract is the most thoroughly studied but still requires a trial with rigorous methodology. Red clover and dong quai do not appear to be efficacious at this time. Preliminary data suggest that ginseng may improve mood and well-being but does not relieve vasomotor symptoms. Wild yam cream is ineffective, and the studies on progesterone cream for vasomotor symptoms are mixed. St. John's wort and kava may help improve mood, but kava has been banned in many countries because of concern of hepatotoxicity. Chastetree is commonly used in menopause, but no clinical trials have evaluated its efficacy.

References

1. Ettinger B, Pressman A: Continuation of postmenopausal hormone replacement therapy in a large health maintenance organization: transdermal matrix patch versus oral estrogen therapy, *Am J Manag Care* 5:779-785, 1999.
2. Rossouw JE, Anderson GL, Prentice RL, et al: Risks and benefits of estrogen plus progestin in healthy postmenopausal women: principal results from the Women's Health Initiative randomized controlled trial, *JAMA* 288:321-333, 2000.
3. Kaunitz AM: Use of combination hormone replacement therapy in light of recent data from the Women's Health Initiative. Available at: http://www.medscape.com/viewarticle/438357, MedGenMed 4(3), 2002.
4. Women's Health Initiative Participant Web Site: National Heart, Lung, and Blood Institute advisory for physicians on the WHI trial of conjugated equine estrogens versus placebo. Available at: www.whi.org/updates/advisory_ea_physicians.asp. Accessed March 18, 2004.
5. Rapp SR, Espeland MA, Shumaker SA, et al: Effect of estrogen plus progestin on global cognitive function in postmenopausal women: the Women's Health Initiative Memory Study: a randomized controlled trial, *JAMA* 289:2663-2672, 2003.
6. U.S. Preventive Services Task Force: Postmenopausal hormone replacement therapy for primary prevention of chronic conditions: recommendations and rationale, *Ann Intern Med* 137:834-839, 2002.
7. Chlebowski RT, Hendrix SL, Langer RD, et al: Influence of estrogen plus progestin on breast cancer and mammography in healthy postmenopausal women: the Women's Health Initiative randomized trial, *JAMA* 289:3243-3253, 2003.

8. Schairer C, Lubin J, Troisi R, et al: Menopausal estrogen and estrogen–progestin replacement therapy and breast cancer risk, *JAMA* 283:485-491, 2000.
9. Olsson HL, Ingvar C, Bladstrom A: Hormone replacement therapy containing progestins and given continuously increases breast carcinoma risk in Sweden, *Cancer* 97:1387-1392, 2003.
10. *Physicians' desk reference,* 54th ed. Montvale, NJ, 2000, Medical Economics Company, pp 3302-3303.
11. Wright JV, Morgenthaler J: *Natural hormone replacement,* Petaluma, CA, 1997, Smart Publications, p 127.
12. Hudson T: *Women's encyclopedia of natural medicine,* Lincolnwood, Ill, 1999, Keats Publishing, pp 298-299.
13. Speroff L, Glass RH, Kase NG: *Clinical gynecologic endocrinology and infertility,* 4th ed, Baltimore, 1989, Williams & Wilkins, p 300.
14. Speroff L, Glass RH, Kase NG: *Clinical gynecologic endocrinology and infertility,* 4th ed, Baltimore, 1989, Williams & Wilkins, p 301.
15. Weiderpass E, Baron JA, Adami HO, et al: Low-potency oestrogen and risk of endometrial cancer. A case-control study, *Lancet* 353:1824-1828, 1999.
16. Kawano H, Yasue H, Hirai N, et al: Effects of transdermal and oral estrogen supplementation on endothelial function, inflammation and cellular redox state, *Int J Clin Pharmacol Ther* 41:346-353, 2003.
17. Nanda S, Gupta N, Mehta HC, et al: Effect of oestrogen replacement therapy on serum lipid profile, *Aust N Z J Obstet Gynaecol* 43:213-216, 2003.
18. Langer RD: Micronized progesterone: a new therapeutic option, *Int J Fertil* 44:67-73, 1999.
19. McAuley JW, Kroboth KJ, Kroboth PD: Oral administration of micronized progesterone: a review and more experience, *Pharmacotherapy* 16:453-457, 1996.
20. Writing Group for the PEPI Trial: The effects of estrogen or estrogen/progestin regimens on heart disease risk factors in postmenopausal women, *JAMA* 273:199-208, 1996.
21. Writing Group for the PEPI Trial: Effects of estrogen or estrogen/progestin regimens on heart disease risk factors in postmenopausal women. The Postmenopausal Estrogen/Progestin Interventions (PEPI) Trial, *JAMA* 274:1676, 1995.
22. Ottoson UB, Johansson BG, Von Schoultz B: Subfractions of high-density lipoprotein cholesterol during estrogen replacement therapy: a comparison between progestogens and natural progesterone, *Am J Obstet Gynecol* 151:746-750, 1985.
23. Hargrove JT, Maxson WS, Wentz AC, et al: Menopausal hormone replacement therapy with continuous daily oral micronized estradiol and progesterone, *Obstet Gynecol* 73:606-612, 1989.
24. Jensen J, Riis BJ, Strom V, et al: Long-term effects of percutaneous estrogens and oral progesterone on serum lipoproteins on serum lipoproteins in postmenopausal women, *Am J Obstet Gynecol* 156:6-71, 1987.
25. Adlercreutz H, Hamalainen E, Gorbach S, et al: Dietary phytoestrogens and the menopause in Japan, *Lancet* 339:1233, 1992.
26. Adachi JD, Sargeant EJ, Sagle MA, et al: A double-blind randomized controlled trial of the effects of medroxyprogesterone acetate on bone density of women taking estrogen replacement therapy, *Br J Obstet Gynaecol* 104:64-70, 1987.
27. Grey A, Cundy T, Evans M, et al: Medroxyprogesterone acetate enhances the spinal bone mineral density response to oestrogen in late post-menopausal women, *Clin Endocrinol* 44:293-296, 1995.
28. Riis BJ, Thomsen K, Strom V, et al: The effect of percutaneous estriol and natural progesterone on postmenopausal bone loss, *Am J Obstet Gynecol* 156:61-65, 1986.
29. McCarty MF: Androgenic progestins amplify the breast cancer risk associated with hormone replacement therapy by boosting IGF-I activity, *Med Hypotheses* 56:213-216, 2001.
30. Komesaroff PA, Black CV, Cable V, et al: Effects of wild yam extract on menopausal symptoms, lipids and sex hormones in healthy menopausal women, *Climacteric* 4:144-150, 2001.
31. Lee JR: Osteoporosis reversal: the role of progesterone, *Int Clin Nutr Rev* 10:384-391, 1990.
32. Leonetti HB, Longo S, Anasti JN: Transdermal progesterone cream for vasomotor symptoms and postmenopausal bone loss, *Obstet Gynecol* 94:225-228, 1999.
33. Wren BG, Champion SM, Willetts K, et al: Transdermal progesterone and its effect on vasomotor symptoms, blood lipid levels, bone metabolic markers, moods, and quality of life for postmenopausal women, *Menopause* 10:13-18, 2003.

34. Cooper A, Spencer C, Whitehead MI, et al: Systemic absorption of progesterone from Progest cream in postmenopausal women, *Lancet* 351:1255-1256, 1998.
35. Wren BG, McFarland K, Edwards L, et al: Effect of sequential transdermal progesterone cream on endometrium, bleeding pattern, and plasma progesterone and salivary progesterone levels in postmenopausal women, *Climacteric* 3:155-160, 2000.
36. Lewis JG, McGill H, Patton VM, et al: Caution on the use of saliva measurements to monitor absorption of progesterone from transdermal creams in postmenopausal women, *Maturitas* 41:1-6, 2002.
37. Farquharson R, Woodbury F: *Guide to therapeutics and materia medica,* Philadelphia, 1882, Lea, p 226.
38. Porcher FP: Report on the indigenous medical plants of South Carolina, Transactions of the American Medical Association, vol II, 1849.
39. Lloyd JU: Vegetable drugs employed by American physicians, *J Am Pharm Assoc* 3:1228-1241, 1912.
40. Stolze H: An alternative to treat menopausal complaints, *Gyne* 3:14-16, 1982.
41. Daiber W: Climacteric complaints: success without using hormones: a phytotherapeutic agent lessens hot flushes, sweating, and insomnia, *Arzt Praxis* 35:1946-1947, 1983.
42. Vorberg G: Therapy of climacteric complaints, *Zeitschrift fur Allgemeinmedizin* 60:626-629, 1984.
43. Petho A: Menopausal complaints: change over of a hormone treatment to a herbal gynecological remedy practical, *Arzt Praxis* 38:1551-1553, 1987.
44. Mielnik J: Extract of *Cimicifuga racemosa* in the treatment of neurovegetative symptoms in women in the perimenopausal period, *Maturitas* 27:S215, 1997.
45. Warnecke G: Influence of a phytopharmaceutical on climacteric complaints, *Die Medizinische Welt* 36:871-874, 1985.
46. Stoll W: Phytopharmaceutical influences of atrophic vaginal epithelium. Double-blind study on *Cimicifuga* versus an estrogen preparation, *Therapeutikon* 1:23-32, 1987.
47. Lehmann-Willenbrock W, Riedel HH: Clinical and endocrinologic examinations concerning therapy of climacteric symptoms following hysterectomy with remaining ovaries, *Zent Bl Gynakol* 110:611-618, 1998.
48. Dog TL, Powell KL, Weisman SM: Critical evaluation of the safety of *Cimicifuga racemosa* in menopause symptom relief, *Menopause* 10:299-313, 2003.
49. Jarry H, Harnischfeger G, Duker E: Studies on the endocrine effects of the contents of *Cimicifuga racemosa.* 2. In vitro binding of compounds to estrogen receptors, *Planta Med* 51:316-319, 1985.
50. Struck D, Tegtmeier M, Harnischfeger G: Flavones in extracts of *Cimicifuga racemosa, Planta Med* 63:289-290, 1997.
51. Kennelly EJ, Baggett S, Nuntanakorn P, et al: Analysis of thirteen populations of black cohosh for formononetin, *Phytomedicine* 9:461-467, 2002.
52. Liske E, Wustenberg P: Therapy of climacteric complaints with *Cimicifuga racemosa:* herbal medicine with clinically proven evidence, *Menopause* 5:250, 1998.
53. Mahady GB: Is black cohosh estrogenic? *Nutr Rev* 61(5 pt 1):183-186, 2003.
54. Nesselhut T, Schellhase C, Dietrich R, et al: Studies of mamma carcinoma cells regarding the proliferative potential of herbal medication with estrogenic-like effects, *Arch Gynecol Obstet* 254:817-818, 1993.
55. Zava DT, Dollbaum CM, Blen M: Estrogen and progestin bioactivity of foods, herbs, and spices, *Proc Soc Exp Biol Med* 217:369-378, 1998.
56. Dixon-Shanies D, Shaikh N: Growth inhibition of human breast cancer cells by herbs and phytoestrogens, *Oncol Rep* 6:1383-1387, 1999.
57. Bodinet C, Freudenstein J: Influence of *Cimicifuga racemosa* on the proliferation of estrogen receptor-positive human breast cancer cells, *Breast Cancer Res Treat* 76:1-10, 2002.
58. Liu J, Burdette JE, Xu H, et al: Evaluation of estrogenic activity of plant extracts for the potential treatment of menopausal symptoms, *J Agric Food Chem* 49:2472-2479, 2001.
59. Jacobson JS, Troxel AB, Evans J, et al: Randomized trial of black cohosh for the treatment of hot flashes among women with a history of breast cancer, *J Clin Oncol* 19:2739-2745, 2001.
60. Maamari R, Schreiber A: *Cimicifuga racemosa* and quality of life. The NAMS Program and Abstract Book, 2001, p 10.

61. Davis VL, Jayo MJ, Hardy ML, et al: Effects of black cohosh on mammary tumor development and progression in MMTV-neu transgenic mice. 94th Annual Meeting of the American Association for Cancer Research, Washington, DC, July 11-14, 2003, abstract R910.
62. Liao JF, Jan YM, Huang SY, et al: Evaluation with receptor binding assay on the water extracts of ten CNS-active Chinese herbal drugs. Proceedings of the National Science Council, Republic of China, Life Sci 19:151-158, 1995.
63. Yoo JS, Jung JS, Lee TH, et al: Inhibitory effects of extracts from traditional herbal drugs on 5-hydroxytryptophan induced diarrhea in mice [abstract], *Saengyak Hakhoechi* 26:355-359, 1995.
64. Jarry H, Metten M, Spengler B, et al: In vitro effects of the *Cimicifuga racemosa* extract BNO 1055, *Maturitas* 44(Suppl 1):S31-S38, 2003.
65. Li JX, Kadota S, Li HY, et al: Effects of *Cimicifuga* rhizome on serum calcium and phosphate levels in low calcium dietary rats and on bone mineral density in ovariectomized rats, *Phytomedicine* 3:379-385, 1996.
66. Wuttke W, Seidlova-Wuttke D, Gorkow C: The *Cimicifuga* preparation BNO 1055 vs. conjugated estrogens in a double-blind placebo-controlled study: effects on menopause symptoms and bone markers, *Maturitas* 44(suppl 1):S67-S77, 2003.
67. Liske E, Wustenberg P: Therapy of climacteric complaints with *Cimicifuga racemosa:* herbal medicine with clinically proven evidence, *Menopause* 5:250, 1998.
68. McGuffin M, Hobbs C, Upton R, et al: *American Herbal Products Association's botanical safety handbook,* Boca Raton, Fla, 1997, CRC Press, p 29.
69. Burke BE, Olson RD, Cusack BJ: Randomized, controlled trial of phytoestrogen in the prophylactic treatment of menstrual migraine, *Biomed Pharmacother* 56:283-288, 2002.
70. Zhu DP: Dong quai, *Am J Chin Med* 15(3-4):117-125, 1987.
71. Belford-Courtney R: Comparison of Chinese and Western uses of *Angelica sinensis, Aust J Med Herb* 5:87-91, 1993.
72. Amato P, Christophe S, Mellon PL: Estrogenic activity of herbs commonly used as remedies for menopausal symptoms, *Menopause* 9:145-150, 2002.
73. Hirata JD, Swiersz LM, Zell B, et al: Does dong quai have estrogenic effects in postmenopausal women? A double-blind, placebo-controlled trial, *Fertil Steril* 68:981-986, 1997.
74. Lo AC, Chan K, Young JH, et al: Danggui (*Angelica sinensis*) affects the pharmacodynamics but not the pharmacokinetics of warfarin in rabbits, *Eur J Drug Metab Pharmacokinet* 20:55-60, 1995.
75. Brown DJ: *Vitex agnus-castus* clinical monograph, *Quarterly Review of Natural Medicine,* Summer: 111-121, 1994.
76. Blumenthal M, Gruenwald J, Hall T, et al, eds: *The complete German Commission E monographs: therapeutic guide to herbal medicine,* Boston, 1998, Integrative Medicine Communications.
77. Second International Symposium on the role of soy in preventing and treating chronic disease. Brussels, Belgium, September 15-18, 1996. Proceedings in *J Am Coll Nutr* 1996.
78. Adlercreutz H, Fotsis T, Bannwart C, et al: Urinary estrogen profile determination in young Finnish vegetarian and omnivorous women, *J Steroid Biochem* 24:289, 1986.
79. Duncan AM, Merz BE, Xu X, et al: Soy isoflavones exert modest hormonal effects in premenopausal women, *J Clin Endocrinol Metab* 84:192-197, 1999.
80. Davis SR, Dalais FS, Simpson ER, et al: Phytoestrogens in health and disease, *Recent Prog Horm Res* 54:185-211, 1999.
81. Tyler VE, Foster SL: *Tyler's honest herbal,* 4th ed, Binghamton, NY, 1999, Hawthorn Herbal Press.
82. Lewis RA: *Lewis' dictionary of toxicology,* Boca Raton, Fla, 1998, CRC Press.
83. Hoffman PC, Combs DK, Brehm NM, et al: Performance of lactating dairy cows fed red clover or alfalfa silage, *J Dairy Sci* 80:3308-3315, 1997.
84. Tice JA, Ettinger B, Ensrud K, et al: Phytoestrogen supplements for the treatment of hot flashes: the Isoflavone Clover Extract (ICE) Study: a randomized controlled trial, *JAMA* 290:207-214, 2003.
85. Baber RJ, Templeman C, Morton T, et al: Randomized placebo-controlled trial of an isoflavone supplement and menopausal symptoms in women, *Climacteric* 2:85-92, 1999.
86. Knight DC, Howes JB, Eden JA: The effect of Promensil, an isoflavone extract, on menopausal symptoms, *Climacteric* 2:79-84, 1999.

87. van de Weijer PH, Barentsen R: Isoflavones from red clover (Promensil) significantly reduce menopausal hot flush symptoms compared with placebo, *Maturitas* 42:187-193, 2002.

88. Fetrow CW, Avila JR: *Complementary & alternative medicines,* Springhouse, Pa, 1999, Springhouse, pp 282-286.

89. McGuffin M, Hobbs C, Upton R, et al: *American Herbal Products Association's botanical safety handbook,* Boca Raton, Fla, 1997, CRC Press, p 81.

90. Wiklund IK, Mattsson LA, Lindgren R, et al: Effects of a standardized ginseng extract on quality of life and physiological parameters in symptomatic postmenopausal women: a double-blind, placebo-controlled trial. Swedish Alternative Medicine Group, *Int J Clin Pharmacol Res* 19:89-99, 1999.

91. Tode T, Kikuchi Y, Hirata J, et al: Effect of Korean red ginseng on psychological functions in patients with severe climacteric syndromes, *Int J Gynaecol Obstet* 67:169-174, 1999.

92. Amato P, Christophe S, Mellon PL: Estrogenic activity of herbs commonly used as remedies for menopausal symptoms, *Menopause* 9:145-150, 2002.

93. Duda RB, Zhong Y, Navas V, et al: American ginseng and breast cancer therapeutic agents synergistically inhibit MCF-7 breast cancer cell growth, *J Surg Oncol* 72:230-239, 1999.

94. Wichtl M: In Bisset NG, editor: *Herbal drugs and phytopharmaceuticals,* Stuttgart, 1994, Medpharm Publishers, pp 112-113.

95. Linde K, Mulrow CD: St John's wort for depression, *Cochrane Database Syst Rev* 2000;(2):CD000448.

96. Liske E, Gerhard I, Wustenberg P: Menopause: herbal combination product for psychovegetative complaints, *TW Gynakol* 10:172-175, 1997.

97. Pittler MH, Ernst E: Efficacy of kava extract for treating anxiety: systematic review and meta-analysis, *J Clin Psychopharmacol* 20:84-89, 2000.

98. Warnecke G: Psychomatic dysfunction in the female climacteric. Clinical effectiveness and tolerance of kava extract WS 1490 [in German], *Fortschr Med* 109:119-122, 1991.

99. Barton DL, Loprinzi CL, Quella SK, et al: Prospective evaluation of vitamin E for hot flashes in breast cancer survivors, *J Clin Oncol* 16:495-500, 1998.

100. Gruenwald J, Skrabal J: Kava ban high questionable: a brief summary of the main scientific findings presented in "In depth investigation on EU member states market restrictions on kava products," *Seminars in Integrative Medicine* 1:199-210, 2003.

101. Wyon Y, Lindgren R, Hammar M, et al: Acupuncture against climacteric disorders? Lower number of symptoms after menopause, *Lakartidningen* 91:2318-2322, 1994.

Integrative Strategies During Pregnancy

The use of dietary supplements and botanicals during pregnancy may be more common than some health care practitioners realize. A recent study of 578 rural-living pregnant women in the eastern United States found that 45% of respondents used herbal medicines and 20% were at least partially nonadherent with prenatal vitamin and mineral use.[1] Women may seek the use of "natural remedies" during pregnancy because they perceive these remedies to be "safer" than conventional drugs. Although it is true that some dietary supplements are milder in both effects and side effects, the indiscriminate use of over-the-counter medicines, prescription drugs, herbal preparations, or nutritional supplements during pregnancy is unwise. The rapid growth of the fetus makes it particularly vulnerable to substances that affect cellular division. Compounds that affect the muscle tone or circulation of the uterus may also lead to adverse consequences. Herbs can act as uterine stimulants, abortifacients, teratogens, and mutagens. It is important for pregnant women to consult a qualified health care practitioner before using any medication. See Table 7-1 for a list of herbs to avoid during pregnancy.

This chapter provides a compilation of some of the most common symptoms that occur during pregnancy and treatments that are either commonly used or those interventions that have some documented evidence of benefit.

STRETCH MARKS

Striae gravidarum (stretch marks) occur in approximately 50% to 90% of pregnant women because of the separation of underlying connective tissue as the uterus enlarges within the abdominal cavity. Dermal collagen is damaged and blood vessels dilate, resulting in the formation of reddish-purple early stretch marks. Collagen remodeling often leads to loss of melanocytes, or pigment-producing cells, which leads to the whitish mature stretch marks. Stretch marks tend to occur primarily on the abdomen, thighs, and breasts. A woman's skin type and genetic history play a significant role in the extent of the striae.

Table **7-1**

*Herbs to avoid during pregnancy**

COMMON NAME	BOTANICAL NAME
Achyranthes root	*Achyranthes bidentata*
Agave plant	*Agave americana*
Alknet root	*Alkanna tinctoria*
Aloe (dried juice)	*Aloe* spp.
American liverleaf herb	*Hepatica nobilis*
American pennyroyal herb	*Hedeoma pulegioides*
Andrographis herb	*Andrographis paniculata*
Angelica root	*Angelica archangelica, A. atrop urpurea, A. sinensis*
Anise fruit (seed)	*Pimpinella anisum*
Arnica herb	*Arnica* spp.
Asafetida gum resin	*Ferula assa-foetida, F. foetida, F. rubricaulis*
Asarabacca rhizome	*Asarum europaeum*
Ashwaganda root	*Withania somnifera*
Barberry root bark	*Berberis vulgaris*
Barley sprouted seed	*Hordeum vulgare*
Basil leaf	*Ocimum basilicum*
Beebalm herb	*Monarda* spp.
Bei mu	*Fritillaria cirrhosa, F. thunbergii*
Beth root	*Trillium erectum*
Birthwort	*Aristolochia clematitis*
Black cohosh root	*Cimicifuga racemosa*
Bladderwrack thallus	*Fucus vesiculosus*
Blazing star root	*Aletris farinosa*
Blessed thistle herb	*Cnicus benedictus*
Bloodroot	*Sanguinaria canadensis*
Blue cohosh root	*Caulophyllum thalictroides*
Blue flag root	*Iris versicolor, I. virginica*
Blue lobelia herb	*Lobelia siphilitica*
Blue vervain herb	*Verbena hastata*
Borage herb	*Borago officinalis*
Bu gu zhi	*Cullen corylifolia*
Buchu leaf	*Barosma betulina, B. crenulata*
Buckthorn fruit	*Rhamnus cathartica*
Bugleweed herb	*Lycopus* spp.
Butterbur rhizome	*Petasites hybridus*
California poppy herb	*Eschscholzia californica*
California spikenard rhizome	*Aralia californica*

*This list is compiled from a variety of sources. It is not exhaustive. Some of the herbs listed (basil, fenugreek) are considered safe when used as a flavoring in food but may be harmful if taken in larger medicinal doses.

Continued

Table 7-1

Herbs to avoid during pregnancy—cont'd

COMMON NAME	BOTANICAL NAME
Camphor distillate	*Cinnamomum camphora*
Canada snakeroot	*Asarum canadense*
Cascara sagrada bark	*Cascara sagrada*
Cassia bark	*Cinnamomum cassia*
Castor seed oil	*Ricinus communis*
Catnip herb	*Nepeta cataria*
Cedar stem	*Thuja occidentalis*
Celandine herb	*Chelidonium majus*
Celery seed	*Apium graveolens*
Chastetree fruit (berry)	*Vitex agnus-castus*
Chinese goldthread rhizome	*Coptis chinensis*
Chinese motherwort	*Leonurus heterophyllus, L. sibiricus*
Chong wei zi	*Leonurus heterophyllus, L. sibiricus*
Chuan huang bai	*Phellodendron amurense, P. chinense*
Chuan jiao	*Zanthoxylum schinifolium, Z. simulans*
Chuan niu xi	*Cyathula officinalis*
Chuan xiong	*Ligusticum chuanxiong*
Cola seed	*Cola nitida*
Coltsfoot flower	*Tussilago farfara*
Comfrey leaf and root	*Symphytum officinale*
Corydalis rhizome	*Corydalis yanhusuo*
Cotton root bark	*Gossypium herbaceum, G. hirsutum*
Culver's root	*Leptandra virginica*
Da huang	*Rheum palmatum*
Di gu pi	*Lycium barbarum, L. chinense*
Dong quai root	*Angelica sinensis*
Dyer's broom herb	*Genista tinctoria*
Elecampane root	*Inula helenium*
Ephedra herb	*Ephedra* spp.
European pennyroyal	*Mentha pulegium*
European vervain	*Verbena officinalis*
False unicorn rhizome	*Chamaelirium luteum*
Fenugreek seed	*Trigonella foenum-graecum*
Feverfew herb	*Tanacetum parthenium*
Forsythia fruit	*Forsythia suspense*
Fritillary bulb	*Fritillaria cirrhosa, F. thunbergii*
Gan cao	*Glycyrrhiza uralensis*
Garlic bulb	*Allium sativum*
Ginger root	*Zingiber officinale*
Goldenseal root	*Hydrastis canadensis*
Goldthread	*Coptis groenlandica*

Table 7-1

Herbs to avoid during pregnancy—cont'd

Common Name	Botanical Name
Gou qi zi	Lycium barbarum, L. chinense
Guggul gum resin	Commiphora mukul
He huan pi	Albizia julibrissin
Hong hua	Carthamus tinctorius
Horehound herb	Marrubium vulgare
Hou po	Magnolia officinalis
Hou po hua	Magnolia officinalis
Huang bi	Phellodendron amurense, P. chinense
Huang lian	Coptis chinensis
Hu lu ba	Trigonella foenum-graecum
Hyssop herb	Hyssopus officinalis
Inmortal root	Asclepias asperula
Ipecac rhizome	Cephaelis ipecacuanha
Jaborandi leaf	Pilocarpus jaborandi
Japanese arisaema tuber	Arisaema japonicum
Job's tears seed	Coix lacryma-jobi
Jujube seeds	Ziziphus spinosa
Juniper berry	Juniperus communis
Kava root	Piper methysticum
Lemongrass herb	Cymbopogon citrates
Lian qiao	Forsythia suspense
Licorice root	Glycyrrhiza spp.
Life root plant	Senecio aureus
Lobelia herb	Lobelia inflata
Lomatium root	Lomatium dissectum
Lovage root	Levisticum officinale
Lycium berry and root bark	Lycium barbarum, L. chinense
Ma huang	Ephedra spp.
Mace seed	Myristica fragrans
Magnolia bark	Magnolia officinalis
Maidenhair fern herb	Adiantum pedatum
Mai ya	Hordeum vulgare
Male fern rhizome	Dryopteris filix-mas
Mandrake root	Podophyllum peltatum
Mimosa tree bark	Albizia julibrissin
Ming dang shen root	Changium smyrnoides
Motherwort herb	Leonurus cardiaca
Mugwort herb	Artemesia vulgaris, A. lactiflora
Mu dan pi	Paeonia suffruticosa
Mu zei	Equisetum hyemale

Continued

Table **7-1**

Herbs to avoid during pregnancy—cont'd

COMMON NAME	BOTANICAL NAME
Myrrh gum resin	*Commiphora molmol, C. myrrha*
Nui xi	*Achyranthes bidentata*
Nutmeg seed	*Myristica fragrans*
Ocotillo stem	*Fouquieria splendens*
Oregon grape root	*Mahonia aquifolium*
Osha root	*Ligisticum porteri*
Parsley leaf and root	*Petroselinum crispum*
Peach seed	*Prunus persica*
Peony root	*Paeonia officinalis*
Phellodendron bark	*Phellodendron amurense, P. chinense*
Pinellia rhizome	*Pinellia ternate*
Pleurisy root	*Asclepias tuberosa*
Prickly ash bark	*Zanthoxylum clava-herculis, Z. americanum*
Psoralea seed	*Cullen corylifolia*
Purslane herb	*Portulaca oleracea*
Quassia bark	*Picrasma excelsa*
Queen of the meadow root/herb	*Eupatorium purpureum*
Qing hao	*Artemesia annua*
Quinine bark	*Cinchona* spp.
Rauwolfia root	*Rauwolfia serpentina*
Red clover flowers	*Trifolium pratense*
Red cedar leaf and berry	*Juniperus virginiana*
Rhubarb rhizome/root	*Rheum palmatum, R. officinale*
Roman chamomile flower	*Chamaemelum nobile*
Rosemary leaf	*Rosmarinus officinalis*
Rou gui	*Cinnamomum cassia*
Rue herb	*Ruta graveolens*
Saffron stigma	*Crocus sativus*
Sage leaf	*Salvia officinalis*
Shi chang pu	*Acorus gramineus*
Seneca snakeroot	*Polygala senega*
Senna leaf	*Senna* spp.
Shepard's purse herb	*Capsella bursa-pastoris*
Spikenard rhizome	*Aralia racemosa*
Southernwood herb	*Artemisia abrotanum*
Suan zao ren	*Ziziphus spinosa*
Sweet Annie herb	*Artemisia annua*
Tansy herb	*Tanacetum vulgare*
Tao ren	*Prunus persica*
Thuja stem	*Thuja occidentalis*
Tian nan xing	*Arisaema triphyllum*

Table **7-1**

Herbs to avoid during pregnancy—cont'd

COMMON NAME	BOTANICAL NAME
Tienchi ginseng	*Panax notoginseng*
Tree peony bark	*Paeonia suffruticosa*
Tricosanthes fruit	*Trichosanthes kirilowii*
Turmeric rhizome	*Curcuma longa*
Uva ursi leaf	*Arctostaphylos uva-ursi*
Vetiver root	*Vetiveria zizanoides*
Virginia snakeroot	*Aristolochia serpentaria*
Watercress leaf	*Nasturtium officinale*
Wild carrot fruit (seed)	*Daucus carota*
Wild indigo root	*Baptisia tinctoria*
Wormseed seed and herb	*Chenopodium ambrosioides*
Wormwood herb	*Artemisia absinthium*
Yan hu suo	*Corydalis yanhusuo*
Yarrow flowers	*Achillea millefolium*
Yellow jasmine herb	*Gelsemium sempervirens*
Yi mu cao	*Leonurus heterophyllus, L. sibiricus*
Yi yi ren	*Coix lacryma-jobi*
Yin chen hao	*Artemisia capillaris*

Although many products are available for treatment of stretch marks, reviewers for the Cochrane Database of Systematic Reviews found only one topical cream helpful in preventing the development of stretch marks in pregnancy. However, this treatment worked only in those women who had developed stretch marks during prior pregnancies. When compared with placebo, treatment with a cream containing *Centella asiatica* extract, alpha tocopherol, and collagen-elastin hydrolysates was associated with fewer women developing stretch marks.[2]

MUSCULAR ACHES AND PAINS

Estrogen and relaxin increase the mobility of the pelvic structure as well as the laxity of the pelvic ligaments. The abdominal muscles stretch, and during the latter part of pregnancy the large rectus abdominis muscles may separate. As a woman's center of gravity shifts forward, she may experience lower back pain. Alterations in her posture occur as the result of decreased muscle tone, increased weight, and enlarging abdomen.

The round ligaments of the uterus extend from the lateral edge of the uterus down through the inguinal canal and terminate in the labia majora. During pregnancy these round ligaments increase in length and diameter, and as they stretch many women have varying degrees of discomfort. Warm baths, leaning into the side of the pain, prenatal yoga, and gentle stretching are common recommendations for reducing round ligament discomfort.

To help reduce back pain, practitioners should encourage women to do pelvic tilt exercises to increase abdominal muscle strength, gently stretch every morning and evening, wear flat shoes with good arch support, sleep on a firm mattress, and soak in a warm bath. Abdominal crunches may be performed during the first trimester but are generally not recommended after that time. The "rocking back arch" is an excellent lower back exercise during the second and third trimesters. The patient kneels on all fours, counts to five as she gently rocks back and forth, and then returns to center and arches the back while exhaling slowly. This exercise can be repeated several times. Over-the-counter ointments and creams that contain camphor, cajeput oil, wintergreen oil, and eucalyptol applied to the lumbosacral area can provide temporary relief.

Prenatal massage is becoming available in many parts of the country. Massage tables are built specifically for women to receive a therapeutic massage even during advanced pregnancy. Many women have reported not only how wonderful the massage feels, but also how great it was to be able to lie on their stomachs for an hour. Pregnant women should be counseled to seek the services of a licensed massage therapist who has experience in providing prenatal massage. Although no studies are available that specifically address prenatal massage and back pain, researchers have found that, when combined with exercise and education, massage is beneficial for those with nonspecific lower back pain.[3]

NAUSEA AND VOMITING OF PREGNANCY

Nausea and vomiting is a common experience for many women (33% to 50%) during early pregnancy. The etiology is not known. Morning sickness usually presents by 4 to 8 weeks' gestation and disappears by week 16. Mild to moderate morning sickness is generally benign, posing no significant risk to mother or baby. The diagnosis of *hyperemesis gravidarum* is made when a woman has nausea and vomiting serious enough to cause a weight loss of at least 5% of the prepregnancy weight, dehydration, electrolyte imbalance, and ketosis. This condition necessitates hospitalization with appropriate treatment.[4]

The cause of nausea and vomiting of pregnancy is probably multifactorial. Numerous hypotheses are suggested in the literature, including vitamin B_6 deficiency, the role of gestational hormones (human chorionic gonadotropin), gastric dysrhythmias, immunologic factors, and psychological factors.[5] Several risk factors are associated with morning sickness: age younger than 20 years, first pregnancy, previous pregnancies with morning sickness, and elevated body mass index.[4]

Nonpharmacologic interventions should be recommended initially. These include eating dry toast or crackers half an hour before rising in the morning and eating small, frequent meals (every 2 to 3 hours) throughout the day. Ensure adequate protein and liquid intake.

Botanicals*

Three published placebo-controlled trials have addressed the safety and efficacy of ginger (*Zingiber officinale*) for morning sickness. The 1990 trial by Fischer-Rasmussen et al[6] randomly assigned 30 pregnant women admitted to the hospital with hyperemesis gravidarum before the 20th week of gestation to receive either 250 mg of powdered ginger

*Excerpt from Coates P, ed: *Encyclopedia of dietary supplements*, 2004, Marcel Dekker.

capsules four times per day or placebo for a 4-day period followed by a 2-day washout and crossover to the other treatment. A scoring system was used to assess the degree of nausea, vomiting, and weight loss before onset of the trial and then as reevaluated on days 5 and 11 after treatment. The relief scores were greater for ginger than placebo with a reduced number of vomiting episodes and degree of nausea. Subjective assessment by the women showed that 70.4% preferred the period when they received ginger; only 14.8% preferred placebo. No adverse effects on pregnancy outcome were noted.

Vutyavanich et al[7] conducted a randomized, double-blind, placebo-controlled study of 70 women (n = 67) with nausea of pregnancy, with or without vomiting, before the 17th week of gestation. The primary outcome was improvement in nausea symptoms. Women received either 250-mg powdered ginger capsules or placebo four times daily for a 4-day period. A visual analog scale (VAS) and Likert scale were used as measuring instruments. The VAS scores decreased (improved) significantly in the ginger group compared with placebo ($P = 0.014$). Vomiting episodes were also significantly decreased ($P < 0.001$). At the 1-week follow up visit, 28 of 32 subjects in the ginger group had improvement of nausea symptoms, whereas only 10 of 35 in the placebo group experienced improvement ($P < 0.001$). Minor side effects were noted in both groups; more heartburn was noted in the ginger group. No adverse effects were noted on pregnancy outcomes.

In 2003, a double-blind placebo-controlled trial randomly assigned 120 women before the 20th week of gestation, who had experienced morning sickness daily for at least a week and had no relief of symptoms through dietary changes, to receive either 125 mg of ginger extract (EV.EXT 35; equivalent to 1.5 g of dried ginger) or placebo four times per day.[8] The nausea experience score was significantly less for the ginger extract group relative to the placebo group after the first day of treatment and this difference was present for each treatment day. For retching symptoms, the ginger extract group had significantly lower symptom scores than the placebo group for the first 2 days only. In contrast to the other published studies, no significant difference was noted between ginger extract and placebo groups for any of the vomiting symptoms. Twenty-one women were excluded from the final analysis because of insufficient data (12 for adverse events and 9 for non-compliance). Adverse events included spontaneous abortion (n = 4 women [3 in the ginger group, 1 in the placebo group]), intolerance of the treatment (n = 4 [all in the ginger group]), worsening of treatment requiring further medical assistance (n = 3 [1 in the ginger group, 2 in the placebo group]), and allergic reaction to treatment (n = 1 [ginger group]). Follow-up of the pregnancies revealed normal ranges of birth weight, gestational age, Apgar scores, and frequencies of congenital abnormalities when the study group infants were compared with the general population of infants born at the Royal Hospital for Women for the year 1999-2000.

Interestingly, the German Commission E and American Herbal Products Association contraindicate the use of ginger during pregnancy. This appears to be based on two concerns. The first is that the inhibition of thromboxane synthetase may affect testosterone binding in the fetus,[9] although inhibition of thromboxane synthetase occurs at doses higher than those used in the studies. The second concern is in vitro evidence that gingerol and shogoal, isolated components of ginger, exhibit mutagenic activity in certain salmonella strains.[10] However, researchers have also found antimutagenic compounds in ginger.[11] Even in large doses, a study in rats failed to find malformations in the offspring of animals who were administered 20 g/L or 50 g/L of ginger tea in their drinking water from gestation days 6 to 15 and then sacrificed at day 20. No gross morphologic malformations were seen in the treated fetuses. Fetuses exposed to ginger tea were found to be significantly heavier than controls and had more advanced skeletal development as determined by measurement of sternal and metacarpal ossification centers. No maternal toxicity was observed in this study, although embryonic loss in the treatment group was almost double that of the controls ($P < 0.05$). Researchers at the Hospital for Sick Children in Toronto, Canada, studied 187 pregnant women who used some form of ginger in the first trimester. They reported that the risk of these mothers having a baby with a congenital malformation was no higher than in a control group.[12] In the published human studies, one spontaneous abortion (among 32 in the ginger group),[7] one spontaneous abortion (of 27 in the crossover design study),[6] and three spontaneous abortions (of 60 in the ginger group)[8] were reported, although one of the three spontaneous abortions in last group occurred in a woman who had not begun taking the treatment. Alhough the total number of women in these clinical trials is small, the rate of spontaneous abortion is not any greater than that seen in the general population. Given the vast numbers of women around the globe who consume ginger during pregnancy, it is unlikely that there is significant risk associated with its use in moderation. It appears reasonable for a woman to use small amounts of ginger, 250 mg four times per day, for the relief of morning sickness.[13]

Raspberry leaf and peppermint teas are also recommended for morning sickness. Peppermint has a long history of quieting a queasy stomach and is safe for use during pregnancy; however, it can aggravate gastroesophageal reflux, another common symptom of pregnancy. Raspberry is not observed to be effective for morning sickness in my experience, but the tea is safe.

Vitamin B_6

Two double-blind, placebo-controlled, randomized clinical trials have been conducted to determine the efficacy of vitamin B_6 during pregnancy. The study by Sahakian et al[14] in 1991 found that 25 mg of vitamin B_6 three times per day was superior to placebo for reducing severe nausea by day 3 of treatment but made little difference for milder cases of nausea. At the completion of therapy, significantly fewer subjects (25.8%) in the pyridoxine group compared with the placebo group (53.6%) had vomiting.

A larger study conducted in 1995 found that only nausea was reduced, not vomiting, when women received 10 mg of pyridoxine hydrochloride three times per day for 5 days. The mean change in nausea scores in the pyridoxine group was significantly greater than those in the placebo group. After 5 days of treatment, 36% of women in the active group had vomiting versus 34% of women in placebo group (33.9%); this difference was not statistically significant.[15]

Potential confounders in all trials studying morning sickness include the natural fluctuation of the condition over time, the quantification of a subjective symptom such as nausea, and a notable placebo effect. The 1995 study used a dose of 30 mg/day versus the 75 mg/day used in the previous study. Thirty mg/day may be insufficient to alter the number of episodes of emesis. Vitamin B_6, at doses used in the aforementioned clinical trials, appears to be safe during pregnancy. The Food and Drug Administration (FDA) categorized the recommended daily allowance dose of 2.2 mg/day as pregnancy category A; if used in doses greater than the recommendation it is classified as FDA pregnancy category C.[16] Although pyridoxine is a water-soluble vitamin, it is associated with toxicity when taken in large doses over time. The majority of toxicity occurs at doses of 500 mg/day or higher, but a few reports of toxicity occurred with prolonged ingestion of 150 mg/day.[17]

Acupuncture

Acupuncture and acupressure have been shown to be useful for alleviating morning sickness. The National Institutes of Health Consensus Development Conference on Acupuncture in 1997 stated "There is clear evidence that needle acupuncture treatment is effective for post-operative and chemotherapy nausea and vomiting, and nausea of pregnancy and post-operative dental pain." Six of seven clinical trials found that acupressure is effective for relieving morning sickness.[18] Acupressure wristbands are popular and readily available. Many women find these a less expensive alternative to acupuncture, which offers a noninvasive and effective remedy for pregnancy-associated nausea and vomiting.

GASTROESOPHAGEAL REFLUX

Heartburn can occur during pregnancy because of increased progesterone reducing the tone of the cardiac (gastroesophageal) sphincter. The refluxing stomach acids irritate the lining of the esophagus, causing heartburn. Hiatal hernias are common in the general population and occur in approximately 20% of pregnant women. Reflux results as a portion of the stomach protrudes above the diaphragm, preventing the proper closure of the cardiac sphincter.

Women should be encouraged to eat small, frequent meals; refrain from eating close to bedtime; and avoid tight-fitting clothes around the abdomen. Some women find it helpful to elevate the head of the bed. Foods and substances that increase stomach acidity or reduce cardiac sphincter tone should be avoided, including cigarettes, alcohol, coffee, peppermint, and chocolate.

Botanicals

A number of herbs are used to soothe esophageal irritation, including several that are safe for use in pregnancy. Two herbs that are readily available are chamomile (*Matricaria recutita*) and marshmallow (*Althaea officinalis*). No significant clinical research has been conducted to evaluate the effectiveness of chamomile teas or extracts for the treatment of gastrointestinal inflammation; however, the herb is widely accepted for this purpose by many authorities. Animal studies have shown that oral administration of (-)-α-bisabolol reduces gastric toxicity induced by acetylsalicylic acid[19] and inhibits the development of ulcers caused by indomethacin, ethanol, and stress.[20] Chamomile, known in Spanish as manzanilla, is one of the most popular herbs used by Mexican Americans and is commonly recommended during pregnancy to ease nausea and heartburn and as a general relaxant.

The leaf and root of marshmallow are rich in mucopolysaccharides that soothe and protect the esophageal lining from irritation. Marshmallow was a food herb for centuries and is considered safe for use during pregnancy. The German health authorities endorse the use of marshmallow root for "mild inflammation of the gastric mucosa."[21] There are no known contraindications to marshmallow; however, because of the high mucilage content, marshmallow may delay the absorption of medications.[22] Prescription medications should be taken at least 30 minutes before using this herb.

CONSTIPATION

Constipation may occur during pregnancy because of hormonal effects, resulting in a decrease in intestinal tone and motility. In addition, as the womb enlarges, the intestines are compressed. Iron supplementation can worsen constipation. Women should be instructed to increase fluid and fiber intake and exercise regularly. Molasses, especially from beets, is a good source of iron and nutrients and is a gentle, safe laxative. The dose is 1 to 2 Tbsp/day until bowels are moving more freely. Flaxseeds can be ground in a coffee grinder and added to cereals to encourage regular bowel movements. Prunes and prune juice have been used to encourage sluggish bowels for centuries and are safe during pregnancy.

Pregnant women should avoid stronger anthraquinone-containing laxatives such as senna, cascara sagrada, and aloe, as they may stimulate uterine contractions.

STRESS, ANXIETY, AND INSOMNIA

Practitioners should evaluate the extent of stressors and anxiety in a woman's life and make recommendations accordingly. As always, practitioners should be mindful that an estimated 4% to 8% of pregnant women experience physical abuse, which might manifest as heightened anxiety, depression, and stress. If abuse is suspected, appropriate referrals should be made. Mild forms of tension are probably best addressed through lifestyle interventions, including gentle, regular exercise; warm baths; journal writing; eliminating or reducing caffeine; and setting priorities and limits on time and responsibilities. Pregnancy and birth may raise issues of fear and loss of control. Encourage women to express their concerns and recommend, as appropriate, childbirth classes that may ease fears and provide support.

Women should be instructed in appropriate sleep strategies. Some women may find that taking a relaxing bath 30 to 60 minutes before bed helps reduce tension and ease the transition to sleep. If desired, a woman may wish to add 5 to 10 drops of an essential oil to the bath for its pleasant aroma. Jasmine, lavender, and vetiver oils have all been used for relaxation. A cup of chamomile tea taken in the evening can also be soothing (see page 101).

Valerian has been used as a mild sleep aid and anxiolytic for centuries. A recent review located 18 experimental studies examining the effects of valerian on human sleep. The majority of studies reported positive effects of valerian on subjective sleep parameters, but objective sleep measures yielded inconsistent results. The two trials comparing valerian with prescription hypnotics were favorable.[28] No contraindications to valerian during pregnancy are found in the literature, including the German Commission E and the *Botanical Safety Handbook*. Valepotriates, key constituents in valerian, given orally for 30 days were innocuous to pregnant rats and their offspring.[29] Occasional use of valerian for sleep appears to be safe. Valerian is often combined with other botanicals for sleep; however, it is probably best to use as a single therapy during pregnancy.

A NOTE ON THE SAFETY OF CHAMOMILE DURING PREGNANCY

The literature contains a great deal of conflicting data on the safety of chamomile during pregnancy. These differences come primarily from extrapolating research on an isolated constituent and then applying it to the whole herb. A 1979 study demonstrated that high doses of α-bisabolol, 3 mL/kg, had a teratogenic effect in animals. This same study also noted the absence of any developmental abnormalities or teratogenic effects with 1-mL/kg doses of α-bisabolol over extended periods of time.[24] Chamomile contains approximately 0.5% essential oil, of which roughly 50% is α-bisabolol. Most women who consume chamomile actually drink the tea. Because of the low water solubility of the essential oil, teas prepared from chamomile flowers contain only 10% to 15% of the oil present in the plant.[25] It would be impossible to drink enough tea to reach the levels cited in the study. Yet reputable books continue to state that "German chamomile is reported to be uterotonic and teratogenic in rats, rabbits, and dogs. This product should be avoided in pregnant and lactating patients."[21] The reference cited for this declaration is the same 1979 study that clearly stated the teratogenicity was found at high doses of an isolated constituent, not the whole plant. The German health authorities[27] and the American Herbal Products Assocation[28] do not consider pregnancy or lactation a contraindication to chamomile.

Kava (*Piper methysticum*) is found in numerous products recommended for anxiety and sleep. Questions of liver toxicity make this herb unsuitable for use during pregnancy.

UPPER RESPIRATORY TRACT INFECTIONS

Minor upper respiratory tract infections can usually be treated at home by increasing fluid intake, getting extra rest, and eating foods rich in vitamin C and zinc (fruits, vegetables, and whole grains). Women should be cautious about the use of over-the-counter medications for alleviating cold symptoms.

Although it is generally best to simply "ride out" the cold, some women may look to herbs to alleviate their symptoms. Marshmallow leaf is rich in mucopolysaccharides that help soothe an irritated throat. The German health authorities endorse its use for alleviating irritation of the mucous membranes of the mouth and throat and the associated dry cough.[30] Marshmallow leaf is considered safe for use during pregnancy.

Many women ask about the use of Echinacea during pregnancy because it is the herb that has been most heavily researched for the treatment of upper respiratory infection. A systematic review of the literature was published in 1999 that included nine treatment trials for acute upper respiratory tract infection and four trials conducted to assess the potential benefit of Echinacea for the prevention of upper respiratory infection. Eight of the treatment trials reported positive results, but three of the four prevention trials found only marginal benefit.[31] This finding is similar to the systematic review published by the Cochrane Collaboration in which 16 trials (eight prevention trials and eight trials on treatment of upper respiratory tract infections) with a total of 3396 participants were evaluated. Variation in preparations investigated and methodologic quality of trials precluded quantitative meta-analysis. Overall, the results suggested that some Echinacea preparations were superior to placebo.[32] Preparations made from the pressed juice of the flowering aerial parts of *Echinacea purpurea* are the most studied and have also yielded the highest number of positive trials.

Questions of bioequivalence between products have been raised with many botanicals, including Echinacea. A recent study in the United States failed to find any benefit of crude Echinacea over placebo in 148 college students being treated for upper respiratory tract infection. An encapsulated mixture of unrefined *E. purpurea* herb (25%) and root (25%) and *E. angustifolia* root (50%) taken in 1-g doses six times on the first day of illness and three times on each subsequent day of illness for a maximum of 10 days was investigated. After controlling for severity and duration of symptoms before study entry, sex, date of enrollment, and use of nonprotocol medications, researchers found no statistically significant treatment effect. Multivariable regression models assessing severity scores over time failed to detect statistically significant differences between the Echinacea and placebo groups.[33]

The assessment of effectiveness of *Echinacea* is further complicated by the fact that different plant parts are used; different extraction methods are used; and some preparations are combined with other herbs or homeopathic remedies—making comparisons between trials difficult. Because the "active" constituents are not known, standardization of products used in clinical trials has been difficult. New investigations have shown that stimulation of macrophages and induction of cytokines are major parts of the mode of action, and that glycoproteins, polysaccharides, and alkamines are part of the activity-relevant constituents.[34] As the basic science builds, products should reflect this knowledge and be prepared and extracted accordingly.

The German Commission E approves the use of Echinacea (*E. purpurea*) as a supportive therapy for colds and chronic infections of the upper respiratory tract and lower urinary tract.[35] The European Scientific Cooperative on Phytotherapy has listed "adjuvant therapy and prophylaxis of recurrent infections of the upper respiratory tract" as a therapeutic indication for *E. pallida* root and *E. purpurea* root and herb and includes infections of the urogenital tract for *E. purpurea* herb.[36]

So is Echinacea safe during pregnancy? Early animal studies failed to demonstrate evidence of mutagenicity or carcinogenicity after 4 weeks of ingestion of the expressed juice of *E. purpurea* at doses that far exceed typical human consumption.[37] A prospective study of 206 pregnant women found no increased risk for fetal malformations when Echinacea was ingested during pregnancy, even during the first trimester.[38] Capsule or tablet formulations, or both, of *Echinacea* were used by 114 (58%) of women, while 76 (38%) of the respondents used tinctures. The dosage of capsules varied from 250 to 1000 mg/day. In tinctures, the percentage of alcohol varied between 25% and 45%. Duration of use, on average, was 5 to 7 days. Most women used either *Echinacea angustifolia* or *E. purpurea* species; only one woman used *Echinacea pallida*. Most women (81%) believed Echinacea was effective for relieving their symptoms. The authors suggest that gestational use of Echinacea during organogenesis is not associated with a detectable increased risk of malformations. Although no evidence of increased risk was noted, the study lacked the statistical power and methodological rigor to determine pregnancy-associated risks with any degree of confidence. There are no contraindications to use during pregnancy or lactation in the British Herbal Compendium, German Commission E monograph, or by the American Herbal Products Association.

URINARY TRACT INFECTION

Urinary tract infection (UTI) is not uncommon during pregnancy, likely occurring because of increased urinary stasis, which provides an excellent medium for bacterial growth. The ureters dilate to accommodate increased urinary output, and both muscle tone and motility decrease. Women should be encouraged to maintain high fluid intake, void after intercourse, and wipe from front to back when going to the bathroom to reduce the risk of bladder infection. Pregnant women can rapidly develop kidney infections; all urinary tract infections should be carefully monitored and treated appropriately.

Cranberry (*Vaccinium macrocarpon*) has been shown to reduce the risk for developing a bladder infection, but the data are insufficient to recommend it for the treatment of an active infection. It was recently shown that the proanthocyanidins present in cranberry prevent the adherence of pathogenic *Escherichia coli* to the lining of the urinary tract.[39] Blueberries and blueberry juice have been shown to exhibit similar activity.[40] The basic science is convincing; however, a recent review concluded that there "is no conclusive evidence to recommend cranberry juice for the prevention of UTIs."[41] Reviewers noted that studies of cranberry juice for UTI prevention were generally of poor quality and that the high number of dropouts or withdrawals may suggest that long-term adherence to drinking cranberry juice may be difficult. A recent study published after this review compared the efficacy of cranberry juice and cranberry tablets with placebo for UTI prevention. One hundred fifty sexually active women aged 21 to 72 years were randomly assigned for 1 year to one of three groups of prophylaxis: placebo juice plus placebo tablets, placebo juice plus cranberry tablets, or cranberry juice plus placebo tablets. Tablets were taken twice daily and 250 mL of juice three times daily. Outcome measures were (1) more than 50% decrease in symptomatic UTIs per year and (2) more than 50% decrease in annual antibiotic consumption. Both cranberry juice and cranberry tablets significantly decreased the number of patients with at least one symptomatic UTI per year compared with placebo. The mean annual cost of prophylaxis was $624 and $1400 for cranberry tablets and juice, respectively.[42] The use of cranberry in tablet form may address the issues of cost and long-term adherence to therapy.

Despite the controversy over effectiveness and compliance, many urologists do accept the rationale for using cranberry for UTI prophylaxis.[43] From a practical point of view it seems appropriate for a woman to drink cranberry juice, if she enjoys it, during pregnancy if she is concerned about the development of UTI. However, recommending cranberry for the *treatment* of a UTI during pregnancy is probably not wise.

Echinacea is approved as an adjuvant treatment for UTIs by a number of authorities (German Commission E and European Scientific Cooperative on Phytotherapy); however, no clinical trials could be found to support this use and therefore it cannot be recommended for UTI in pregnancy. Uva ursi (*Arctostaphylos uva-ursi*) is another herb that is commonly recommended for the treatment and prevention of UTIs. Although some clinical research indicates a reduction in recurrence of bladder infection,[44] both the German Commission E and the American Herbal Products Association contraindicate the use of this herb during pregnancy.

Acupuncture significantly reduced the recurrence of UTIs in a 6-month trial of 67 adult women. Patients were divided into three groups and given acupuncture, sham acupuncture, or no treatment. In the acupuncture group 85% were free of cystitis during the 6-month observation period compared with 58% in the sham group and 36% in the control group.[45] This research is intriguing but needs confirmation by other studies before it can be formally recommended, given the expense of treatment and lack of understanding for a mechanism of action.

VAGINAL INFECTIONS
Vaginal Candidiasis

As the pH of the vagina becomes more alkaline during pregnancy, overgrowth of *Candida* spp. can occur. Progesterone enhances the adherence of *Candida* to the vaginal walls, while estrogen increases local glucose, providing ample substrate for growth. (If yeast infections are recurrent, gestational diabetes and HIV should be ruled out.) Women should be instructed to avoid bubble baths and refrain from douching during pregnancy. Clotrimazole is rated category B for pregnancy; however, the other topical azole creams are rated category C.

Lactobacillus recolonization (by yogurt or capsules) shows promise for the treatment of yeast vaginitis and bacterial vaginosis with little potential for harm. Because infection is associated with a disruption of the normal commensal microflora in the vagina, primarily a loss of lactobacilli, the exogenous application of lactobacilli to the host as probiotic agents may serve as an alternative management regimen to antimicrobial treatment.[46]

Although a substantial amount of basic science is available about the "hows and whys" for using *L. acidophilus* for the prevention and treatment of vaginal candidiasis, clinical trials are few. Given the safety and relatively low cost of this type of therapy, the lack of more rigorous inquiry into its effectiveness is disappointing.

A randomized, double-blind, placebo-controlled trial of HIV-positive women compared weekly intravaginal application of *L. acidophilus* tablets or clotrimazole. Vaginal candidiasis (VC) was defined as a vaginal swab positive for *Candida* species in the presence of signs or symptoms of vaginitis and the absence of a diagnosis of *Trichomonas vaginalis* or bacterial vaginosis. Thirty-four episodes of VC occurred among 164 women followed up for a median of 21 months. The relative risk of having an episode of VC was 0.4 in the clotrimazole arm and 0.5 in the *L. acidophilus* arm. The estimated median time to first episode VC was longer for clotrimazole and *L. acidophilus* when compared with placebo.[47]

One small open study found that women who consumed 8 ounces of *L. acidophilus*–containing yogurt per day had a threefold decrease in infections compared with control subjects. The mean number of infections during the 6-month trial was 2.54 in the control group and 0.38 in the yogurt group. Candidal colonization in the vagina and rectum decreased from a mean of 3.23 per 6 months in the control group to 0.84 per 6 months in the yogurt group.[48]

Eating yogurt enriched with *L. acidophilus* seems a sensible approach for maintaining a healthy vaginal flora; finding a quality *L. acidophilus* product may prove difficult. A recent analysis of 20 probiotic products labeled to contain *Lactobacillus* species found that 30% of products were contaminated with other organisms and 20% contained no viable organisms. None of the products contained what they claimed on the label.[49]

Adherence to epithelial cells varies greatly among the *Lactobacillus* species and among different strains belonging to the same species,[50] making the need for basic science and appropriate formulation of products necessary before this therapy can be fully integrated into a treatment regimen.

Bacterial Vaginosis

Bacterial vaginosis (BV) is a disorder of the vaginal ecosystem characterized by a shift in the vaginal flora from the normally predominant *Lactobacillus* to one dominated by sialidase enzyme–producing mixed flora. It is the most common cause of abnormal vaginal discharge in adult women.[51] Studies have shown that spontaneous abortion, preterm labor, premature birth, preterm premature rupture of the membranes, amniotic fluid infection, postpartum endometritis, and postcesarean wound infections are increased because of infection with BV during pregnancy.[52] BV-associated endotoxins induce cytokine production in the vaginal fluid,[53] may activate the prostaglandin system, leading to preterm labor.[5]

Treatment of asymptomatic abnormal vaginal flora and BV with oral clindamycin early in the second trimester significantly reduces the rate of late miscarriage and spontaneous preterm births.[54] A review of antibiotic prophylaxis in pregnancy found a risk reduction in preterm delivery in pregnant women with a previous preterm birth associated with BV during the current pregnancy, but no risk reduction in pregnant women with previous preterm birth without BV during the pregnancy.[55] This review found that vaginal antibiotic prophylaxis during pregnancy did not prevent infectious pregnancy outcomes and may increase the risk of adverse effects such as neonatal sepsis.

Lactobacillus

L. acidophilus, the dominant bacteria in a healthy vaginal ecosystem, helps maintain the normal pH of the vagina through the production of lactic acid. The presence and dominance of *Lactobacillus* in the vagina are associated with a reduced risk of BV. The mechanisms appear to involve antiadhesion factors, by-products such as hydrogen peroxide, bacteriocins lethal to pathogens, and perhaps immune modulation or signaling effects.[56] Studies evaluating the efficacy of *L. acidophilus* for the treatment of BV in both pregnant and nonpregnant women have been conducted.

Women may be able to normalize vaginal flora partially by consuming products that contain live *L. acidophilus*. A crossover study of 46 women found that daily ingestion of 150 mL of yogurt, enriched with live *L. acidophilus*, was associated with an increased prevalence of colonization of the rectum and vagina by the bacteria when compared with ingesting pasteurized yogurt that had not been enriched. The authors noted reduced episodes of BV in the small study.[57] Only 7 of the original 46 participants completed the study, however, raising the question of whether this long-term treatment is feasible for the general population.

Two small studies used intravaginal yogurt for the treatment of BV in pregnancy. One open randomized study compared the intravaginal application of yogurt to acetic acid tampons or no treatment in pregnant women with documented BV. The yogurt group used 10 to 15 mL of commercially available yogurt containing more than 100 million/mL of

L. acidophilus twice daily for 7 days, with the regimen repeated 1 week later. Clinical improvement was significantly better in the yogurt group compared with the acetic acid group and control subjects receiving no therapy.[58]

An uncontrolled trial of 22 pregnant patients with documented BV found that 10 mL of commercially available yogurt containing more than 100 million/mL of *L. acidophilus* applied intravaginally twice daily for 7 days and then repeated in 1 week was an effective treatment. At 4 and 6 weeks after the second treatment, 90.9% and 86.4% of patients, respectively, had negative findings for criteria of BV.[59]

More rigorous research is needed to assess this low-cost treatment for BV because it can have significant health implications for both the pregnant and nonpregnant woman. The development of vaginal tablets with optimal strains of *Lactobacillus* is crucial for making this treatment, if found effective, practical to use. As mentioned previously, adherence to epithelial cells varies greatly among the *Lactobacillus* species and among different strains belonging to the same species.[51] Four strains of lactobacilli—*L. acidophilus* (61701 and 61880), *L. crispatus* (55730), and *L. delbrueckii* subsp. delbrueckii (65407) demonstrated the greatest inhibitory activity against the BV-associated bacterial species in one series.[60]

THREATENED MISCARRIAGE

An evaluation for threatened miscarriage, ectopic pregnancy, vaginal or cervical lesions, endometrial infection, or molar pregnancy should be performed if a woman has uterine irritability or vaginal bleeding during the first trimester. Two herbs are commonly recommended in herb books as being useful for the prevention of threatened miscarriage.

Black Haw and Cramp Bark (*Viburnum prunifolium* or *V. opulus*)

Indigenous North American women used black haw and cramp bark for the prevention of miscarriage. Numerous early American physicians wrote of its use in "preventing abortion and miscarriage: whether threatened from accidental cause or criminal drugging."[61] *Gunn's New Family Physician* (1869) extolled the tonic effects of black haw on the uterus and its effectiveness in preventing miscarriage. *King's American Dispensatory* states that black haw "acts promptly in spasmodic dysmenorrhea, especially with excessive flow...cramps of limbs attending pregnancy yield to both black haw and cramp bark. It is considered almost specific for cramps in the legs, not dependent on pregnancy, especially when occurring at night. *The condition for which black haw is most valued is threatened abortion.*"[62] It is likely because of this high praise that black haw was officially entered into the United States Pharmacopoeia in 1882 and remained in the National Formulary until 1960.

Herbalists practicing in the United States and United Kingdom commonly recommend black haw and cramp bark for painful menstrual cramps, threatened miscarriage, leg cramps, tension headaches, afterbirth pains, and muscle spasm. However, despite the praise from those physicians of old and contemporary practitioners of botanical medicine, the antispasmodic effects of the Viburnums have not been evaluated in clinical trials. The most recent data are almost 40 years old. An in vitro study with an active glycoside from *V. prunifolium* noted relaxation in both animal and human uteri.[63] Scopoletin, a substance found in the bark of black haw, exerted antispasmodic effects on the uterine muscle. In addition to test tube studies, animal research demonstrated complete relaxation of uterine tissue in rats with administration of extracts from black haw, cramp bark (*V. opulus*), *V. carlcephalum*, and *V. chenaulti*. *V. chenaulti* actually had twice the uterine relaxant activity of the others. Four other constituents in black haw and cramp bark were found to exert uterine relaxant properties.[64]

No adverse events in pregnancy could be found in the literature, and no known constituents that would sound an alarm; however, given the widespread use of this botanical by herbalists for menstrual cramping and threatened miscarriage, some basic science would be welcomed.

PREECLAMPSIA

Preeclampsia is a hypertensive condition that can develop during pregnancy, principally after 20 weeks' gestation, and is generally associated with proteinuria, albuminuria, edema, and excessive weight gain. Preeclampsia is seen mainly in women pregnant for the first time and those with a prior history of hypertension or vascular disease (Box 7-1). In the United States, an estimated 26 (3%) of 1000 births are complicated by preeclampsia and 0.56 of 1000 births by eclampsia.[65]

The true pathogenesis of preeclampsia is likely multifactorial and may involve genetic, immunologic, and dietary factors. Preeclampsia is thought to start with a placental trigger followed by a systemic response in the mother that produces the clinical signs and symptoms of the disorder (Box 7-2).[66]

Treatments

Aspirin. A recent systematic review of all randomized trials showed an acceptable safety profile and a significant but moderate reduction in the risk of preeclampsia

Box 7-1

Risk factors for preeclampsia

- Familial disposition
- Young maternal age
- Nulliparity
- African-American women (African-American > Hispanic > White)
- Previous history of preeclampsia
- Diabetes
- Hypertension
- Renal disease
- Obesity
- Hydatidiform mole
- Dietary deficiencies (protein, certain vitamins)
- Diethylstilbestrol (DES)—in utero exposure may predispose to the development of preeclampsia in adulthood
- Sickle cell trait

Box 7-2

Signs and symptoms of preeclampsia

- Blood pressure ≥140/90 mm Hg on two occasions at least 6 hours apart or an increase in systolic pressure >30 mm Hg or diastolic 15 mm Hg
- Edema
- Proteinuria >300 mg/24 hours
- Albuminemia
- Blood pressure increases of 30 mm Hg systolic or 15 mm Hg diastolic from prepregnancy blood pressure
- Rapid excessive weight gain (>5 pounds in 1 week)
- Hyperreflexia
- Visual disturbances
- Headache

---

regardless of gestation at trial entry or dose of acetylsalicylic acid. Thirty-nine trials (30,563 women) were included, and 45 trials (more than 3000 women) excluded. Use of antiplatelet drugs was associated with a 15% reduction in the risk of preeclampsia (32 trials, 29,331 women; relative risk, 0.85; 95% confidence interval, 0.78-0.92). An 8% reduction in the risk of preterm birth and a 14% reduction in the risk of fetal or neonatal death for women receiving antiplatelet drugs were also noted. Small for gestational age babies were reported in 25 trials (20,349 women), with no overall difference between the groups. No significant differences were observed in other measures of outcome.[67]

A growing body of evidence now indicates that the earlier aspirin treatment is started, the greater the reduction in risk of preeclampsia. Stronger effects are noted with higher doses (80 to 150 mg/day) than lower doses in the protection against preeclampsia and the prevention of severe fetal growth retardation.[68] In a double-blind, controlled trial, 341 pregnant women at high risk for hypertension because of obesity, family or personal history of gestational hypertension or preeclampsia, or a history of miscarriage were randomly assigned to treatment with 100 mg of aspirin or placebo at one of three times (on awakening, 8 hours later, or at bedtime) starting at 12 to 16 weeks of gestation. Compared with placebo, morning administration of aspirin had no effect on blood pressure. However, blood pressure reduction was highly statistically significant when aspirin was given 8 hours later and to a greater extent at bedtime. Compared with placebo, aspirin given at bedtime reduced the incidence of preeclampsia (1.7% vs. 14.3%), gestational hypertension (6.8% vs. 30.4%), intrauterine growth retardation (3.4% vs. 16.1%), and preterm delivery (0% vs. 17.9%; $P < 0.001$ for all).[69]

Calcium. A review of 11 studies showed a modest reduction of hypertension with calcium supplementation. A modest reduction in the risk of preeclampsia was also noted with calcium supplementation (2 g/day). The effects were greatest for women at high risk of hypertension and those with low baseline calcium intake. The reviewers concluded that calcium supplementation appears to be beneficial for women at high risk of gestational hypertension and in communities with low dietary calcium intake.[70] A mechanism of action for calcium in preeclampsia has not yet been fully elucidated.

Antioxidants. Lipid peroxidation has been put forth as contributing to the pathogenesis of preeclampsia. Various research has suggested that antioxidant nutrients are excessively used by the body in an attempt to counteract the cellular changes mediated by free radicals in preeclampsia.[71] Some studies have shown that antioxidant levels (carotenoids,[72] vitamin C, or vitamin E[73,74]) are decreased in women with pregnancy-induced hypertension and preeclampsia, whereas others have failed to find significant differences in levels between those with preeclampsia and control groups.[75,76]

Research is needed to clarify the therapeutic and prophylactic role, if any, of antioxidant nutrients in preeclampsia. Are certain antioxidants more effective than others? If there is a beneficial effect, optimal dosage recommendations are needed. Doses of 1 g/day of vitamin C and 400 International Units/day of vitamin E have been used in some of the trials addressing this issue. Most prenatal vitamins do not provide these levels of vitamins. Women who are at high risk may wish to consider supplementing with a higher-potency prenatal multivitamin.

Essential fatty acids. One hypothesis postulates that prostaglandins play a role in the progression of preeclampsia. Two clinical trials have been conducted on essential fatty acids to determine the efficacy of supplementation for the prevention and treatment of preeclampsia.

A partial double-blind, placebo-controlled study assessed the efficacy of evening primrose oil, fish oil, and magnesium for the prevention of preeclampsia. One hundred fifty pregnant women were randomly assigned to one of three treatment groups: placebo, mixture of evening primrose and fish oil (containing 37 mg gamma-linolenic acid, 18 mg eicosapentaenoic acid, and 10 mg docahexaenoic acid), or 1000 mg/day of magnesium for 4 months. Blood pressure, proteinuria, edema, eclampsia symptoms, and birth weights were assessed. Hypertension was highest in the placebo group; the magnesium-supplemented group had the lowest rate of hypertension. Preeclamptic symptoms were greater in the placebo group than either of the active treatment groups.[77] Another small study of 47 pregnant women (average 34 to 35 weeks' gestation) with preeclampsia failed to find a reduction in symptoms when given either 4000 mg/day of evening primrose oil or placebo.[78]

The numbers in both studies are too small to draw any conclusions about the efficacy of evening primrose oil for either the prevention or treatment of preeclampsia. What is the optimal form of essential fatty acid supplementation? Optimal dose? When should it be initiated? It may be a case of "too little, too late" when preeclampsia is diagnosed late in pregnancy.

Herbal diuretics. Herbalists often recommend the use of herbal diuretics for pregnancy-induced hypertension and preeclampsia. Dandelion (*Taraxacum officinale*), leaf or root, is the most common herb recommended for this purpose. It may be found in combination with nervines and uterine tonics. The rationale for herbalists' choice of diuretic therapy for a woman with hypertension and edema is understandable. However, preeclampsia is generally characterized by intravascular depletion and vasoconstriction, making the use of diuretics a poor choice for treatment. Medications that effectively reduce hypertension during pregnancy include hydralazine, labetalol, and methyldopa. Nifedipine is often used to manage severe hypertension in pregnancy.

Herbal antihypertensives. Hawthorne flowers, leaves, and berries often find their way into herbal antihypertensive formulas, including those designed for pregnancy-induced hypertension. Some postulate that the mild hypotensive activity of hawthorne is due to the inhibition of angiotensin-converting enzyme.[79] Laboratory studies also indicate that flavonoids induce endothelium-dependent, nitric oxide–mediated relaxation.[80] Reductions in systolic and diastolic blood pressure in human beings are small, however, both in clinical trials and clinical patients.[81] Hawthorne is a rich source of naturally occurring antioxidants, which may have some role in reducing oxidative stress, although the role of lipid peroxidation is still debated in the pathogenesis of preeclampsia. Hawthorne is not contraindicated during pregnancy, but no evidence has demonstrated efficacy for the prevention or treatment of eclampsia.

Sodium restriction. Although low-salt diets are sometimes recommended as a treatment for preeclampsia in lay books, they have not proved effective for preeclampsia with or without proteinuria.[82]

PARTUS PREPARATORS AND LABOR AIDS

Over the centuries pregnant women have used and midwives have recommended herbs to facilitate labor. Blue cohosh root (*Caulophyllum thalictroides*), black cohosh root (*Cimicifuga racemosa*), cotton root bark (*Gossypium* spp), partridge berry (*Mitchella repens*), raspberry leaf (*Rubus* spp), and others were used to ensure a timely and efficient birth. Depending on the practitioner, herbs were used up to a month before the expected due date. When herbs are used in this way they are referred to as *partus preparators*.

Blue Cohosh

Blue cohosh was official in the United States Pharmacopoeia from 1882 to 1905 for labor induction and then in the National Formulary from 1916 to 1950. Weak dilutions of blue cohosh fluid extract were shown to increase tone in excised guinea pig uteri in one older study. The tonic contraction lasted up to 1 hour in some specimens. However, in vivo studies in cats and dogs failed to demonstrate uterine activity.[83] In vitro research in the 1950s demonstrated that caulosaponin, a glycoside present in the root of blue cohosh, has a stimulating effect on smooth muscle of the uterus and small intestine in vitro and a vasoconstricting action on coronary blood vessels in vivo.[84]

The American Herbal Products Association states that blue cohosh root should not be used during pregnancy. Several case reports have noted adverse birth outcomes in infants born to women who were ingesting blue cohosh. In 1998 the *Journal of Pediatrics* described an infant born with severe congestive heart failure associated with acute anterolateral myocardial infarction who required mechanical ventilation for 20 minutes after delivery. The baby had a mitral regurgitation murmur, cardiomegaly, pulmonary edema, enlarged liver, and abnormal liver function. The infant required ventilator support for 3 weeks and was hospitalized for 1 month. The child was still receiving digoxin therapy at 2 years of age but was developing normally at last report. The researchers ruled out other possible causes of myocardial infarction. They concluded it was caused by the maternal ingestion of three times the amount of blue cohosh recommended by her midwife 4 weeks before delivery.[85]

A case report from New Zealand described myocardial toxicity in a baby born to a woman taking a partus preparator mixture that included blue and black cohosh before delivery. The authors did not describe the dosage, preparation, or treatment length.[86]

Two other poorly described case reports can be found in the FDA Special Nutritionals Adverse Event Monitoring System database. One describes an infant who had a stroke after consuming an undisclosed amount of blue cohosh tincture and an infant born with aplastic anemia after maternal ingestion of an undescribed blue cohosh product.[87]

Blue cohosh unquestionably contains some potentially harmful constituents. The plant is featured in standard textbooks on North American poisonous plants.[88] The rhizome is known to contain the piperidine alkaloids N-methylcytisine, baptifoline, and anagyrine. N-methylcytisine has peripheral effects similar to nicotine.[89] Toxic effects include coronary vasoconstriction, tachycardia, hypotension, and respiratory depression.[90] Rao et al reported a case of nicotinic toxicity in a woman who attempted to induce an abortion by ingesting large quantities of a tincture of blue cohosh along with slippery elm tea.[91] Concentrations of N-methylcytisine ranging from 5 to 850 ppm have been found in dietary supplements containing blue cohosh.[92] In vitro studies have demonstrated that extracts of the whole rhizome or pure N-methylcytisine (at 20 ppm) induce major malformations in cultured rat embryos at concentrations of 20 ppm[93]; however, neither the National Institute of Environmental Health Sciences nor the Environmental Protection Agency recognizes this test as an appropriate screen for human reproductive risk.

Another constituent of the plant, the quinolizidine alkaloid anagyrine, has been associated with toxicity and teratogenicity in livestock.[94] The congenital deformity that occurs after maternal ingestion of anagyrine in lupine is called *crooked calf disease*. Although anagyrine is a known teratogen in livestock, its status as teratogenic in human beings is unkown. Some researchers have postulated that the teratogenic effects only occur after metabolism by microflora in the ruminant gut. One case report describes an infant born with skeletal dysplasia and vascular anomalies after maternal consumption of anagyrine-containing goat milk.[95] Anagyrine is present in blue cohosh rhizome at a concentration of 2 to 390 ppm. Researchers at the FDA have recommended that pregnant women avoid ingesting any amount of anagyrine until more is known about its potential teratogenicity in human beings.[92] The American Herbal Products Association's *Botanical Safety Handbook* categorizes blue cohosh as a "class 2b" herb (not to be used during pregnancy because of its potential abortifacient activity) but goes on to state that *Caulophyllum* may used in small doses as a parturifacient near term to induce childbirth under the supervision of a qualified practitioner.[28]

What does this all mean? Studies of isolated constituents in vitro and in vivo provide intriguing insights into understanding the pharmacologic properties of a botanical; however, many factors must be accounted for when considering the potential benefit or toxicity when whole herbs are taken orally. Was the herb accurately identified? What method of extraction/administration was used? How well are the constituents absorbed across the gastrointestinal barrier? How are the constituents metabolized and excreted? What is the serum concentration of key constituents when the herb is taken in the usual and customary manner, and how well do they cross the placental barrier?

Teratogenicity can be hard to identify because hundreds of babies must be carefully examined and monitored to identify even a small increased incidence of birth anomalies. Fetal alcohol syndrome is a classic example. It has been present for hundreds, if not thousands, of years, yet the association of alcohol consumption during pregnancy with this syndrome was not recognized until 1972.

Was blue cohosh responsible for the myocardial infarction and congestive heart failure that occurred in the infant whose mother purportedly consumed blue cohosh during her final month of pregnancy? One simply cannot say. Whole-organism studies would help clarify the question of teratogenicity. Although abnormal birth outcomes in animals will not predict the risk in human beings, the absence of birth anomalies is a reassuring finding.

Despite the shortcomings of published case reports, the chemistry and pharmacology of the plant are reasonably well known. The human case reports, flawed as they are, paint a picture that is consistent with the evidence provided by the in vitro and animal studies. At this time, it does not seem wise for practitioners to recommend, or for women to consume, blue cohosh during pregnancy.

Cotton Root Bark (*Gossypium herbaceum*)

Cotton root bark has been used in Ayurvedic and indigenous North American medicine as an emmenagogue and abortifacient because of its uterine stimulant properties. The plant's activity was common knowledge among physicians in the southern states by the 1840s. One early medical journal discussed the use of the plant as an abortifacient, adding that it was highly "valued by the female slaves."[96] This medical reference is a chilling reminder of the abuse suffered by women of color in early America. Many attempted to terminate their pregnancies, which were brought about by rape. Lloyd Pharmaceutical Company and later Eli Lilly marketed cotton root bark as an oxytocic and emmenagogue. It was official as a parturifacient in the United States Pharmacopoeia from 1860 to 1880. Cotton root bark is still used to stimulate uterine contractions during labor in some pockets of the Southwest. Because of its antiprogesterone effect and subsequent reduction of corpus luteum activity, it can cause abortion. No clinical studies have evaluated the oxytocic activity of cotton root bark.

Research has focused primarily on one isolated compound found in the plant. Gossypol is a polyphenolic bisesquiterpene present in the subepidermal glands found throughout the plant and in the seed. Animal studies have shown that fetal implantation can be impaired by gossypol.[97] Gossypol has been shown to exert antifertility activity in both men and women. In China it was tested experimentally as a contraceptive with 12,000 men.[98] Antifertility activity exceeding 99% efficacy has been noted. Research continues to seek improved systems of delivery and methods to reduce adverse effects. The primary serious side effect is hypokalemia. In addition to contraception in women, some evidence exists that gossypol is useful in the treatment of endometriosis and uterine fibroids.[99] This is probably caused by the induction of amenorrhea and endometrial changes that result in infertility. One report in the literature states that endometrial atrophy occurred in all cases (67 women), with complete recovery of the endometrium occurring within 6 months of cessation of gossypol treatment.[98]

Raspberry Leaf (*Rubus idaeus, R. occidentalis*)

Raspberry leaf has been used as a "family" medicine for centuries. The fruits of the black and red raspberry shrubs are enjoyed as food, and the leaves are used as an astringent for a variety of conditions, principally diarrhea. Raspberry leaf tea has also been used as a uterine tonic for at least two centuries in the United States and it remains a popular "pregnancy tea." Many herb books promote the use of raspberry leaf to prevent miscarriage, ease morning sickness, and ensure a timely birth. A survey of 172 certified nurse-midwives found that of the 90 midwives who used herbal preparations, 63% recommended red raspberry leaf.[100]

A study recently published in an Australian medical journal suggests that raspberry leaf is safe when used during pregnancy. A retrospective observational design was used. Labor and birth outcomes of 57 Australian women who had used raspberry leaf products during pregnancy were compared with 51 control subjects randomly selected from hospital records of women who had not consumed raspberry leaf. The groups did not significantly differ in age, weight, parity, ethnicity, and type of prenatal care. The majority (59%) of women began to take raspberry from 30 to 34 weeks onward, followed by 28% starting at 35 to 39 weeks. Thirteen percent began using raspberry products between 8 and 28 weeks. Seventy-five percent of those drinking the tea consumed between 1 and 3 cups per day. Of those taking raspberry leaf in tablet form, six tablets per day was the most common dose. Six women discontinued raspberry leaf products because of taste (2 women), diarrhea (1 woman), Braxton Hicks contractions (1 woman), labor (1 woman), and a decision to switch to castor oil (1 woman).

Maternal safety outcomes assessed included maternal diastolic blood pressure before labor and, if the birth was vaginal, blood loss. Infant safety outcomes included duration of gestation, 5-minute Apgar score, and likelihood of infant transfer to neonatal special care or intensive care. Labor outcomes included length of stages of labor, likelihood of medical augmentation, need for epidural, occurrence of meconium staining, and percentage of normal deliveries. No differences were found between groups in any outcomes.[101]

This preliminary review led to the implementation of a randomized, double-blind, placebo-controlled study of 192 low-risk, nulliparous women to determine the effect and safety on labor and birth outcomes of raspberry leaf tablets (two tablets of 1.2 g per day) consumed from 32 weeks' gestation until labor. Raspberry leaf, consumed in tablet form, caused no adverse effects for mother or baby, but contrary to popular belief did not shorten the first stage of labor. Clinically significant findings were a shortening of the second stage of labor (mean difference, 9.59 minutes) and a lower rate of forceps deliveries between the treatment group and the control group (19.3% vs 30.4%). No significant relation was found between tablet consumption and birth outcomes.[102]

No contraindications are found in the literature, except for Brinker,[103] who states that women with a history of rapid labor should avoid raspberry leaf during pregnancy. However, given the recently reported findings of the randomized trial, this precaution seems somewhat unnecessary—at least at the dose of raspberry leaf used in the study.

COMMENT ON PARTUS PREPARATORS

That a healthy woman needs to take an herb 1 month before her due date to ensure a timely childbirth is a disconcerting idea. Women are very capable of bringing a baby into the world without taking herbs or drugs to "prepare" for the event. Practitioners would better serve their clients by helping them psychologically prepare for birth. This can be done through childbirth classes, journal writing, or other meaningful experiences. But if a woman wants to take an herb, raspberry leaf appears to be the safest.

References

1. Glover DG, Amonkar M, Rybeck BF, et al: Prescription, over-the-counter, and herbal medicine use in a rural, obstetric population, *Am J Obstet Gynecol* 188:1039-1045, 2003.
2. Young GL, Jewell D: Creams for preventing stretch marks in pregnancy, *Cochrane Database Syst Rev* 2:CD000066, 2002.
3. Furlan AD, Furlan AD, Brosseau L, et al: Massage for low back pain, *Cochrane Database Syst Rev* 2:CD001929, 2002.
4. Cashion C: Endocrine and metabolic disorders. In Lowdermilk DL, Perry SE, Bobak IM, eds. *Maternity and women's health care,* 7th ed, St. Louis, 2000, Mosby, pp 861-886.
5. von Dadelszen P: The etiology of nausea and vomiting of pregnancy. In Koren G, Bishai R, eds: *Nausea and vomiting of pregnancy: state of the art,* vol 1, Toronto, 2000, The Hospital for Sick Children, pp 5-14.
6. Fischer-Rasmussen W: Ginger treatment of hyperemesis gravidarum, *Eur J Obstet Gynecol Reprod Biol* 38:19-24, 1990.
7. Vutyavanich T, Kraisarin T, Ruangsri RA: Ginger for nausea and vomiting in pregnancy: randomized, double-masked, placebo-controlled trial, *Obstet Gynecol* 97:577-582, 2001.
8. Willetts KE, Ekangaki Abie, Eden JA: Effect of a ginger extract on pregnancy-induced nausea: a randomised controlled trial, *Aust N Z J Obstet Gynaecol* 43:139-144, 2003.
9. Backon J, Fischer-Rasmussen W: Ginger in preventing nausea and vomiting of pregnancy; a caveat due to its thromboxane synthetase activity and effect on testosterone binding, *Eur J Obstet Gynecol Reprod Biol* 42:163-164, 1991.
10. Nagabhushan M: Mutagenicity of gingerol and shogoal and antimutagenicity of zingerone in salmonella/microsome assay, *Cancer Lett* 36:221-223, 1987.
11. Fulder S, Tenne M: Ginger as an anti-nausea remedy in pregnancy; the issue of safety, *Herbalgram* 38:47-50, 1991.
12. Portnoi G, Chng LA, Karimi-Tabesh L, et al: Prospective comparative study of the safety and effectiveness of ginger for the treatment of nausea and vomiting in pregnancy, *Am J Obstet Gynecol* 189:1374-1377, 2003.
13. Muller JL, Clauson KA: Pharmaceutical considerations of common herbal medicine, *Am J Managed Care* 3:1753-1770, 1997.
14. Sahakian V, Rouse D, Sipes S, et al: Vitamin B6 is effective therapy for nausea and vomiting of pregnancy: a randomized, double-blind placebo-controlled study, *Obstet Gynecol* 78:33-36, 1991.
15. Vutyavanich T, Wongtrangan S, Ruangsri R: Pyridoxine for nausea and vomiting of pregnancy: a randomized, double blind, placebo-controlled trial. *Am J Obstet Gynecol* 173:881-884, 1995.
16. Briggs GG, Freeman RK, Yaffe SJ: *Drugs in pregnancy and lactation,* 5th ed, Baltimore, 1998, Williams & Wilkins, pp 920-928.
17. Cohen M, Bendich A: Safety of pyridoxine—a review of human and animal studies, *Toxicol Lett* 34:129-139, 1986.
18. Fugh-Berman A: Acupressure for nausea and vomiting of pregnancy, *Alt Ther Women's Health* 1:9-16, 1999.
19. Torrado S, Torrado S, Agis A, et al: Effect of dissolution profile and (-)-alpha-bisabolol on the gastrotoxicity of acetylsalicylic acid, *Pharmazie* 50:141-143, 1995.
20. Szelenyi I, Isaac O, Thiemer K: Pharmacological experiments with compounds of chamomile. III. Experimental studies of the ulcerprotective effect of chamomile, *Planta Med* 35:218-227, 1979.
21. Blumenthal M, Gruenwald J, Hall T, et al, eds: *The complete German Commission E monographs: therapeutic guide to herbal medicine,* Boston, 1998, Integrative Medicine Communications.
22. DeSmet PGAM, Keller K, Hansel R, et al, eds: *Adverse effects of herbal drugs 2,* Berlin, 1993, Springer-Verlag.
23. Habersang S, Leuschner F, Isaac O, et al: Pharmacological studies with compounds of chamomile IV. Studies on toxicity of (-)-α-bisabolol, *Planta Med* 37:115, 1979.
24. *The Lawrence Review of natural products: chamomile,* St. Louis, Facts and Comparisons, 1991.
25. Hale T: *Medications and mothers' milk,* 8th ed, Amarillo, TX, 1999, Pharmasoft Medical Publishing, pp 131-132.

26. Deleted in proof.
27. Pallesen S, Bjorvatn B, Nordhus IH, et al: Valerian as a sleeping aid? [in Norwegian], *Tidsskr Nor Laegeforen* 122:2857-2859, 2002.
28. McGuffin M, Hobbs C, Upton R, et al: *American Herbal Products Association's botanical safety handbook,* Boca Raton, Fla, 1997, CRC Press.
29. Tufik S, Fujita K, Seabra M de L, et al: Effects of a prolonged administration of valepotriates in rats on the mothers and their offspring, *J Ethnopharmacol* 41:39-44, 1994.
30. Deleted in proof.
31. Barrett B, Vohmann M, Calabrese C: Echinacea for upper respiratory infection, *J Fam Pract* 48:628-635, 1999.
32. Melchart D, Linde K, Fischer P, et al: Echinacea for preventing and treating the common cold. In The Cochrane Library, Oxford, 2001, Cochrane Database Rev 2000(2): CD000530.
33. Barrett BP, Brown RL, Locken K, et al: Treatment of the common cold with unrefined echinacea. A randomized, double-blind, placebo-controlled trial, *Ann Intern Med* 137:939-946, 2002.
34. Bauer R. New knowledge regarding the effect and effectiveness of Echinacea purpurea extracts [in German], *Wien Med Wochenschr* 152:407-411, 2002.
35. Deleted in proof.
36. *European Scientific Cooperative on Phytotherapy monographs on the medicinal uses of plant drugs,* Exeter, UK, 1999, ESCOP.
37. Mengs U, Clare CB, Poiley JA: Toxicity of Echinacea purpurea. Acute, subacute and genotoxicity studies, *Arzneim-Forsch/Drug Res* 41:1976-1981, 1991.
38. Gallo M, Sarkar M, Au W, et al: Pregnancy outcome following gestational exposure to Echinacea: a prospective controlled study, *Arch Intern Med* 160:3141-3143, 2000.
39. Howell AB, Vorsa N, Der Marderosian A, et al: Inhibition of the adherence of p-fimbriated *Escherichia coli* to uroepithelial-cell surfaces by proanthocyanidin extracts from cranberries, *N Engl J Med* 339:1085-1086, 1998.
40. Ofek I, Goldhar J, Zafriri D, et al: Anti-*Escherichia coli* adhesin activity of cranberry and blueberry juices, *N Engl J Med* 324:1599, 1991.
41. Jepson RG, Mihaljevic L, Craig J: Cranberries for preventing urinary tract infections, *Cochrane Database Syst Rev* 3:CD001321, 2001.
42. Stothers L: A randomized trial to evaluate effectiveness and cost effectiveness of naturopathic cranberry products as prophylaxis against urinary tract infection in women, *Can J Urol* 9: 1558-1562, 2002.
43. Krieger JN: Urinary tract infections: what's new? *J Urol* 168:2351-2358, 2002.
44. Larsson B, Jonasson A, Pianu S: Prophylactic effect of UVA E in women with recurrent cystitis: a preliminary report, *Curr Ther Res Clin Exp* 53:441-443, 1993.
45. Aune A, Alraek T, LiHua H, et al: Acupuncture in the prophylaxis of recurrent lower urinary tract infection in adult women, *Scand J Prim Health Care* 1:37-39, 1998.
46. Reid G: Probiotics for urogenital health, *Nutr Clin Care* 5:3-8, 2002.
47. Williams AB, Yu C, Tashima K, et al: Evaluation of two self-care treatments for prevention of vaginal candidiasis in women with HIV, *J Assoc Nurses AIDS Care* 12:51-57, 2001.
48. Hilton E, Isenberg HD, Alperstein P, et al: Ingestion of yogurt containing *Lactobacillus acidophilus* as prophylaxis for candidal vaginitis, *Ann Intern Med* 116:353-357, 1992.
49. Berman S: American Public Health Association 130th Annual Meeting, Philadelphia, November 9-13, 2002, Abstract 37244.
50. Mastromarino P, Brigidi P, Macchia S, et al: Characterization and selection of vaginal *Lactobacillus* strains for the preparation of vaginal tablets, *J Appl Microbiol* 93:884-893, 2002.
51. Myziuk L, Romanowski B, Johnson SC: BVBlue test for diagnosis of bacterial vaginosis, *J Clin Microbiol* 41:1925-1928, 2003.
52. McGregor JA, French JI: Bacterial vaginosis in pregnancy, *Obstet Gynecol Surv* 55(5 suppl 1): S1-S19, 2000.
53. Mattsby-Baltzer I, Platz-Christensen JJ, Hosseini N, et al: IL-1beta, IL-6, TNF-alpha, fetal fibronectin, and endotoxin in the lower genital tract of pregnant women with bacterial vaginosis, *Acta Obstet Gynecol Scand* 77:701-706, 1998.

54. Ugwumadu A, Manyonda I, Reid F, et al: Effect of early oral clindamycin on late miscarriage and preterm delivery in asymptomatic women with abnormal vaginal flora and bacterial vaginosis: a randomised controlled trial, *Lancet* 361:983-988, 2003.
55. Thinkhamrop J, Hofmeyr GJ, Adetoro O, et al: Prophylactic antibiotic administration in pregnancy to prevent infectious morbidity and mortality, *Cochrane Database Syst Rev* 4:CD002250, 2002.
56. Reid G, Burton J: Use of Lactobacillus to prevent infection by pathogenic bacteria, *Microbes Infect* 4:319-324, 2002.
57. Shalev E, Battino S, Weiner E, et al: Ingestion of yogurt containing *Lactobacillus acidophilus* compared with pasteurized yogurt as prophylaxis for recurrent candidal vaginitis and bacterial vaginosis, *Arch Fam Med* 5:593-596, 1996.
58. Neri A, Sabah G, Samra Z: Bacterial vaginosis in pregnancy treated with yoghurt, *Acta Obstet Gynecol Scand* 72:17-19, 1993.
59. Tasdemir M, Tasdemir I, Tasdemir S, et al: Alternative treatment for bacterial vaginosis in pregnant patients: restoration of vaginal acidity and flora, *Arch AIDS Res* 10:239-241, 1996.
60. McLean NW, Rosenstein IJ: Characterisation and selection of a *Lactobacillus* species to re-colonise the vagina of women with recurrent bacterial vaginosis, *J Med Microbiol* 49:543-552, 2000.
61. Rusby HH: *Viburnum (Viburnum prunifolium* L.). In Bull Pharm, July 1891.
62. Felter HW, Lloyd JU: *King's American dispensatory,* 18th ed, 3rd rev, vol II. Portland, Ore, 1983, Eclectic Medical Publications, pp 2059-2062.
63. Evans WE, Harne WG, Krantz JC: A uterine principle from *Viburnum prunifolium, J Pharmacol Exp Ther* 75:174-177, 1942.
64. Jarboe CH, Schmidt CM, Nicholson JA, et al: Scopoletin, an antispasmodic component of *Viburnum opulus* and *V. prunifolium, J Med Chem* 10:488-491, 1967.
65. Saftlas AF, Olson DR, Franks AL, et al: Epidemiology of preeclampsia and eclampsia in the United States, 1979-1986, *Am J Obstet Gynecol* 163:460-465, 1990.
66. Working Group on High Blood Pressure in Pregnancy: Report of the National High Blood Pressure Education Program Working Group on High Blood Pressure in Pregnancy, *Am J Obstet Gynecol* 183:S1-S22, 2000.
67. Duley L, Henderson-Smart D, Knight M, et al: Antiplatelet drugs for prevention of pre-eclampsia and its consequences: systematic review, *BMJ* 322:329-333, 2001.
68. Klockenbusch W, Rath W: Prevention of pre-eclampsia by low-dose acetylsalicylic acid—a critical appraisal [in German], *Z Geburtshilfe Neonatol* 206:125-130, 2002.
69. Hermida RC, Ayala DE, Iglesias M: Administration time-dependent influence of aspirin on blood pressure in pregnant women, *Hypertension* 41(3 pt 2):651-656, 2003.
70. Atallah AN, Hofmeyr GJ, Duley L: Calcium supplementation during pregnancy for preventing hypertensive disorders and related problems, *Cochrane Database Syst Rev* 1:CD001059, 2002.
71. Madazli R, Benian A, Gumustas K, et al: Lipid peroxidation and antioxidants in preeclampsia, *Eur J Obstet Gynecol Reprod Biol* 85:205-208, 1999.
72. Palan PR, Mikhail MS, Romney SL: Placental and serum levels of carotenoids in preeclampsia, *Obstet Gynecol* 98:459-462, 2001.
73. Kharb S: Vitamin E and C in preeclampsia, *Eur J Obstet Gynecol Reprod Biol* 93:37-39, 2000.
74. Akyol D, Mungan T, Gorkemli H, et al: Maternal levels of vitamin E in normal and preeclamptic pregnancy, *Arch Gynecol Obstet* 263:151-155, 2000.
75. Ben-Haroush A, Harell D, Hod M, et al: Plasma levels of vitamin E in pregnant women prior to the development of preeclampsia and other hypertensive complications, *Gynecol Obstet Invest* 54:26-30, 2002.
76. Regan CL, Levine RJ, Baird DD, et al: No evidence for lipid peroxidation in severe preeclampsia, *Am J Obstet Gynecol* 185:572-578, 2001.
77. D'Almeida A, Carter JP, Anatol A, et al: Effects of a combination of evening primrose oil (gamma linolenic acid) and fish oil (eicosapentaenoic + docahexaenoic acid) versus magnesium, and versus placebo in preventing pre-eclampsia, *Women Health* 19:117-131, 1992.
78. Moodley J, Norman RJ: Attempts at dietary alteration of prostaglandin pathways in the management of pre-eclampsia, *Prostaglandins Leukot Essent Fatty Acids* 37:145-147, 1989.

79. Stitcher O, Meier B: Hawthorn (*Crataegus*): biological activity and new strategies for quality control. In Lawson LK, Bauer R, eds: *Phytomedicines of Europe: chemistry and biological activity*, Washington, DC, 1998, American Chemical Society, pp 241-262.

80. Kim SH, Kang KW, Kim KW, et al: Procyanidins in crataegus extract evoke endothelium-dependent vasorelaxation in rat aorta, *Herz* 24:465-474, 1999.

81. Tauchert M, Ploch M, Hubner WD: Efficacy of hawthorn extract LI 132 in comparison with captopril: multicentre double-blind study on 132 patients with cardiac insufficiency of NYHA grade II, *Munch Med Wschr* 136:27-33, 1994.

82. Knuist M, Bonsel, Zondervan HA, et al: Low sodium diet and pregnancy-induced hypertension: a multi-centre randomised controlled trial, *Br J Obstet Gynaecol* 105:430-434, 1998.

83. Pilcher JD: The action of certain drugs on the excised uterus of the guinea pig, *J Pharm Exp Ther* 8:110-111, 1916.

84. Ferguson HC, Edwards LD: A pharmacological study of a crystalline glycoside of *Caulophyllum thalictroides*, *J Am Pharm Assoc* 43:16-21, 1954.

85. Jones TK, Lawson BM: Profound neonatal congestive heart failure caused by maternal consumption of blue cohosh herbal medication, *J Pediatr* 132:550-552, 1998.

86. Gunn TR, Wright IM: The use of black and blue cohosh in labor, *NZ Med J* 109:410-411, 1996.

87. FDA/CFSAN resources page, Food and Drug Administration, http://vm.cfsan.fda.gov/~dms/aems.html. Accessed September 2000.

88. Lampe KF, McCann MA: *AMA handbook of poisonous and injurious plants*, Chicago, 1985, American Medical Association.

89. Barlow RB, McLeod LJ: Some studies on cytosine and its methylated derivatives, *Br J Pharm* 5:161-174, 1969.

90. Scott CC, Chen KK: The pharmacological action of n-methylcytisine, *J Pharmacol Exp Ther* 79:334, 1943.

91. Rao RB, Hoffman RS, Desiderio R, et al: Nicotinic toxicity from tincture of blue cohosh (*Caulophyllum thalictroides*) used as an abortifacient, *J Toxicol Clin Toxicol* 36:455, 1998.

92. Betz JM, Andrzejewski D, Troy A, et al: Gas chromatographic determination of toxic quinolizidine alkaloids in blue cohosh *Caulophyllum thalictroides* (L.), *Phytochem Anal* 9:232-236, 1998.

93. Kennelly EJ, Flynn TJ, Mazzola EP, et al: Detecting potential teratogenic alkaloids from blue cohosh rhizomes using an in vitro rat embryo culture, *J Nat Prod* 62:1385-1389, 1999.

94. Panter KE, James LF, Gardner DR: Lupines, poison-hemlock and Nicotiana spp: toxicity and teratogenicity in livestock, *J Nat Toxins* 8:117-134, 1999.

95. Ortega JA, Lazerson J: Anagyrine-induced red cell aplasia, vascular anomaly, and skeletal dysplasia, *J Pediatr* 111:87-89, 1987.

96. Bouchelle EF: Medicinal properties of cotton plant, *Am J Med Sci* 1:275, 1841.

97. De Smet PAGM, Keller K, Hansel R, et al, eds: Gossypol. In *Adverse effects of herbal drugs*, vol 2. Berlin, 1993, Springer-Verlag, p 195-207.

98. Evans WC: *Trease and Evans' pharmacognosy*, 14th ed, London, 1996, WB Saunders, pp 326.

99. Wu DF: An overview of the clinical pharmacology and therapeutic potential of gossypol as a male contraceptive agent and in gynaecological disease, *Drugs* 38:333-341, 1989.

100. McFarlin BL, Gibson MH, O'Rear J, et al: A national survey of herbal preparation use by nurse-midwives for labor stimulation. Review of the literature and recommendations for practice, *J Nurse Midwifery* 44:205-216, 1999.

101. Parsons M, Simpson M, Ponton T: Raspberry leaf and its effect on labour: safety and efficacy, *J Aust Coll Midwives* 12:20-25, 1999.

102. Simpson M, Parsons M, Greenwood J, et al: Raspberry leaf in pregnancy: its safety and efficacy in labor, *J Midwifery Womens Health* 46:51-59, 2001.

103. Brinker F: *Herb contraindications and drug interactions*, Sandy, Ore, 1997, Eclectic Institute.

Lactation, Breastfeeding, and the Postpartum Period

B reastfeeding is the optimal form of nourishment for a newborn baby. A policy statement by the American Academy of Pediatrics recommends exclusive breastfeeding as the ideal nutrition for the first 6 months of life, followed by introduction of iron-enriched solid foods during the second half of the first year. The group also encourages breastfeeding for at least 12 months and longer if desired by both mother and baby.[1]

Although the benefits of breastfeeding may be self-evident, they are also increasingly demonstrated by science. Researchers have documented numerous benefits associated with breastfeeding, including the superior nutritional composition of breast milk,[2] positive immunologic effects,[3] and reduced incidence of feeding intolerance and necrotizing enterocolitis in preterm infants,[4] as well as significant psychological benefit for both mother and infant.

Healthy People 2010 reaffirms the U.S. Surgeon General's goals to increase the use of breastfeeding in the United States to 75% of infants at the time of hospital discharge and to increase the use of breastfeeding at the age of 6 months to 50%.[5]

DURING PREGNANCY

The decision to breastfeed is almost always made while a woman is pregnant; most women have made their choice by the time they are in the last trimester of pregnancy.[6] Many factors influence the mother's decision, including her attitude toward and knowledge of breastfeeding, demographic specifics, support from the baby's father, and the attitude of the woman's health care provider.[7] It is extremely important that a woman receive enough information during prenatal visits for her to make a truly informed decision about whether to breastfeed her baby.

A woman should undergo a careful and thorough breast examination to help determine her ability to provide milk to her newborn. During pregnancy, the weight of a woman's breast normally doubles. Women who fail to note an increase in breast size during pregnancy are more likely to have difficulty with lactation.[8] Women with inverted nipples may also experience difficulty with lactation because it is harder for the infant to latch onto the breast. Milk cups, also known as breast shells, may be used during the last months of pregnancy to apply steady pressure around the base of the nipple in hope of causing it to project forward. Although these devices are widely recommended, studies have shown that they do not increase the likelihood of a woman's ability to nurse for longer than 6 weeks after birth.[9]

Previous breast surgery can affect a woman's ability to nurse. If surgery involved cutting tissue surrounding the areola, the incision may have severed the milk ducts or nerve supply necessary for lactation. Breast reduction or enlargement may also negatively affect a woman's ability to breastfeed.[10] Tubular breasts, severe differences in breast size, and a history of breast irradiation have also been linked to poor lactation.[8] For all these reasons, a woman should have her breasts carefully examined during pregnancy.

BIRTH

The United Nations Children's Fund, along with the World Health Organization, inaugurated the Baby-Friendly Hospital Initiative worldwide in 1991. Baby-Friendly USA was created in 1997 to carry out this campaign in the United States. This program centers on 10 Steps to Healthy Breastfeeding that are to be followed by hospitals and clinics where maternity services are offered (Box 8-1).[11]

Although these initiatives represent important steps in the right direction, at the end of 1998 only 17 hospitals and birth centers in the United States had been designated "baby-friendly." A woman should be encouraged to visit the facility where she will give birth and inquire about the breastfeeding policies of the institution.

Box **8-1**

Steps to healthy breastfeeding

- Have a written breastfeeding policy that is routinely communicated to all health care staff.
- Train all health care staff in the skills necessary to implement this policy.
- Inform all pregnant women about the benefits and management of breastfeeding.
- Help mothers start breastfeeding within 1 hour of delivery.
- Show mothers how to breastfeed and how to maintain lactation even if they should be separated from their infants.
- Give newborn infants no food or drink other than breast milk unless medically indicated.
- Practice rooming-in, allowing mothers and infants to remain together 24 hours a day.
- Encourage breastfeeding on demand.
- Give no artificial teats or pacifiers to breastfeeding infants.
- Foster the establishment of breastfeeding support groups and refer mothers to them at the time of hospital discharge.

Adapted from Kyenka-Isabrrye M: UNICEF launches the Baby-Friendly Hospital Initiative, *Am J Matern Child Nursing* 17:177-179, 1992.

BREASTFEEDING
Positioning the Baby

A variety of techniques can be used to enhance the breastfeeding experience. Correct positioning reduces the risk of physical discomfort to the mother and enhances the transfer of milk to the baby.

The cradle position is used most often by nursing mothers (Figure 8-1). The mother sits in a comfortable chair and places a pillow on her lap to lift the baby to the height of her breast. The baby is supported by the mother's arm that is closest to the nursing breast. The baby's body is turned to face the breast, with the head, shoulders, and hips in proper alignment. While the baby is learning to suckle, the mother uses her other hand to support the breast, with the thumb on top and four fingers underneath, well behind the areola so as not to interfere with the baby's feeding.

When ready, the mother lightly touches her nipple to the baby's lips to stimulate suckling. The baby should take the entire nipple and at least half an inch of the surrounding areola and breast into the mouth. This is necessary to ensure adequate milk intake because the baby must compress the large storage reservoirs beneath the areola to effectively drain them. Also, nipple tenderness will be diminished if the baby takes an ample amount of breast tissue into the mouth while suckling.

Other positions include the cross-cradle, reclining, and football holds. The last two options work well for women who have had cesarean deliveries. The breastfeeding mother should feel comfortable with at least two positions to ensure a successful nursing experience once she has been discharged from the birth facility.

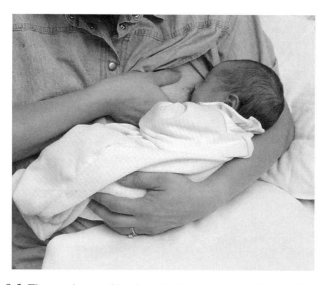

Figure **8-1 The mother in this photo is demonstrating the cradle position while breastfeeding.** (*From Murray SM, McKinney ES, Gorrie TM:* Foundation of maternal-newborn nursing, *ed 3, Philadelphia, 2001, WB Saunders.*)

Feeding Schedules

Knowing how often to nurse a newborn is not as easy as one might assume. A newborn commonly nurses 8 to 12 times a day for 10 to 15 minutes per breast, although this varies from baby to baby.[1] A woman may interpret frequent nursing as a sign that her milk supply is insufficient. During the first few weeks of a baby's life, the interval between nursing sessions may be just an hour. The health care provider should explain that this is normal as long as the baby has frequent wet diapers (six to eight per day by day 5) and is gaining weight. Frequent feeding is important to prevent weight loss, increase breast-milk production, and reduce the risk of jaundice. A newborn should not go longer than 5 hours between feedings. Older babies can wait for longer periods between feedings as they learn to suckle more efficiently.

During the first few days of life, the baby will be taking in colostrum from the breast. This yellowish fluid is filled with antibodies, vitamin A, minerals, and other beneficial substances. Colostrum is sufficient nutrition for the newborn, and supplementation is not necessary. The milk supply usually arrives 3 to 5 days after birth. The more the baby suckles, the more milk is produced. When the baby nurses, the pituitary gland is stimulated to release the hormone prolactin, which signals the milk glands to discharge milk. The pituitary gland also releases the hormone oxytocin, which stimulates the "letdown" reflex that forces milk through the breast. Many women feel a tingling sensation when this letdown occurs, and milk leakage is common if the baby is not at the breast.

Crying is a late sign of hunger, so parents should be alert to earlier hunger cues: The baby may suck on fingers, flex arms or legs, make mouthing movements, or turn the head from side to side. A baby normally nurses from both breasts during a feeding. The first breast is usually nursed more vigorously than the second, so the starting breast should be alternated from one feeding to the next. Nursing from just one breast increases the risk of engorgement in the breast that is not emptied. Use of a bottle should be avoided until breastfeeding is well established; suckling the breast is more difficult for the infant than sucking a bottle nipple, and a bottle preference may develop.

Adequate Milk Production

Inadequate milk production is the No. 1 reason nursing is discontinued and other foods and liquids are added to the infant's diet before 4 months of age.[12] In a small percentage of women, milk production is inadequate, and the baby experiences weight loss or poor weight gain as a result. Seeking out a lactation consultant who is generally well trained in nursing difficulties and who will spend time with the mother and baby is often beneficial.

Health care providers should be alert to slow weight gain and development and should thoroughly review the clinical picture. The mother's breasts should be examined, her medications, alcohol, and cigarette consumption reviewed, and, if necessary, her thyroid and pituitary hormones checked; a discussion of stress should be undertaken as well. An observation of nursing technique should be conducted. The baby should be checked for gastroesophageal reflux, neurologic disorders, a short frenulum, urinary tract infection, congenital heart disease, and allergies, depending on the clinical picture.

Despite adequate weight gain and development, many women believe that they are not producing enough milk to satisfy their babies. This may be more a result of infant growth spurt than of poor milk supply. Infant growth spurts occur in normal, healthy infants with appropriate weight gain. These spurts normally occur during the first 12 to16 weeks of life and are characterized by a fussy baby who feeds constantly but pulls away from the breast while nursing and is irritable before and after being fed. This irritability is more likely the result of the discomfort of rapid growth than of a feeling of hunger.[13] After the growth spurt, which usually lasts 3 to 7 days, the baby again becomes content with 8 to 12 feedings per 24 hours. During the growth spurt the mother should make sure that the baby is positioned correctly during breastfeeding and is fed on demand. Both baby and mother need plenty of extra rest.

Infant Weight Gain

Because a nursing mother cannot measure the amount of milk her newborn is ingesting, the most accurate assessment of breastfeeding volume is the baby's weight. Loss of as much as 10% from birth weight is considered acceptable. The breastfed baby should regain the birth weight by 10 to 14 days of age. Weight gain of 1 oz per day for the first 2 months of life is normal. An inadequate supply of breast milk should be suspected if a baby does not gain 5 to 7 oz per week during the first 2 months of life. A knowledgeable professional should examine the baby by 4 or 5 days of age. Early intervention can help ensure adequate transfer of breast milk to the baby, proper positioning, and early detection of any serious health problems that might exist. A wait-and-see approach often spells failure for the nursing mother. Incremental weight gain normally declines between the third and twelfth months of life.

Stool and Voiding Patterns

A newborn baby should pass a black-green (meconium) stool during the first day of life. The baby may pass several of these stools before the mother's milk arrives, usually by day 5. The stools then change from black-green to yellow and take on the consistency of yogurt with seedy curds. Babies should have four or more yellow stools per day during the first 2 months of life. Fewer stools should raise the suspicion of an inadequate milk supply.[14] Once a baby reaches the age of 2 to 3 months, stool frequency varies greatly. Some babies continue to pass stools several times a day, whereas others go several days or up to a week before passing a large, loose stool. Newborns should pass stools more frequently: A 2-week-old who only passes stools once every 3 or 4 days should be carefully examined. A newborn may only urinate one or two times in a 24-hour period during the first 2 or 3 days of life. Once the mother's milk arrives, the infant should have six to eight wet diapers per day, soiled with light-yellow or colorless urine. The presence of reddish urate crystals in the diaper is normal during the first of days of life, but this phenomenon signifies inadequate milk intake in an older infant.[14]

Jaundice in the Breastfed Newborn

Jaundice is a yellowing of the skin and whites of the eyes caused by the buildup of a metabolic product called bilirubin. Jaundice may be the result of breast milk itself or of inadequate milk intake. Breast milk jaundice usually begins around 7 days of age and can last for several weeks, even as a baby is thriving and gaining weight and appears healthy. It is believed that a substance in human breast milk increases the absorption of bilirubin across the intestinal wall. This excessive unconjugated bilirubin causes the yellow discoloration of the skin and eyes. As long as the baby is gaining weight and appears healthy, there is no reason to discontinue nursing or to supplement breast milk with other liquids.

Sometimes, however, the diagnosis of breast milk jaundice is made in a baby who is not getting enough milk. A recommendation of more frequent nursing will not help if the baby is not able to efficiently remove milk from the breast. One way to determine whether the baby is not getting enough milk is to weigh the baby before and after nursing on a scale that is accurate to within 2 g. The prenursing weight is subtracted from the postnursing weight to yield the amount, in milliliters, of breast milk the baby has taken in during the feeding (breast milk weighs approximately 1 g/mL). If the baby is not taking in enough milk, the mother should use a good electric pump to express her remaining milk. This supply can be fed to the baby until he or she learns to nurse more effectively.

BREASTFEEDING PROBLEMS AND SOLUTIONS
Nipple Pain and Superinfection

Nipple pain is a common problem in breastfeeding mothers. During the first few days of nursing, the nipple can become sore due to the baby's suckling. This soreness usually improves by the end of the first week. Nipples that remain sore or become cracked should be evaluated and treated. Abnormal sucking, improper nursing technique, or both must be corrected as early as possible. The baby is nursed first on the least sore breast and then placed on the other breast when he or she is sucking less vigorously. The mother should be encouraged to nurse more frequently but for shorter periods. If nursing is simply too painful, she can use a pump to express her milk until the nipples have healed.

It is common for health professionals to recommend the use of a nipple ointment to help soothe sore or cracked nipples. While these creams may help soothe and heal cracked nipples, little evidence exists to support the benefit of such ointments and creams to prevent *sore* nipples. The authors of one randomized study found no difference between nursing mothers who used a nipple ointment (n = 123) and those who did not (n = 96) with regard to the incidence of sore and cracked nipples and duration of breastfeeding.[15] Interestingly, it was noted that the incidence of sore nipples was increased when babies were given pacifiers and bottle-fed before hospital discharge.

The best prevention involves teaching new mothers proper breastfeeding techniques. Breast shells and application of lanolin in association with instruction in breastfeeding technique have been found more effective than moist wound dressings in treating cracked nipples.[16] Breast shells protect the nipple from contact with clothing, which can further irritate the skin.

Green tea **(Camellia sinensis).** Tea is an established natural remedy for sore or cracked nipples. It was found in one study that teabags applied four times daily were as effective as water compresses and superior to no treatment in women with sore nipples 36 hours after delivery.[17] One advantage of tea over a simple water compress involves the prevention of infection. The antimicrobial activity of water extracts of *C. sinensis* has been long known and was first documented in a Western medical journal more than 90 years ago.[18] The antimicrobial effects are direct (bacteriostatic and bactericidal) and indirect (by way of inhibition of certain bacterial enzymes).[19] Tea is bactericidal to *Staphyloccus aureus* at concentrations lower than those found in a typical cup of tea.[20] Topical preparations containing tea were shown to be as effective as oral antibiotics (cephalexin) for *S. aureus* infection of the skin in one randomized clinical trial.[21] This finding is consistent with previous work demonstrating antimicrobial effects of *C. sinensis*, including preliminary data suggesting that compounds within the herb have some effect against methicillin-resistant *S. aureus*.[22] It is likely that many compounds within tea are active, but the principal ones are thought to be catechins. Teabags are readily available in many households, so this is an inexpensive and easy-to-use treatment.

TEAS

Tea, a familiar drink, is a substance we may not consider an herb, let alone an herbal remedy. It has been used medicinally as a "tonic" (stimulant and digestive remedy) in many parts of Asia for 5,000 years.

Tea remains popular throughout the world and is still the most frequently consumed beverage after water. The word *tea*, although commonly used to describe the infusion that results when the dried leaves and leaf buds of the shrub *Camellia sinensis* are steeped in boiling water for 5 to 15 minutes, is also used as a generic term to describe any infusion made from other plants (e.g., herbal teas, red tea). Green tea is one of the three main types of tea prepared from *C. sinensis*.

Around the world, approximately 2.5 million tons of tea are manufactured annually. Black tea, which accounts for nearly 80% of production, is prepared by drying and then fermenting the leaves. This is the type of tea most widely drunk in Europe, India, and North America. Oolong, a specialty tea that is only partly fermented, accounts for just 2% of production and is drunk mostly in southeastern China and Japan.

Green tea accounts for nearly 20% of production and is consumed mainly in China and Japan. The leaves are steamed or pan-fried, then dried without fermentation. By dry weight, approximately 36% of green-tea leaves is polyphenols—principally flavonols (mostly catechins), flavonoids, and flavondiols. About 4% is plant alkaloids, including caffeine, theobromine, and theophylline. Other constituents include proteins, carbohydrates, phenolic acids, minerals (including fluoride and aluminum), and fiber. The precise composition of green tea (and all teas) varies with the geographic origin of the leaf, the time of harvest, and the manufacturing process. The constituents of black tea differ from those of green tea as a result of the oxidation process that occurs during fermentation; however, both are considered healthy additions to the diet.

When green tea is taken for medicinal purposes, 1 or 2 tsp of the dried herb are steeped in a cup of boiling water for about 15 minutes. While many prefer to drink their green tea "straight," recent research shows that the addition of milk does not alter its medicinal properties.

Continued

TEAS—CONT'D

The medicinal use of green tea has not been reported to carry adverse side effects. A cup of black or green tea contains 10 to 80 mg of caffeine, depending on the type of tea and the method of preparation. Excessive caffeine consumption may cause nervousness, insomnia, and irregularities in heart rate. Herbal handbooks advise pregnant women, nursing mothers, and patients with cardiac problems to limit their intake of tea.[22a] This is likely due to the presence of caffeine.

The consumption of teas (infusions) made from the African red bush (*Aspalathus linearis*) has long been a popular pastime in South Africa. The Afrikaans name for red bush, *rooibos*, is becoming increasingly familiar to consumers in the United States. Many tea drinkers have embraced red tea because it is caffeine-free and lower in tannins than black or green tea but carries similar health benefits.

Data on *rooibos* are accumulating. It has been demonstrated that *rooibos* is rich in many of the ingredients of interest in the area of cancer prevention among the natural constituents of plants that protect the body against oxidants.[22b] Many scientists believe it is important that antioxidants come from rich mixtures of biologically active compounds in plants rather than from isolated synthetic antioxidants: Studies of the isolated synthetic antioxidant β-carotene did not show this substance to be protective against cancer. The results of studies of mixtures of herbal constituents, as found in teas, appear promising, however.

Red tea contains significant levels of antioxidants, which may explain its apparent health-promoting properties. Polyphenol antioxidants such as flavonoids are present in similar amounts in red and green tea. The antioxidant effect of green tea is thought to be conferred in part by these phenolic components.

Studies comparing *rooibos* with other teas have revealed that *rooibos* contains levels of known antioxidants similar to those of green tea. However, *rooibos* appears to contain active antioxidant components that are not present in green and other teas, such as additional polyphenols, including certain flavonols and flavones. These antioxidants may account for the association of teas with anticancer and other beneficial effects. These effects are seen over long periods of tea consumption. Botanically, as a legume, *rooibos* contains other plant chemicals that may help account for its observed short-term effects in calming the nervous and gastrointestinal systems.

The method of preparation of *rooibos* can influence its activity; the water-soluble component of *rooibos* also appears to be therapeutically active. Because *rooibos* contains no caffeine, unlike green and other teas, larger amounts of *rooibos* can be consumed without side effects. Red tea is more appropriate for children and others who must limit their caffeine intake. Studies of red tea indicate that consumption of this beverage is an effective way of obtaining the benefits of many of the plant chemicals that appear to help protect against cancer.

Calendula (Calendula officinalis). Herbalists often recommend calendula ointment to encourage healing and retain moisture in chafed nipples. Animal studies have shown that ointment containing 5% calendula extract speeds the healing of wounds.[23] The ointment has mild antibacterial properties that may help prevent infection of the nipple. Many calendula-based creams and ointments are available commercially, including those sold as 10% homeopathic dilutions. Although no case reports of adverse effects from the topical use of calendula have been published, the use of some nipple creams, especially papaya cream, has been associated with an increased risk of mastitis.[24]

Nipple Infection

If nipple pain is severe or does not respond to the aforementioned remedies, bacterial or yeast infection should be suspected. One study demonstrated that women with babies younger than 1 month of age who complained of moderate to severe nipple pain and presented with deep cracks or discharge had a 64% chance of having an infection, most caused by *S. aureus*.[25] A randomized trial of women with *S. aureus*–infected nipples found that after 5 to 7 days of treatment, only 8% of the women showed improvement with "optimal breastfeeding treatment alone," 16% experienced improvement with the use of topical mupirocin, 29% improved with topical fusidic acid, and 79% showed improvement with oral antibiotics ($P < 0.0001$). Mastitis developed in 12% to 35% of mothers who were not treated with systemic antibiotics, compared with 5% of mothers treated with systemic antibiotics ($P < 0.005$).[26]

Bottom line: preventing infection is key! Topical antimicrobials may be used but if infection does not rapidly clear, the use of oral antibiotics may be necessary.

Candida albicans *and thrush.* A woman with infection of the nipple caused by the yeast *C. albicans* characteristically presents with breast pain before and after nursing that is described as deep, burning, shooting, or stabbing. A statistically significant correlation ($P < 0.05$) was found between nipple candidiasis and three factors: vaginal candidiasis ($P = 0.001$), previous antibiotic use ($P = 0.036$), and nipple trauma ($P = 0.001$).[27] Medical therapies have not been thoroughly evaluated, but standard antifungal therapies such as nystatin are commonly used to treat thrush.

Tea tree oil (Melaleuca alternifolia). Tea tree essential oil is the most popular herbal preparation used for the treatment of yeast and fungal infections. In one study 25 subjects with acquired immunodeficiency syndrome and fungal infections of the mouth and throat who had failed to respond to therapy with fluconazole (400 mg/day for at least 14 days) were randomly assigned to receive an alcohol-free mouthwash containing tea tree oil (Breath-Away [Melaleuca]; Idaho Falls, Idaho). Participants were instructed to swish a small amount of the preparation around the mouth for 30 to 60 seconds, then expel it. They were told not to rinse their mouths for at least 30 minutes afterward and repeat four times a day. Fifteen of 25 subjects (60%) demonstrated a response to the mouthwash after 4 weeks: 28% were cured, and 32% had fewer signs and symptoms of infection. However, the authors noted that the response at the end of 2 weeks was not impressive and that for best results, tea tree oil must be used for at least 4 weeks.[28]

Among infants with candidiasis or thrush, a healthy baby with an intact immune system would likely respond more quickly to tea tree oil therapy than a sicker infant. Also, a baby would be unable to spit the rinse out, and safe doses for very young babies are not known. Several case reports describe ataxia and drowsiness in young children who have consumed 10 mL or less of the essential oil of tea tree. Although this amount is obviously greater than that which would be found in a diluted mouthwash, the oral application of tea tree oil in infants with thrush is probably best avoided until more information about efficacy, safety, dosage, and most appropriate form of administration becomes available. If a mother chooses to apply tea tree oil to the nipple area after nursing, she should wash the breast before nursing again.

Grapefruit seed extract. Grapefruit seed extract, which is used to treat a variety of bacterial and fungal infections, is growing in popularity as a treatment for thrush. It is also recommended as a wash for pacifiers and toys to prevent reinfection. Several sources recommend mixing four or five drops of grapefruit seed extract in 1 cup of water, then applying it with the finger into the child's mouth four to six times a day. The antimicrobial activity and purity of commercial grapefruit seed extract have been subjects of controversy. The authors of one in vitro study noted both bactericidal activity and toxicity of grapefruit seed extract at a dilution of 1:128. The same extract lacked toxicity but was reported to retain bactericidal activity at a dilution of 1:512. The researchers stated that the antibacterial effects resulted from disruption of the bacterial membrane, resulting in cell lysis, after direct contact with the extract.[29]

However, a study of six commercial grapefruit seed extracts found that five contained benzethonium chloride, a synthetic antimicrobial often used in cosmetics and other topical preparations, as well as the preservatives triclosan and methylparaben.[30] The one extract that contained none of these additives was devoid of antimicrobial activity. This information is consistent with the findings of other researchers, who have found benzethonium chloride[31] and triclosan[32] in samples of liquid and powdered grapefruit seed extract. In summary, it is unclear whether grapefruit seed extract has antimicrobial activity (antifungal activity has not been documented) and that considerable adulteration of this "natural" product with synthetic antimicrobial/preservative agents seems to be widespread. Toxicity at even lower dilutions has been suggested. For all of these reasons, practitioners should avoid recommending this extract for the treatment of oral thrush in the infant or nipple thrush in the mother.

Myrrh (Commiphora molmol). Limited data suggest that tincture of myrrh is efficacious in the treatment of oral candidiasis. German health authorities have approved the use of myrrh for inflammations of the oral and pharyngeal mucosa. Local antiseptic activity is well documented,[33] and myrrh can be found in toothpaste and mouthwash products throughout the United States. One German pediatric textbook recommends that a diluted tincture of myrrh (1:1) be applied with a cotton swab to areas of thrush.[34] A dilution of 1:2 or 1:3 is generally recommended because myrrh tinctures are generally prepared with 80% to 90% alcohol to appropriately extract the gum resin. Although only very small amounts of the tincture are used in the mouth, the alcohol may irritate the tissue if the tincture is used undiluted. Myrrh appears to be quite safe when used in this fashion; oral doses of up to 3 g/kg have been shown to cause no significant harm. Likewise, long-term administration of 100 mg/kg per day was not associated with side effects.[35]

Breast Engorgement

Cabbage leaf. The application of cabbage leaves to the breasts is a popular treatment for engorgement. Fresh, cool, dry cabbage leaves are applied to the breasts for 3 or 4 hours after nursing, after which fresh leaves are applied. Three different studies have been published in which cabbage leaves or cabbage-leaf extracts were used in an attempt to relieve breast engorgement; no significant benefit was noted.[36]

Jasmine (Jasminum sambac). Topical application of jasmine flowers is traditionally used in southern India to suppress lactation. Sixty women in Vellore, India, whose babies were stillborn or died within 24 hours of birth were randomly assigned to receive bromocriptine, 2.5 mg every 8 hours for 5 days, or to have jasmine flowers (strung on a

50-cm thread) taped to each breast.[37] Flowers were replaced daily for 5 days. Paracetamol (acetaminophen) was permitted to relieve breast pain. Prolactin levels were assessed 24 hours after delivery and after 72 hours of treatment. Breast engorgement was rated on a 4-point scale, and milk production was evaluated by means of manual expression.

Although bromocriptine and jasmine flowers each achieved a significant reduction in serum prolactin, the decrease was significantly greater with bromocriptine. Lactation scores were similar between groups after 72 hours of treatment. Bromocriptine failed to suppress lactation in one woman; jasmine flowers failed in two. Two women in the bromocriptine group demonstrated rebound lactation on 2-week follow-up. Consumption of analgesics was similar between groups. This interesting study would have been improved by the use of a placebo group.

In lactating mice, topical contact with jasmine flowers inhibited milk production and caused regressive changes in breast parenchyma.[37a]

Proteolytic enzymes. Three studies reported that proteolytic enzymes were effective in reducing breast engorgement. Cochrane reviewers found that proteolytic enzymes (Danzen and bromelain/trypsin combination) significantly improved the symptoms of engorgement.[38] Serrapeptase, a proteolytic enzyme found in the proprietary product Danzen, is grown from bacterial cultures (*Serratia marcescens*). A randomized, placebo-controlled study of 70 women with breast engorgement found that serrapeptase was superior to placebo for improvement of breast pain, breast swelling, and induration. "Marked" improvement was found in 23% of the treatment group and in 3% of the placebo group, whereas moderate to marked improvement was reported by 86% of the patients in the treatment group, compared to 60% of those taking placebo ($P < 0.05$).[39]

Products containing various proteolytic enzymes (usually combinations of bromelain and trypsin with other enzymes such as pancreatin or papain) have been used in Europe for more than 30 years for the reduction of postoperative inflammation and pain. Bromelain is the best-studied proteolytic enzyme. Research suggests that it is absorbed systemically after oral ingestion and produces antiinflammatory, analgesic, immunomodulatory, and antiedema effects in vivo.[39] Although the results are inconsistent, studies (placebo-controlled and comparisons with nonsteroidal antiinflammatory drugs) in patients with rheumatic diseases suggest that oral therapy with proteolytic enzymes produces specific analgesic and antiinflammatory effects.[40] Proteolytic enzymes appear to be very well tolerated, although they may interact with anticoagulant medications[41] and increase the absorption and tissue levels of various antibiotics, including amoxillin, tetracycline, chloramphenicol, and penicillin.[42] It may be reasonable for a woman to use bromelain (or a combination of proteolytic enzymes) to relieve engorgement. The best approach likely remains prevention through frequent nursing accompanied by the application of warm compresses or showers before feedings.

Mastitis

Mastitis is inflammation of the breast that may or may not involve infection. Clinicians generally use the term *mastitis* to describe an infection of the breast that involves fever of 38.5°C (101.3° F) or higher, chills, flulike illness, and a tender, red, wedge-shaped area of the breast.[43] Common causes include cracked nipples, inadequate milk removal, infrequent feeding, rapid weaning, and blocked milk ducts. Therefore a breastfeeding woman should empty her breasts frequently, nursing from the affected side first. If this is too painful, she should nurse from the unaffected breast first, switching to the affected side after milk let-down. The practitioner should reassure a woman with mastitis that there is no evidence of harm to a healthy term infant who drinks milk from an affected breast. It is also critical to explain that a sudden decrease in breastfeeding frequency will increase the stasis of milk and increase the risk of abscess development.[44]

Palliative measures include the application of hot packs before nursing to encourage milk flow, followed by cold compresses after nursing to reduce pain and inflammation. Some women find that massaging the breast, starting with the blocked area and moving toward the nipple, is helpful. If the friction is too uncomfortable, gentle massage with a food-grade oil (e.g., olive, canola, sunflower) may be helpful. Ibuprofen is not detected in breast milk at doses up to 1.6 g/day and is considered safe for the relief of pain during breastfeeding.[45]

If symptoms are mild and have been present for less than 24 hours, many authorities recommend conservative management (compresses, frequent nursing, ibuprofen). If the symptoms are more severe or do not improve within 12 to 24 hours, appropriate antimicrobial medication should be initiated. Cultures of breast milk are not routinely taken. The World Health Organization suggests that breast milk culture and sensitivity testing "be undertaken if there is no response to antibiotics within two days, if the mastitis recurs, if it is hospital-acquired mastitis, or in severe or unusual cases."[43] The most common pathogen in infective mastitis is penicillin-resistant *S. aureus*, followed by *Streptococcus* species and *Escherichia coli*.[46] Dicloxacillin (500 mg, four times a day) is generally considered the first-line treatment; cephalexin or clindamycin is recommended for women who are allergic to penicillin.

Some women contract *Candida* mastitis, which typically presents with shooting pains in the breast during nursing. The nipples may appear shiny and flaky, bear white patches, or be persistently cracked. *Candida* mastitis is more likely to develop in women with a history of antibiotic use, nipple trauma, diabetes, or steroid use and those who are taking estrogen-containing oral contraceptives. Treatment is directed at both mother and baby. One survey showed that the most common initial treatment was oral nystatin for the infant and nystatin cream for the mother's breasts, followed by oral nystatin for the infant and oral fluconazole for the mother. Treatment of recurrent or persistent infection most commonly involved the administration of nystatin to both mother and infant, followed by oral nystatin for the infant and oral fluconazole for the mother or oral fluconazole for both.[47]

Insufficient Milk Supply

When the amount of maternal milk supply is in question, the first step is a thorough physical examination and history, as noted earlier in this chapter. Galactagogues (or lactagogues) are substances believed to aid in the initiation, maintenance, or augmentation of milk production. Common indications include increase of milk production after maternal or infant illness or separation, reestablishment of milk supply after weaning, and induction of lactation in a woman who did not give birth to the infant being nursed (e.g., adoption).

A variety of medications and botanicals have been used as galactagogues. Maternal milk production is a complex process. Dopamine agonists inhibit, whereas dopamine antagonists increase, prolactin and milk production. Although some act as dopamine antagonists, the mechanism of action for others is not known.

Drugs used as galactagogues

Metoclopramide. Metoclopramide is the most studied medication for the induction or augmentation of lactation.[48] The drug, a dopamine antagonist, is commonly used as an antiemetic agent and in the treatment of gastroesophageal reflux in infants. Metoclopramide is detected in breast milk after oral administration; however, it has been shown to be undetectable or well below therapeutic levels in infants who are exposed to the drug through breast milk.[49] No side effects have been noted in the babies of lactating mothers taking metoclopramide.[48] Maternal side effects include fatigue, agitation, diarrhea, and rare but dangerous extrapyramidal side effects, such as headache, confusion, severe agitation, and depression. If extrapyramidal side effects are noted, the drug should be discontinued immediately. Acute dystonic reactions do occur but are extremely rare. The drug is contraindicated in patients taking anticonvulsant or antidepressant medications, as well as in those with poorly controlled hypertension. The dose is generally 10 mg three times a day but may be increased to 15 mg three times a day after 3 to 5 days. Metoclopramide is generally administered for 1 to 2 weeks and the dose is then tapered over 5 to 7 days.

Domperidone. Domperidone, a dopamine antagonist, is prescribed outside the United States as an antiemetic and in the treatment of gastroesophageal reflux. Domperidone was shown to be safe and effective for the augmentation of milk production in a randomized, controlled clinical trial of women with premature newborns.[50] Serum prolactin levels are significantly increased by domperidone. Some believe that the drug is less likely than metoclopramide to cross the blood-brain barrier or enter into breast milk.[51] The dose is 10 to 20 mg three times a day for 3 to 8 weeks; most women respond during the first week of treatment. The drug is well tolerated. Side effects, which are generally mild, include dry mouth, gastrointestinal cramping, and headache. Headache is generally resolved by a reduction in dosage.

Sulpiride and chlorpromazine. The dopamine antagonists sulpiride and chlorpromazine are primarily used as antipsychotic agents. Both drugs have been shown to increase milk supply by increasing prolactin-releasing hormone from the hypothalamus. Sulpiride is not available in the United States. Extrapyramidal side effects occur with both of these drugs.

Human growth hormone. Subcutaneous administration of 0.1 International Unit/kg per day of human growth hormone was shown to increase milk volume after 7 days in 16 healthy lactating women. No changes in milk composition were noted and no side effects reported. Confirmatory studies are needed. This research is interesting, but the treatment is expensive and somewhat impractical in clinical practice.

Botanical galactagogues. Around the world and throughout history, women have used certain herbs and foods to enhance their milk supply. Scientific evaluation of most of these herbs has not been undertaken, but many are widely recommended. Herbs commonly mentioned in the literature include aniseed, borage, caraway seed, cinnamon, comfrey, dill, fennel seed, fenugreek, goat's rue, marshmallow, milk thistle, blessed thistle, nettle, raspberry leaf, and chastetree.

Aniseed, caraway seed, cinnamon, dill, and fennel seed are all aromatic spices that can be easily and safely added to foods. For example, a woman seeking to use one of these herbs might add some dill to a tuna salad, put cinnamon in applesauce, add anise to sugar cookies, or eat a half-teaspoon of candied fennel seed after a meal. Although no studies have been conducted to support the use of these herbs as lactagogues, their addition to the diet is certainly not harmful. Raspberry and nettle are both benign and can be freely consumed by nursing mothers. It is inappropriate to recommend comfrey or borage for internal use to nursing mothers because these herbs contain pyrrolizidine alkaloids, which have the potential to cause liver damage. These alkaloids have been shown to cross into breast milk.[52]

HERBS TO BE AVOIDED DURING BREASTFEEDING

These herbs are generally recognized as unsafe for consumption during lactation. This list should not be considered exhaustive because many herbs have not been adequately studied in this area.

- Aloes, powdered leaf (*Aloe* spp.)
- Black cohosh (*Cimicifuga racemosa*)
- Bladderwrack (*Fucus vesiculosus*)
- Blue cohosh (*Caulophyllum thalictroides*)
- Borage (*Borago officinalis*)
- Buckthorn fruit (*Rhamnus cathartica*)
- Bugleweed leaf (*Lycopus* spp.)
- Cinchona bark (*Cinchona* spp.)
- Cola seed (*Cola nitida*)
- Coltsfoot leaf (*Tussilago farfara*)
- Comfrey leaf and root (*Symphytum officinale*)
- Ephedra (*Ephedra* spp.)
- Guarana (*Paullinia cupana*)
- Jasmine flower (*Jasminum grandiflorum*)
- Kava (*Piper methysticum*)
- Madder root (*Rubia tinctorum*)
- Ma huang (*Ephedra sinica*)
- Pulsatilla (*Anemone pulsatilla*)
- Queen of the meadow root and herb (*Eupatorium purpureum*)
- Senecio (*Senecio aureus*)
- Wormwood (*Artemesia absinthium*)

Fenugreek (Trigonella foenum-graecum). Fenugreek has been treasured as a spice and medicine throughout India and the Middle East for thousands of years. The seeds are used to relieve intestinal gas, upset stomach, respiratory congestion, and, topically, for the treatment of wounds and skin inflammations. Fenugreek has a substantial reputation for increasing breast milk in nursing mothers.[53] Drunk as an infused tea, fenugreek seeds are quite safe. The Food and Drug Administration has placed the herb on its "Generally Recognized as Safe" list. The American Herbal Products Association gives it a rating of 1, meaning that the herb can be safely consumed when used appropriately and that it is not contraindicated during lactation. The American Herbal Products Association does recommend caution in using more than 5 g of seeds per day,[54] although doses of 30 to 40 g/day have been shown to be safe in studies involving diabetic patients. No double-blind studies have been conducted to validate its historical use as a lactagogue. The tea is prepared by steeping one-fourth teaspoon of powdered seeds (roughly 1 g) in 8 oz of water for 10 minutes. One cup of the tea is drunk three times a day. Some women prefer to take the herb in capsule form. Fenugreek can cause diarrhea and bloating in larger doses.[55] Allergic reactions are rare. The taste and odor of fenugreek are similar to those of maple syrup, and this odor can be imparted to the urine. In a child, this could mistakenly lead a practitioner to consider the diagnosis of maple syrup–urine disease (branched-chain hyperaminoaciduria), a rare inherited metabolic disorder.

Goat's rue (Galega officinalis). The dried leaves of goat's rue were first presented to the French Academy by Gillet-Damitte in 1873 after the observation that goat's rue increased milk production in cows by 35% to 50%. Remington later confirmed the lactogenic activity of goat's rue in 1913.[56] Maternal ingestion of a lactation tea containing extracts of licorice (*Glycyrrhiza glabra*), fennel, anise, and goat's rue was linked to drowsiness, hypotonia, lethargy, emesis, and poor suckling in two breastfed neonates; an evaluation for infection yielded negative results, and symptoms and signs resolved after discontinuation of the tea and a 2-day break from breastfeeding.[57] The tea was not tested for contaminants or adulterants, and no other adverse event reports have been made in Europe and South America, where the herb is also used as a hypoglycemic agent. Goat's rue is known to be toxic to sheep at doses as low as 0.8 g/kg, although the animals quickly adapt to the plant and can subsequently consume as much as 10 times this amount after repeated exposure.[58] Although goat's rue is less popular in the United States as a lactagogue, several products contain it in combination with other herbs. The tea is generally prepared by steeping 1 tsp of dried leaves in 8 oz of water for 10 minutes, with one cup taken two or three times a day.

Milk thistle (Silybum marianum). Milk thistle, best known for its liver-protectant effects, has historically been used as a lactagogue throughout Europe. The plant was once known as St. Mary's thistle in honor of the Virgin Mary. Early Christians believed that the white veins in the leaves were symbolic of the Virgin's breast milk. No randomized controlled trials have been conducted to validate the use of this herb as a lactagogue. The American Herbal Products Association gives it a rating of 1, meaning that the herb may be safely consumed when used appropriately and that its use is not contraindicated during lactation.[54] The tea is prepared by simmering 1 tsp of crushed seeds in 8 oz of water for 10 minutes, one to three cups taken daily. Notably, this is not a standardized extract but, rather, a crude water preparation of the seeds. Milk thistle standardized extract is a potent preparation of the herb that is typically used in individuals with liver disorders.

Chastetree berry (Vitex agnus-castus). Vitex was recommended as a lactagogue 20 centuries ago in ancient Greece. Dioscorides and Pliny both recommended consumption of the seeds to "bring down the milk."[59] The most widely quoted study was conducted by Mohr in 1954. The trial compared vitamin B_1 (102 women), the *Vitex* seed extract Alyt (353 women), and no treatment (362 women). The study's methodologic limitations included its short duration and unblinded nature, a lack of lactation protocols, and a lack of statistical measures and significance testing. Although little can be drawn from the study, sustained use of *Vitex* in the postpartum period was noted to cause early return of the menses.[60] This is important to consider because the period of amenorrhea associated with lactation offers protection against breast and ovarian cancer. In vitro data show that *Vitex* fruit extract actually inhibits prolactin by way of dopamine-agonist activity.[61] Animal studies have revealed that subcutaneous injection of *Vitex* for 14 days after delivery was associated with increasing cumulative mortality in suckling rats. The authors also noted a reduction of "milk spots," indicating a reduced milk supply. This was thought to be a result of prolactin inhibition.[62] Lactogenic activity may be related to dose. An open placebo-controlled study of 20 healthy male subjects found that thyroid-releasing hormone–induced prolactin secretion increased with a 120-mg dose and decreased with a 480-mg dose.[63] The manufacturer of Agnolyt (Madaus AG, Cologne, Germany), the most heavily studied German chastetree product, notes that its use is contraindicated during lactation.[62] At this time, there is no reason to recommend *Vitex* as a lactagogue. (See Chapters 3 and 6 for other uses.)

POSTPARTUM MOOD DISORDERS

Having a baby is a life-changing event, bringing joy, happiness, stress, and fatigue into a new mother's life. Many women have unrealistic expectations about motherhood and are unprepared for the reality that quickly unfolds after birth. Changes in work schedules and home routines can be stressful. A woman often describes feelings of loss—the loss of who she was before the baby, the loss of control over time, the loss of certain freedoms, the loss of "alone" time with her partner, and the loss of the body she had before her pregnancy.

These issues should be raised during pregnancy and again after delivery. The practitioner should make it very clear to the mother that she may speak freely about her feelings. She may not recognize that her feelings and emotions are more extreme than normal. Even if she does recognize that she is depressed or anxious, the mother may be reluctant to admit this to family or friends. A woman may worry that if she tells a health care provider about her feelings, someone may try to take her baby away. If the provider who assisted her in the delivery is not her primary care provider, she may not know where to go for guidance and help. Opportunities to inquire about sleep, mood, relationships, and sense of self should not be missed during postpartum visits and well-baby appointments.

Women can be subject to any mood disorder during the postpartum period; however, this chapter focuses only on postpartum depression. The following mood disorders are most described in the literature.

Maternity blues, which presents as mild depression and mood lability during the week after the birth, occurs in as many as 50% of new mothers. Tearfulness, irritability, nervousness, insomnia, and poor concentration are common. It is important to reassure the mother that these feelings are common and help dispel the myth that good mothers are always joyful and happy after a birth. She should not feel guilty if she is not as happy as she expected. The "baby blues" are short-lived and generally resolve without treatment.

The diagnosis of *postpartum depression* is used to cover all depressive disorders in the postpartum period, both those that occur during that time and as preexisting conditions. The postpartum period is generally defined as the year following a birth. Postpartum depression is diagnosed when a woman reports 2 weeks of dysphoric mood or lack of interest or pleasure in usual activities, in addition to at least four of the following symptoms: sleep disturbance, guilt, fatigue, impaired concentration, appetite disturbance, psychomotor activation or retardation, low self-esteem, feelings of hopelessness and worthlessness, and suicidal ideation.[65]

Postpartum psychosis is a serious mental illness that occurs in roughly 1 or 2 per 1000 births, generally within weeks of delivery. Patients may experience delusional thinking, auditory hallucinations, agitation, and inability to sleep and may demonstrate bizarre behavior. Health care providers should be aware that women with a history of bipolar disorder are at increased risk for postpartum psychosis.[66] A history of bipolar illness increases the risk of postpartum psychosis by as much as 25%, and previous episodes of postpartum psychosis further increase the risk to 50% to 75%.[67] Recognition of the disorder and urgent treatment are essential.

The syndrome of *postpartum panic disorder* is characterized by recurrent, unexpected episodes of at least four of the following symptoms: shortness of breath, heart palpitations, tremulousness, lightheadedness, paresthesias, hot flushes or chills, nausea, diaphoresis, chest tightness, choking sensation, and cognitive symptoms of derealization and depersonalization, losing control or "going crazy," impending doom, or fear of dying.[65]

In *postpartum obsessive-compulsive disorder*, the new mother is plagued by obsessive thoughts and compulsive behaviors. An obsessive thought is one that cannot be controlled and returns frequently in unwanted patterns. Compulsive behaviors occur in the form of repetitive rituals that dominate one's life. Women may experience repetitive, intrusive thoughts of harming their babies or become hypervigilant in protecting their infants.[68]

Posttraumatic stress disorder occurs in 3% to 5% of women as a result of birth trauma.[69] The disorder is characterized by reexperience of the event, avoidance of reminders of the stressor, numbing of responsiveness, and symptoms of increased arousal.

Postpartum Depression

Postpartum depression occurs in as many as 18% of new mothers. Although the hormonal changes that occur after childbirth are believed to play a role in postpartum depression, no specific hormonal cause has been identified. As in any suspected case of depression, an appropriate examination and thorough history should be undertaken. Thyroid testing should be performed to rule out hypothyroidism (Box 8-2).

Treatment strategies

The black rose blooms and we know postnatal depression means mothers in despair; energy gone underground, flatness and grayness above ground; devastation, silence, withdrawal from life ... It is like the night of the soul, the extinguishing of a flame. How the baby perceives this withdrawal as the cloud moves over the sun, we can only guess.—Vivienne Welburn, *Postnatal Depression*[71]

This vivid portrayal of postpartum depression by Welburn allows one to feel the intensity of the disorder. It is clear why appropriate and effective treatments should be promptly initiated.

Psychotherapy. A survey of experts in the field of depression in women found that most preferred psychotherapy over medication during pregnancy and lactation.[72] This is likely due to concerns over the long-term effects of antidepressant medications in nursing

Box **8-2**

Factors associated with postpartum depression
• Prenatal depression • Low self-esteem • Child care stress • Prenatal anxiety • Life stress • Low level of social support • Poor marital relationship • History of depression • Difficult infant temperament • Maternity blues • Single marital status • Unplanned/unwanted pregnancy • Low socioeconomic status

Adapted from Beck CT: Revision of the postpartum depression predictors inventory, *J Obstet Gynecol Neonatal Nurs* 31:394-402, July-August 2002.

infants. Research indicates that counseling is as effective as treatment with fluoxetine.[73] Although short-term improvement in mood does occur with counseling, its long-term effects have been called into question. Women with postpartum depression (n = 193) were randomly assigned to receive routine primary care, nondirective counseling, cognitive-behavioral therapy, or psychodynamic therapy. The women and their children were assessed $4\frac{1}{2}$, 18, and 60 months after delivery. All three treatments had a significant benefit with regard to maternal reports of early difficulties in relationships with the infants; counseling yielded better infant emotional and behavior ratings at 18 months and more sensitive early mother-infant interactions. The treatments had no significant impact on maternal management of early infant behavior problems, security of the infant-mother attachment, infant cognitive development, or any child outcome at 5 years.[74] In this same study, all three treatments had a significant impact, compared with control, at $4\frac{1}{2}$ months on maternal mood (Edinburgh Postnatal Depression Scale), although only psychodynamic therapy produced a rate of reduction in depression (Structured Clinical Interview for *Diagnostic and Statistical Manual of Mental Disorders DSM-III-R*) significantly superior to that of the control. The benefit of treatment was no longer apparent 9 months after delivery, and treatment did not reduce the incidence of subsequent episodes of postpartum depression. The short-term benefits to maternal mood were not superior to spontaneous remission in the long term.[75] These findings are consistent with those of other studies of counseling in depression revealing significant short-term, but not long-term, benefit.[76]

Counseling remains a reasonable option for women with postpartum depression, especially those who are breastfeeding and do not wish to take antidepressant medications. Practitioners should realize, however, that this type of therapy is often unavailable, cost-prohibitive, or problematic as a result of child care difficulties.

Exercise. Research suggests that regular exercise improves mood.[77] A pilot study was conducted in England as health care workers sought innovative ways of addressing the high incidence of postpartum depression seen in their district. Believing that exercise may have a beneficial effect on depression, they set up a project to make fitness activities more affordable and available to their client base. After an initial survey of local mothers had indicated support, a pilot "swim, gym and crèche (baby care facility)" scheme was set up in a leisure center in partnership with other agencies. The response from the pilot group was positive and suggested that the participants were benefiting mentally and physically from the exercise and the social aspects of the group.[78] This is an excellent example of community interventions that may provide an environment for physical and social support. When on-site child care is provided, new mothers are able to exercise and visit with each other with their babies safe nearby.

Antidepressant medications. Many women are reluctant to take antidepressant medication, especially when they are breastfeeding. The use of these medications in lactating women remains controversial. Although some data demonstrate no direct influence of such medications on the infant, their long-term effects on neurodevelopment remain uncertain. Methodologically sound long-term studies on this topic have not been published. As a result, many providers recommend that mothers stop breastfeeding while taking antide-pressant medications because many drugs are secreted into breast milk. However, most experts agree that if the mother wants to continue breastfeeding, the risks of ongoing severe depression may outweigh the potential risks of medication.

Cochrane reviewers concluded that postnatal depression could be effectively treated with fluoxetine; however only one clinical trial met the criteria for inclusion in their review.[79] They stressed that "more trials with a longer follow-up period are needed to compare different antidepressants in the treatment of postnatal depression, and to compare antidepressant treatment with psychosocial interventions. This is an area that has been neglected despite the large public health impact." One study included in the Cochrane review, by Appleby et al.,[73] showed that both fluoxetine and cognitive-behavioral counseling given as a course of therapy were effective treatments for non-psychotic depression in postnatal women. They found no additional benefit to the provision of both counseling and medication and suggested that, after an initial session of counseling, women should choose which therapy they prefer. Obviously the choice of counseling would be a wise one for many women, especially those who are breastfeeding. However, as previously mentioned, this type of therapy is often unavailable, cost-prohibitive, or problematic as a result of child care difficulties, leaving many women with more severe depression little choice but to take medication.

A review of 15 studies in which serum levels of drugs in nursing infants were obtained revealed that amitriptyline, nortriptyline, desipramine, clomipramine, dothiepin, and sertraline were not found in quantifiable amounts in nursing infants and that no adverse effects were reported.[80] Cognitive and psychomotor development appears to be normal in infants exposed to fluoxetine,[81] and infants exposed to sertraline demonstrated no neurologic or developmental abnormalities at 1-year follow-up.[82] With the limited data currently available, if a woman's depression is severe enough to require medication and the woman wishes to continue breastfeeding a healthy term baby, sertraline is generally considered the first-line therapy. Some providers prefer tricyclic antidepressants because of their long history of use. They may also be a better choice in women who are more agitated than somnolent. The collective serum level data suggest that infants older than 10 weeks are at low risk for adverse effects of tricyclic antidepressants, and no evidence supports accumulation. As a class, however, many practitioners still prefer the selective serotonin reuptake inhibitors (SSRIs), likely because of the danger of overdose with tricyclics and their side effect profile. Many women object to the excessive sedation, and weight gain can be bothersome with tricyclics, especially at a time when a woman is trying to lose the weight she gained during pregnancy.

Hormone therapy. Numerous researchers have postulated that the sudden postpartum decrease in estrogen level leads to the maternal blues and marked increase in the incidence of psychosis that occurs in the first weeks after birth. The theory has some biologic foundation; estrogen is known to affect neurotransmitter mechanisms in the brain. Research findings at this time should be considered preliminary, but some small studies have shown that estrogen is superior to placebo in certain reproductive-related mood disorders, including postpartum depression,[83] especially in women with documented estradiol deficiency.[84]

Long-acting norethisterone enanthate is associated with an increased risk of postnatal depression. It and other long-acting progestogen contraceptives should be used with caution in the postnatal period, especially in women with a history of depression. The role of progesterone in the prevention and treatment of postpartum depression has yet to be evaluated in a randomized, placebo-controlled trial.[85]

St. John's wort (Hypericum perforatum). St. John's wort is the most heavily studied botanical for depression. Through 2002, 34 controlled clinical trials involving more than 3000 patients showed the effectiveness of St. John's wort in the treatment of mild to moderate depression. No studies of the efficacy of this herb in the treatment of postpartum depression have been published, and its safety in lactating women has not been evaluated. According to the German Commission E and the American Herbal Products Association, the use of St. John's wort during pregnancy or lactation is not contraindicated. Maternal administration of 180 mg/kg hypericum before and throughout gestation did not affect long-term growth or physical maturation of exposed mouse offspring.[86] No adverse effects were noted in the offspring of animals given as much as 1.5 g/kg per day of hypericum.[87] No genotoxic properties or chromosomal aberrations have been found on in vitro or animal testing.[88]

In one published case report, low levels of hyperforin were found in the breast milk of a woman who had been taking 300 mg, three times a day, of a standardized extract of St. John's wort while nursing. However, hyperforin and hypericin were undetectable in the baby's plasma. No adverse effects were noted in the mother or the infant.[89]

Omega-3 fatty acids. A growing body of evidence demonstrates the many health benefits of fish. Intervention trials in human subjects show that omega-3 fatty acids may have positive effects in the treatment of various psychiatric disorders.[90] One study revealed an inverse relationship between fish consumption and postpartum depression in women from 23 countries. A sample of the data is shown in Table 8-1. The authors of the research report analyzed 14,532 subjects and found that higher omega-3 fatty acid content in breast milk and greater seafood consumption were both associated with lower rates of postpartum depression.[91] Researchers also discovered that the breast milk of women who eat large amounts of fish contains high levels of the fatty acid docosahexaenoic acid (DHA). Although this study is interesting and its findings are consistent with current thinking

Table 8-1

Incidence of postpartum depression by country and fish consumption

COUNTRY	FISH CONSUMED PER WOMAN PER YEAR (LB)	% OF WOMEN REPORTING YEAR
South Africa	8.6	24.5
United States	48.1	11.1
Singapore	81.1	0.5

that omega-3 fatty acids have a beneficial effect on mood, a recent study failed to show any beneficial influence on self-ratings of depression, diagnostic measures of depression, or information processing among breastfeeding women given 200 mg/day of DHA or placebo for 4 months after delivery.[92] Some argue that this dose is not sufficient. However, laboratory testing showed a significant increase in the DHA levels of the women taking the supplement, and a recent trial of 36 patients with major depression who were given a much higher dose, 2 g/day of DHA or placebo, for 6 weeks failed to show any significant effect.[93] Other experts argue that eicosapentaenoic acid (EPA), another fatty acid in fish, is more important than DHA in alleviating depressive moods. A study providing 1 g/day of EPA as an adjunct therapy to antidepressant medication found it beneficial in those patients who failed to demonstrate a full treatment response.[94] EPA was significantly superior to DHA in relieving positive symptoms (delusions, hallucinations, bizarre behaviors) of schizophrenia in a small pilot study.[95] More rigorous research in this area is needed to determine the best product and dose to study in clinical trials.

Pregnant women, lactating women, and young children must be careful about the amounts of certain types of fish they consume because of the presence of methyl mercury. The U.S. Food and Drug Administration (FDA) recommends that these populations limit their consumption of tuna and other cooked fish to 12 oz per week. Some states have established their own guidelines. According to guidelines issued by the FDA in March 2001, members of the aforementioned populations should not eat shark, swordfish, king mackerel, or tilefish (also called golden or white snapper) because these fish contain more than 1 ppm of methyl mercury, an amount the FDA considers unsafe. Halibut, salmon, and other seafoods are low in mercury and can be safely enjoyed several times a week. For those who do not like fish or who are concerned about the presence of methyl mercury (and other pollutants), most fish oil capsules appear to be free of this heavy metal. A recent study of 20 fish oil supplements taken off the shelf revealed that none contained detectable mercury (<1.5 ppb).[96] Fish oil supplements contain both DHA and EPA. The dose generally recommended is 1 to 3 g/day, although the optimal dose is not yet known.

SAMe. Derived from the sulfur-containing amino acid methionine and adenosine triphosphate, SAMe (S-adenosyl-L-methionine) is a natural substance that plays an important role in many of the body's biochemical processes. SAMe is the most important methyl donor in transmethylation reactions occurring in the central nervous system. Levels of SAMe in the serum and cerebrospinal fluid are reported to be low in some patients with depression. A recent review by the Agency for Healthcare Research and Quality concluded that SAMe is likely more effective than placebo in relieving symptoms of depression, and no statistically significant difference in outcomes occurred when SAMe was compared with conventional antidepressant pharmacologic treatment.[97] The reviewers did note that a possible publication bias may have tempered the strength of the conclusions reported.

The standard dosage of SAMe used in depression is 400 to 1200 mg/day, taken in the morning before breakfast, starting with 400 mg/day and increasing by 200 mg every 3 to 5 days until therapeutic results are achieved. The product must be enteric-coated. The onset of action for SAMe in depression is much shorter than that of conventional antidepressants. Taking the product later in the day can cause insomnia. The dose may be reduced if agitation occurs. Taking the dose with food can reduce the incidence of gastric upset in susceptible patients. SAMe is contraindicated in patients with bipolar disorder.

No studies of SAMe in the treatment of postpartum depression could be located. No contraindications to use in pregnancy or lactation were found, either. In fact, the Agency for Healthcare Research and Quality report included the finding that SAMe is likely more effective than placebo in relieving pruritus and reducing the bilirubin level in women with cholestasis during pregnancy.[97] Given the safety profile, the use of SAMe for postpartum depression, especially in breastfeeding women, should be subjected to rigorous research.

References

1. American Academy of Pediatrics Work Group on Breastfeeding: Breastfeeding and the use of human milk, *Pediatrics* 100:1035-1039, 1997.
2. Wagner CL, Anderson DM, Pittard WB: Special properties of human milk, *Clin Pediatr* 35:283-293, 1996.
3. Wright AL, Bauer M, Naylor A, et al: Increasing breastfeeding rates to reduce infant illness at the community level, *Pediatrics* 101:837-844, 1998.
4. Lucas A, Cole TJ: Breast milk and neonatal necrotizing enterocolitis, *Lancet* 336:1519-1523, 1990.
5. Office of Disease Prevention and Health Promotion: *Healthy People 2000,* DHHS publication No.(PHS) 91-50212, Washington, DC, US Government Printing Office, 1990.
6. Sarett HP, Bain KR, O'Leary JC: Decision on breastfeeding or formula feeding and trends in infant-feeding practices, *Am J Dis Child* 37:719-723, 1983.
7. Losch M, Dungy CI, Russell D, et al: Impact of attitudes on maternal decisions regarding infant feeding, *J Pediatrics* 6:507-514, 1995.
8. Neifert M, DeMarzo S, Seacat J, et al: The influence of breast surgery, breast appearance, and pregnancy-induced breast changes on lactation sufficiency as measured by infant weight gain, *Birth* 17:31-38, 1990.
9. The MAIN Trial Collaborative Group: Preparing for breastfeeding: treatment of inverted and non-protractile nipples in pregnancy, *Midwifery* 10:200-214, 1994.
10. Neifert M: Breastfeeding after breast surgical procedure or breast cancer, *NAACOG's Clinical Issues in Perinatal and Women's Health Nursing* 3:673-682, 1992.
11. Kyenka-Isabrrye M: UNICEF launches the Baby-Friendly Hospital Initiative, *Am J Matern Child Nursing* 17:177-179, 1992.
12. Chute G: Breastfeeding, *NAACOG's Clinical Issues in Perinatal and Women's Health Nursing* 3:647-644, 1992.
13. Lampl M, Veldhuis JD, Johnson ML: Saltation and stasis: a model of human growth, *Science* 258:801-803, 1992.
14. Neifert M: Early assessment of the breastfeeding infant, *Contemp Pediatr* 13:142-166, 1996.
15. Centuori S, Burmaz T, Ronfani L, et al: Nipple care, sore nipples, and breastfeeding: a randomized trial, *J Hum Lact* 15:125-130, 1999.
16. Brent N, Rudy SJ, Redd B, et al: Sore nipples in breast-feeding women: a clinical trial of wound dressings vs conventional care, *Arch Pediatr Adolesc Med* 152:1077-1082, 1998.

17. Lavergne NA: Does application of tea bags to sore nipples while breastfeeding provide effective relief? *J Obstet Gynecol Neonatal Nurs* 26:53-58, January-February 1997.
18. McNaught JG: On the action of cold or lukewarm tea on *Bacillus typhosus, J R Army Med Corps* 7:372-373, 1906.
19. Hamilton-Miller JMT: Antimicrobial properties of tea *(Camellia sinensis L.) Antimicrob Agents Chemother* 39:2375-2377, 1995.
20. Yam TS, Shah S, Hamilton-Miller JM: Microbiological activity of whole and fractionated crude extracts of tea (Camellia sinensis), and of tea components, *FEMS Microbiol Lett* 152:169-174, 1997.
21. Sharquie KE, al-Turfi IA, al-Salloum SM: The antibacterial activity of tea in vitro and in vivo (in patients with impetigo contagiosa), *J Dermatol* 27:706-710, 2000.
22. Yam TS, Hamilton-Miller JM, Shah S: The effect of a component of tea *(Camellia sinensis)* on methicillin resistance, PBP2' synthesis, and beta-lactamase production in *Staphylococcus aureus, J Antimicrob Chemother* 42:211-215, 1998.
22a. McGuffin M, Hobbs C, Upton R, et al: *American Herbal Products Association's botanical safety handbook*, Boca Raton, Fla, CRC Press, 1997, p 22.
22b. Inanami O, Asanuma T, Inukai N, et al: The suppression of age-related accumulation of lipid peroxides in rat brain by administration of Rooibos tea *(Aspalathus linearis), Neurosci Lett* 196:85-88, 1993.
23. Klouchek-Popova E, Popov A, Pavlova N, et al: Influence of the physiological regeneration and epithelialization using fractions isolated from *Calendula officinalis, Acta Physiol Pharmacol Bulg* 8:63-67, 1982.
24. Kinlay JR, O'Connell DL, Kinlay S: Risk factors for mastitis in breastfeeding women: results of a prospective cohort study, *Aust N Z J Public Health* 25:115-120, 2001.
25. Livingstone VH, Willis CE, Berkowitz J: *Staphylococcus aureus* and sore nipples, *Can Fam Phys* 42:654-659, 1996.
26. Livingstone V, Stringer LJ: The treatment of *Staphyloccocus aureus* infected sore nipples: a randomized comparative study, *J Hum Lact* 15(3):241-246, 1999.
27. Tanguay KE, McBean MR, Jain E: Nipple candidiasis among breastfeeding mothers. Case-control study of predisposing factors, *Can Fam Phys* 40:1407-1413, 1994.
28. Vazquez JA, Zawawi AA: Efficacy of alcohol-based and alcohol-free melaleuca oral solution for the treatment of fluconazole-refractory oropharyngeal candidiasis in patients with AIDS, *HIV Clin Trial* 3:379-385, 2002.
29. Heggers JP, Cottingham J, Gusman J, et al: The effectiveness of processed grapefruit-seed extract as an antibacterial agent. II. Mechanism of action and in vitro toxicity, *J Altern Complement Med* 8:333-340, 2002.
30. von Woedtke T, Schluter B, Pflegel P, et al: Aspects of the antimicrobial efficacy of grapefruit seed extract and its relation to preservative substances contained, *Pharmazie* 54:452-456, 1999.
31. Takeoka G, Dao L, Wong RY, et al: Identification of benzethonium chloride in commercial grapefruit seed extracts, *J Agric Food Chem* 49:3316-3320, 2001.
32. Sakamoto S, Sato K, Maitani T, et al: Analysis of components in natural food additive "grapefruit seed extract" by HPLC and LC/MS [in Japanese], *Eisei Shikenjo Hokoku* 114:38-42, 1996.
33. El Ashry ES, Rashed N, Salama OM, et al: Components, therapeutic value and uses of myrrh, *Pharmazie* 58:163-168, 2003.
34. Schilcher H: *Phytotherapy in paediatrics: handbook for physicians and pharmacists*, Stuttgart, 1997, Medpharm Scientific Publishers, p 29.
35. Rao RM, Khan ZA, Shah AH: Toxicity studies in mice of *Commiphora molmol* oleo-gum-resin, *J Ethnopharmacol* 76:151-154, 2001.
36. Snowden HM, Renfrew MJ, Woolridge MW: Treatments for breast engorgement during lactation, *Cochrane Database Syst Rev* 2: CD000046, 2001.
37. Shrivastav P, George K, Balasubramaniam N, et al: Suppression of puerperal lactation using jasmine flowers *(Jasminum sambac), Aust N Z J Obstet Gynecol* 28:68-71, 1988.
37a. Abraham M, Devi NS, Sheela R: Inhibiting effect of jasmine flowers on lactation, *Indian J Med Res* 69:88-92, 1979.
38. Kee WH, Tan SL, Lee V, et al: The treatment of breast engorgement with serrapeptase (Danzen): a randomised double-blind controlled trial, *Singapore Med J* 30:48-54, 1989.

39. Lotz-Winter H: On the pharmacology of bromelain: an update with special regard to animal studies on dose-dependent effects. *Planta Med* 56:249-253, 1990.
40. Leipner J, Iten F, Saller R: Therapy with proteolytic enzymes in rheumatic disorders, *BioDrugs* 15:779-789, 2001.
41. Metzig C, Grabowska E, Eckert K, et al: Bromelain proteases reduce human platelet aggregation in vitro, adhesion to bovine endothelial cells and thrombus formation in rat vessels in vivo, *In Vivo* 13:7-12, 1999.
42. Bratman S: Proteolytic enzymes for chronic pain conditions, *Alt Ther Women Health* 4:25-32, 2002.
43. *Mastitis: causes and management,* Geneva, 2000, World Health Organization Department of Child and Adolescent Health and Development WHO/FCH/CAH/0013.
44. Marshall BR, Hepper JK, Zirbel CC: Sporadic puerperal mastitis: an infection that need not interrupt lactation, *JAMA* 233:1377-1379, 1975.
45. Hale T. *Medications and mother's milk,* ed 9. Texas, 2000, Pharmasoft Medical Publishing, pp 345-346.
46. Thomsen AC, Espersen T, Maigaard S: Course and treatment of milk stasis, noninfectious inflammation of the breast, and infectious mastitis in nursing women, *Am J Obstet Gynecol* 149:492-495, 1984.
47. Brent NB: Thrush in the breastfeeding dyad: results of a survey on diagnosis and treatment, *Clin Pediatr* 40:503-506, 2001.
48. Gabay MP: Galactagogues: medications that induce lactation, *J Hum Lact* 18:274-279, 2002.
49. Kaupilla AM, Arvel P, Koivisto M, et al: Metoclopramide and breastfeeding transfer into milk and the newborn, *Eur J Clin Pharmacol* 25:819-823, 1983.
50. DaSilva OP, Knoppert DC, Angelini MM, et al: Effect of domperidone on milk production in mothers of premature newborns: a randomized double-blind, placebo controlled trial, *Can Med Assoc J* 164:17-21, 2001.
51. Hofmeyer GJ, Van Iddekinge B: Domperidone and lactation, *Lancet* 1:647, 1983.
52. Panter KE, James LF: Natural plant toxicants in milk: a review, *J Anim Sci* 68:892-904, 1990.
53. Mabey R, editor: *The new age herbalist.* London, 1988, Gaia Books, p 93.
54. McGuffin M, Hobbs C, Upton R, et al, editors: *American Herbal Products Association's botanical safety handbook*, Boca Raton, Fla, 1997, CRC Press, p 53.
55. Sharma RD, Raghuram TC, Rao NS: Effects of fenugreek seeds on blood glucose and serum lipids in type 1 diabetes, *Eur J Clin Nutr* 44:301-306, 1990.
56. Remington JP, editor: *The dispensatory of the United States of America*, ed 20, Philadelphia, 1918, Lippincott-Raven.
57. Rosti L, Nardini A, Bettinelli ME, et al: Toxic effects of a herbal tea mixture in two newborns, *Acta Paediatr* 83:683, 1994.
58. Keeler RF, Baker DC, Evans JO: Individual animal susceptibility and its relationship to induced adaptation of tolerance in sheep to *Galega officinalis L, Vet Hum Toxicol* 30:420-423, 1988.
59. Snow JM: *Vitex agnus-castus* L. (Verbenaceae) *Prot J Bot Med* 20-23, Spring 1996.
60. Mohr H: Clinical investigations of means to increase lactation, *Dtsche Medizin Wochenschr* 79:1513-1516, 1954.
61. Sliutz G, Speiser P, Schultz AM, et al: *Agnus castus* extracts inhibit prolactin secretion of rat pituitary cells, *Horm Metab Res* 25:253-255, 1993.
62. Agnolyt [package insert], Cologne, Madaus.
63. Merz PG, Gorkow C, Schroedter A, et al: The effects of a special *Agnus castus* extract (BP1095E1) on prolactin secretion in healthy male subjects, *Exp Clin Endocrinol Diabetes* 104:447-453, 1996.
64. Deleted in proof.
65. *Diagnostic and Statistical Manual of Mental Disorders*, ed 4, Washington DC, 1994, American Psychological Association.
66. Beck CT: Predictors of postpartum depression: an update, *Nurs Res* 50:275-285, 2001.
67. Pedersen CA: Postpartum mood and anxiety disorders: a guide for the nonpsychiatric clinician with an aside on thyroid associations with postpartum mood, *Thyroid* 9:691-697, 1999.
68. Sichel DA, Cohen LS, Dimmock JA, et al: Postpartum obsessive compulsive disorder: a case series, *J Clin Psychiatr* 54:156-159, 1993.

69. Czarnocka J, Slade P: Prevalence and predictors of post-traumatic stress symptoms following childbirth, *Br J Clin Psychol* 39:35-51, 2000.
70. Beck CT: Revision of the postpartum depression predictors inventory, *J Obstet Gynecol Neonatal Nurs* 31:394-402, 2002.
71. Welburn V: *Postnatal depression*, Manchester, UK, 1980, Manchester University Press.
72. Altshuler LL, Cohen LS, Moline ML, et al: The Expert Consensus Guideline Series. Treatment of depression in women, *Postgraduate medicine*, New York: McGraw-Hill, 2001, pp 1-107.
73. Appleby L, Warner R, Whitton A, et al: A controlled study of fluoxetine and cognitive-behavioural counselling in the treatment of postnatal depression, *BMJ* 314:932-936, 1997.
74. Murray L, Cooper PJ, Wilson A, et al: Controlled trial of the short- and long-term effect of psychological treatment of post-partum depression. 2. Impact on the mother-child relationship and child outcome, *Br J Psychiatr* 182:420-427, 2003.
75. Cooper PJ, Murray L, Wilson A, et al: Controlled trial of the short- and long-term effect of psychological treatment of post-partum depression. 1. Impact on maternal mood, *Br J Psychiatr* 182:412-419, 2003.
76. Bower P, Rowland N, Hardy R: The clinical effectiveness of counselling in primary care: a systematic review and meta-analysis, *Psychol Med* 33:203-215, 2003.
77. Ernst E, Rand JI, Stevinson C: Complementary therapies for depression: an overview, *Arch Gen Psychiatr* 55:1026-1032, 1998.
78. Wilkinson J, Phillips S, Jackson J, et al: "Mad for Fitness": an exercise group to combat a high incidence of postnatal depression, *J Fam Health Care* 13:44-48, 2003.
79. Hoffbrand S, Howard L, Crawley H: Antidepressant treatment for post-natal depression (Cochrane Review). In *The Cochrane Library*, issue 2. Oxford, UK, 2003, Update Software.
80. Wisner KL, Perel JM, Findling RL: Antidepressant treatment during breast-feeding, *Am J Psychiatr* 153:1132-1137, 1996.
81. Yoshida K, Kumar R, Smith B, et al: Psychotropic drugs in breast milk: no evidence for adverse effect on prepulse modulation of startle reflex or on cognitive levels in infants, *Dev Psychobiol* 32:249-256, 1998.
82. Stowe ZN: A follow up of infants breastfed on sertraline, Melbourne, June 1996, presented at the Collegium Internationale Neuro-Psychopharmacologicum Conference.
83. Grigoriadis S, Kennedy SH: Role of estrogen in the treatment of depression, *Am J Ther* 9:503-509, 2002.
84. Ahokas A, Kaukoranta J, Wahlbeck K, et al: Estrogen deficiency in severe postpartum depression: successful treatment with sublingual physiologic 17beta-estradiol: a preliminary study, *J Clin Psychiatr* 62:332-336, 2001.
85. Lawrie TA, Herxheimer A, Dalton K: Oestrogens and progestogens for preventing and treating postnatal depression (Cochrane Review). In *The Cochrane Library*, issue 2. Oxford, UK, 2003, Update Software.
86. Rayburn WF, Gonzalez CL, Christensen HD, et al: Effect of prenatally administered hypericum (St John's wort) on growth and physical maturation of mouse offspring, *Am J Obstet Gynecol* 184:191-195, 2001.
87. Mills S, Bone K: *Principles and practice of phytotherapy*, London, 2000, Churchill Livingstone, pp 548-549.
88. Okpanyi SN, Lidzba H, Scholl BC, et al: Genotoxicity of standardized Hypericum extract, *Arzneimittelforschung* 40(8 Pt 2):851-855, 1990.
89. Klier CM, Schafer MR, Schmid-Siegel B, et al: St. John's Wort (*Hypericum perforatum*): is it safe during breastfeeding? *Pharmacopsychiatry* 35:29-30, 2002.
90. Haag M: Essential fatty acids and the brain, *Can J Psychiatr* 48:195-203, 2003.
91. Hibbeln JR: Seafood consumption, the DHA content of mothers' milk and prevalence rates of postpartum depression: a cross-national, ecological analysis, *J Affect Disord* 69(1-3):15-29, 2002.
92. Llorente AM, Jensen CL, Voigt RG, et al: Effect of maternal docosahexaenoic acid supplementation on postpartum depression and information processing, *Am J Obstet Gynecol* 188:1348-1353, 2003.

93. Marangell LB, Martinez JM, Zboyan HA, et al: A double-blind, placebo-controlled study of the omega-3 fatty acid docosahexaenoic acid in the treatment of major depression, *Am J Psychiatr* 160:996-998, 2003.
94. Peet M, Horrobin DF: A dose-ranging study of the effects of ethyl-eicosapentaenoate in patients with ongoing depression despite apparently adequate treatment with standard drugs, *Arch Gen Psychiatr* 59:913-919, 2002.
95. Peet M, Brind J, Ramchand CN, et al: Two double-blind placebo-controlled pilot studies of eicosapentaenoic acid in the treatment of schizophrenia, *Schizophr Res* 49:243-251, 2001.
96. Product Review: *Omega-3 fatty acids (EPA and DHA) from fish/marine oil.* Available at www.consumerlabs.com. Accessed January 2004.
97. Agency for Healthcare Research and Quality: *S-adenosyl-l-methionine for treatment of depression, osteoarthritis, and liver disease.* AHRQ publication no. 02-E033, August 2002. Available at: www.ahrq.gov/clinic/epcsums/samesum.htm. Accessed January 2004.

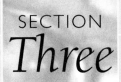

SECTION

Three

The Nervous System

Women are disproportionately affected by headache, depression, and anxiety. Effective integrative medical approaches are available to treat these conditions. Many of these problems have become more common, more commonly diagnosed, and more frequently diagnosed in younger patients. New and effective pharmacologic interventions are now available; however, concerns about the safety and side effects of these treatments have arisen. This, in part, has fueled research on the safety and efficacy of St. John's wort and S-adenosyl-L-methionine (SAMe) for depression.

Data have become available that provide an informed basis for decision making by practitioners and consumers about the appropriate and safe use of these dietary supplements for nervous system conditions in the ambulatory care setting.

This section presents chapters on the general problem of headaches, on migraine headache specifically, and on depressive disorders, insomnia, cognitive disorders, and dementia.

Headaches

Headaches are one of the most common pain conditions for which medical attention is sought. Headaches are typically classified as primary or secondary. Primary headache disorders include migraine (see Chapter 10), tension-type headache, and cluster headache. Secondary headaches result from other organic disturbances such as infections and metabolic disorders.

Although most headaches are not serious, some signal dangerous medical conditions such as cerebral aneurysm, brain tumor, stroke, meningitis, or encephalitis. A severe headache that comes on suddenly—especially if it is accompanied by numbness, loss of consciousness, dizziness, slurred speech, seizures, or fever—must be evaluated immediately by an appropriately trained medical professional.

TENSION-TYPE HEADACHES

An estimated 88% of women and 69% of men experience a tension-type headache sometime during their lifetimes.[1] Approximately 820 workdays are lost annually for every 1000 persons as a result of tension-type headaches,[2] compared with 270 days lost annually per 1000 persons as a result of migraines. More than 45 million Americans live with chronic recurrent headaches. For some, these headaches are simply a nuisance; for others, tension-type headaches create a significant reduction in their quality of life.

It is estimated that only 15% of people who experience tension-type headaches seek medical attention (see "Self-Help Ideas for Handling Headaches"). This may be due in part to the very nature of the name *tension-type headache*. This term has fostered the widely held belief that this type of headache is purely psychological in nature. This chapter provides a discussion of the physiologic basis, diagnosis, and treatment of tension-type headaches.

SELF-HELP IDEAS FOR HANDLING HEADACHES

During times of heightened stress, the number and severity of headaches may increase. Several self-care strategies are useful in obtaining relief from headache pain.

- Relax with 5 minutes of deep abdominal breathing. If possible, lie down, close your eyes, and place one hand on your abdomen. Focus on the rise and fall of your hand as you breathe deeply.
- Stretch the muscles of the back, shoulders, and neck. While sitting in a chair, gently drop your chin toward your chest and hold for a count of 10. Slowly raise your head. Now reach your right hand around the back of the chair and look over your right shoulder. Hold for a count of 10. Slowly release the right hand and repeat the same movement on the left. Now lift your shoulders up toward your ears, hold for a count of three, and then relax the shoulders. Perform this movement twice and repeat the entire routine two or three times. Make sure to take deep, slow breaths throughout.
- If you are having problems sleeping, you may want to try valerian (*Valeriana officinalis*), one of the most widely used herbal sleep aids in the world. German health authorities recognize the use of valerian for restlessness and sleep problems caused by stress or nervous conditions. Valerian is not habit-forming and appears to be quite safe when used appropriately. Don't take it with prescription sleeping medications, however.
- Take a 5-minute walk to help relieve a tension headache. Exercise releases endorphins, the body's natural painkillers, thereby relieving head pain.
- Peppermint compresses are an old and effective treatment for tension headaches. Add two to four drops of peppermint oil to a cup of cold water. Dip a cloth into the fragrant water and apply it to the painful area for 10 to 15 minutes.
- Limit your intake of monosodium glutamate (a.k.a. MSG), alcohol, and caffeine. However, don't just suddenly stop drinking caffeine-containing drinks, or you might experience "rebound" headaches. Wean yourself off caffeine slowly.
- Calcium and magnesium, 1,000 and 500 mg/day, respectively, may help reduce muscle tension. Take these supplements in divided doses, morning and night.
- Warm baths relax tense muscles and can ease aches and pains. Add some essential oils to further enhance the medicinal effects of the bath. Eucalyptus, mint, rosemary, ginger and sage are all excellent for relaxing tight muscles. Enhance the effect by turning down the lights and putting on some soft music.
- Add 2 T of dried ginger to a saucepan of water and simmer for 10 minutes. Put the warm water in a small tub big enough for your feet. Soak your feet in while drinking a cup of chamomile tea in a quiet room for 10 to 15 minutes.
- During stressful periods, it is extremely important to schedule personal time for exercise and relaxation. Try a yoga or Pilates class. Ever dream of signing up for martial arts? Grab a friend (two- or four-legged) and go for a 30-minute walk. Whatever you do, just remember to move on a regular basis.

Physiologic Basis

Although the tension-type headache is the most common type of head pain, its physiologic basis remains unclear. It is been thought for many years that tension-type headaches are muscular in origin because myofascial pain tends to be dull and achy, poorly localized, and radiating, whereas pain originating from cutaneous structures is normally sharp, localized, and nonradiating. Increased myofascial tenderness and muscle firmness are two of the most prominent abnormal findings in patients with chronic tension-type headache.[3,4] What causes and sustains this muscle firmness and myofascial tendernesshas become a matter of debate. From the findings of experimental research and clinical studies it appears that myofascial nociception is a key component of episodic tension-type headache; however, central sensitization appears to predominate in the chronic form.[5] (*Nociception* refers to the detection of noxious stimuli by the nervous sytem. The receptors involved in pain detection are referred to as *nociceptors*.) Central sensitization is best described as an increased excitability of central nervous system neurons that results from prolonged nociceptive input from the periphery. Central sensitization has been shown to play a significant role in chronic myofascial pain.[6] Increased tenderness in patients with chronic tension-type headaches may be a result of sensitization of spinal dorsal-horn neurons induced by prolonged sensory input from pericranial myofascial tissues.[7]

Role of nitric oxide. Nitric oxide (NO) is involved in the development of central sensitization[8] and nitric oxide synthase (NOS) inhibitors, which reduce the level of NO, also have been shown to reduce central sensitization in animal studies of persistent pain.[9,10] In light of these data, the role of NO as a mediator in tension-type headaches is being explored. Inhibition of NO was found to effectively reduce both pain and muscle firmness in a small randomized double-blind crossover study of 16 patients with chronic tension-type headaches. Patients were administered intravenous infusions of 6 mg/kg L-NMMA (NG-monomethyl-L-arginine hydrochloride, an inhibitor of NOS) or placebo for 2 days, separated by at least 1 week, in a randomized fashion. Headache intensity was measured on a 100-mm visual-analog scale at baseline and 30, 60, and 120 minutes after start of treatment. L-NMMA reduced pain intensity significantly more than did placebo ($P = 0.01$).[11,12]

Medications

In addition to NOS inhibitors, established medications for chronic myofascial pain and tension-type headache may be effective, partly because they reduce sensitivity.[13] The documented analgesic effect of the tricyclic antidepressant amitriptyline in patients with chronic myofascial pain is thought to be due to a reduction in the transmission of painful stimuli from myofascial tissue, rather than a reduction in overall pain sensitivity.[14]

Practitioners should always inquire about long-term use of nonsteroidal antiinflammatory drugs (NSAIDs) by patients who have chronic headaches as the frequent use of these medications may lead to persistent headaches. Studies indicate that an increase in NOS activity is associated with a hyposerotonergic state. This state may contribute to central sensitization in chronic tension-type headache patients, particularly in those who engage in analgesic abuse.[15]

Additional basic scientific research is necessary to more accurately clarify the mechanism underlying both episodic and chronic tension-type headaches. This information is essential for the design and tailoring of effective treatments for the millions of patients who continue to suffer from episodic and chronic tension-type headaches.

Evaluation and Diagnosis

A thorough history and physical examination should be undertaken for the evaluation of headache. The history should include appropriate exploration of secondary causes of headache, including depression, medication (prescription and over-the-counter [OTC]), substance abuse, and neurological disorders. It is essential that the provider determine whether the headaches are episodic or chronic because the clinical management will differ accordingly.

The physical examination should include a comprehensive neurologic evaluation that includes observation for cranial nerve defects, cerebellar dysfunction, papilledema, absence of venous pulsation on fundoscopic examination, visual-field defects, and motor and sensory deficits. Abnormal findings could indicate intracranial irregularitis, and appropriate diagnostic studies should be performed before a definitive diagnosis of tension-type headache is made. The following recommendations were proposed as diagnostic criteria for neuroimaging: focal neurologic finding on physical examination, headache starting after exertion or Valsalva's maneuver, acute onset of severe headache, headache awakens patient at night, change in well-established headache pattern, new-onset headache in a patient older than 35 years, and new-onset headache in a patient who has human immunodeficiency virus infection or a previously diagnosed cancer.[16]

Careful palpation of the head in a patient with tension-type headache often reveals tenderness in the pericranial muscles, the occipital region, and the trapezius. Palpation of the temporomandibular joint should also be performed, as this joint is often involved in the development of headaches.

PRIMARY DIAGNOSTIC CRITERIA FOR TENSION-TYPE HEADACHE

1. Headache features at least two of the following characteristics:
   - Bilateral pain
   - Pressure
   - Mild to moderate pain
   - No increase in pain on physical exertion
2. *And* no more than one of the following:
   - Sensitivity to light
   - Sensitivity to sound
3. *And* neither of the following*:
   - Nausea
   - Vomiting
4. *And* a duration of 30 minutes to 7 days

Subdivision Diagnosis

Episodic (<15 days/mo) *or* chronic (>15 days/mo for >6 mo)
2. Associated *or* not associated with coexisting pericranial muscle tenderness[†]

Adapted from the Headache Classification Committee of the International Headache Society.
Classification and diagnostic criteria for headache disorders, cranial neuralgia and facial pain, *Cephalgia* 8 (Supp 7):29–34, 1988.
*Chronic tension-type headache may include one of these symptoms.
[†]Diagnosed on the basis of manual palpation or electromyographic studies.

Treatment

Over-the-counter and prescription medications. Tension-type headaches are most commonly self-treated with OTC analgesics. Research has confirmed the effectiveness of both ibuprofen and acetaminophen. However, a large randomized, controlled trial revealed that ibuprofen was superior to acetaminophen in relieving headache pain. The study assigned patients with tension-type headache to receive a single-dose treatment consisting of placebo, 400 mg of ibuprofen, or 1000 mg of acetaminophen. Participants taking ibuprofen achieved pain relief faster than did those taking acetaminophen or placebo, and more participants taking ibuprofen experienced complete relief of headache than did those taking placebo or acetaminophen.[18]

Careful inquiry should be made regarding the frequency of OTC analgesic use. The use of pain relievers more than twice weekly places the patient at risk for chronic daily headache. Analgesics can be augmented with a sedating antihistamine such as promethazine or diphenhydramine, or an antiemetic such as metoclopramide. Analgesics combined with butalbital or opiates can be useful in relieving tension-type pain, but all of these options carry an increased risk of causing chronic daily headache.[19]

Drug and behavioral treatments are effective in relieving episodic tension-type headache but are only moderately effective in the treatment of chronic tension-type headache.[20] Although the best evidence supports the use of analgesia plus amitriptyline,[21] other antidepressant medications may be equally effective. Amitriptyline, at doses ranging from 10 to 75 mg 1 hour before bedtime, is the most researched of the prophylactic agents used for chronic tension-type headache. Double-blind, randomized, controlled studies have demonstrated a reduction in both frequency and severity of headaches.[22,23] The side effects (dry mouth, orthostasis, weight gain) can lead to nonadherence to therapy in some patients. To minimize side effects, patients should start with a dose of 10 mg before bedtime and increase gradually, if necessary.

Selective serotonin-reuptake inhibitors have fewer side effects than the tricyclic antidepressants, making them a treatment option for some patients. Both paroxetine and fluoxetine have demonstrated efficacy in the prophylaxis of chronic tension-type headache in small studies.[24,25] A comparative trial showed that amitriptyline and fluoxetine were equally effective in reducing the number of days with headache pain each month[25]; however, other studies have shown that fluoxetine has a slower onset of action. Fluoxetine should be started at 10 mg/day and gradually increased if necessary.

In addition to relieving the symptoms of depression, substances that modulate both the serotonin and norepinephrine pathways can be helpful to patients with pain. Both serotonin and norepinephrine neural circuits directly modulate the descending pathways and are an integral part of the complex system that controls pain perception.[26] Amytriptyline may be especially effective in chronic pain conditions because of its ability to affect both serotonin and norepinephrine at low doses. Other medications that inhibit serotonin and norepinephrine reuptake may prove useful in patients with chronic pain and in those with the dual diagnosis of pain and depression. Preliminary data suggest that venlafaxine is effective in the prophylaxis of both migraine and chronic tension-type headaches,[27] although a rigorous clinical trial is needed.

When antidepressant medication is prescribed to a patient with chronic tension-type headache, the practitioner should explain the rationale for the use of such drugs, especially in the patient without depression. A patient may believe that the physician thinks the pain is completely psychogenic. Explaining that the chemicals involved in pain and depression are similar and reassuring the patient that you know the pain is real will go a long way toward cementing a solid relationship between provider and patient and increasing the likelihood of adherence with therapy.

Botanical medicine

Willow bark. The best known of the botanical remedies for the treatment of headache is willow (Figure 9-1). The Greek physician Hippocrates prescribed the bitter powdered bark to alleviate headache, relieve labor pains, and reduce fever. Native Americans regularly used willow to treat fever and pain. The Rev. Edmund Stone reported the first study of willow in 1763 after he successfully treated 50 parishioners afflicted with rheumatic fever.[29] In 1829, Henri Leroux, a French pharmacist, isolated salicin, a precursor that can be metabolized to salicylic acid. In 1860, Kolbe and Lautemann synthesized salicylic acid. From 1860 to 1898, salicylic acid was widely used as a medicine; however, the acid burned the mouth. Sodium was added to form sodium salicylate, which still tasted horrible but did not cause the burning sensation imparted by salicylic acid. Meanwhile, Swiss pharmacist Johann Pagenstecher distilled meadowsweet flowers (*Spiraea salicifolia*) and obtained and characterized a substance called salicylaldehyde. Hoffman, a chemist working for Bayer pharmaceutical company, was dissatisfied with the stomach distress experienced by his arthritic father while taking sodium salicylate. In an effort to find a less unpleasant

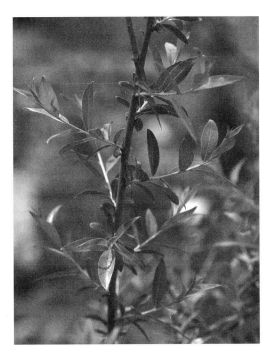

Figure **9-1 Willow bark.** (*Courtesy Martin Wall Botanical Services.*)

way to administer salicylic acid, Hoffman reinvestigated the acetylation reaction first conducted by the French chemist Gerhardt in 1853. He found that acetylsalicylic acid worked as effectively as sodium salicylate but that it was much gentler on the stomach. The synthetic material, called aspirin ("a" for the acetyl group and "spirin" for the botanical genus *Spiraea,* or meadowsweet) was shown to have the desirable properties of salicylic acid but lacked the strong acidity and the unpleasant taste of its sodium salt. Aspirin remains one of the most effective OTC analgesics available.

No current clinical trials have been conducted to evaluate the effectiveness of willow bark in the treatment of tension-type headache, although two randomized, double-blind, placebo-controlled studies have shown that willow bark extract (standardized to provide 240 mg/day salicin) is effective in the treatment of lower back pain[29] and osteoarthritis.[30] Some data suggest that willow bark, taken in the dosages used in clinical trials, does not adversely affect the stomach mucosa.[31]

Controversy continues regarding the effect of willow bark on platelet aggregation. A recent clinical trial revealed that the herb does not significantly affect platelets compared with aspirin. Thirty-five patients with chronic lower back pain were given willow bark extract (240 mg/day salicin) or placebo in a randomized, double-blind trial. Another 16 patients with stable chronic ischemic heart disease were given 100 mg/day acetylsalicylic acid. The mean maximal arachidonic acid–induced platelet aggregation was 61% for willow, 78% for placebo, and 13% for acetylsalicylic acid. Acetylsalicylic acid had a significant inhibitory effect on platelet aggregation compared with willow bark extract ($P = 0.001$). Daily consumption of willow bark extract (240 mg/day salicin) has only a small inhibitory effect on platelets.[32]

Depending on the time of harvest and species, total salicylates in willow bark range from 1.5% to 11%.[33] This means that a 1000-mg dose of willow bark may contain anywhere from 15 to 110 mg of salicylates. Because of this variation, standardized products are highly recommended. Both the German Commission E and the *British Herbal Compendium* list headache as an indication for the administration of willow bark.

Lavender (Lavandula angustifolia). Lavender flower has a long history of use as a sedative, antispasmodic, digestive aid, and treatment for depression, nervousness, and headache. German health authorities endorse the use of lavender for the treatment of restlessness and difficulty sleeping. Lavender is often combined with other herbs for the relief of tension-type headache. Research information for lavender in this arena is scarce. Lavender essential oil has been shown to enhance sleep in geriatric nursing patients.[34] The use of lavender in aromatherapy for headaches is also a common practice and quite safe. Patients are instructed to place 3 or 4 drops of lavender essential oil in one cup of cold water and apply to the forehead for 10 to 15 minutes.

Peppermint (Mentha piperitax). Research has shown that 10% peppermint oil in ethanol applied to the forehead and temples compares favorably with acetaminophen in terms of its ability to relieve headache symptoms.[35]

Scullcap (Scutellaria lateriflora). Scullcap is found in many herbal formulations for headache relief. It was officially recognized as a tranquilizer in the *United States Pharmacopoeia* until 1916. In addition to its tranquilizing effects, early herbalists believed that it could be used to treat convulsions, uterine spasms, and rabies. Today, herbalists use scullcap in combination with other herbs for the treatment of insomnia, headache, stress, and tension. It is generally considered a "nervine tonic/relaxant." Virtually no scientific data exist for the evaluation of *S. lateriflora.* However, a related Asian species, *S. baicalensis,* has documented antiinflammatory activity, which may provide some biological plausibility for the effect reported with *S. lateriflora.*

Valerian (Valeriana officinalis). Valerian has been used for at least 10 centuries as a calmative and sedative. It was listed as a tranquilizer in the *United States Pharmacopoeia* from 1820 to 1942. Valerian is an effective, non–habit-forming anxiolytic[36] and is useful for the treatment of insomnia.[37] Valerian is often included in herbal formulations as a relaxant for those with headaches caused by stress.

Wood betony (Stachys officinalis). Herbalists have valued the well-known European garden betony for its sedative and astringent properties for centuries. Virtually no research has been conducted on this herb. Betony does contain roughly 15% tannin, which would explain its historical use in the treatment of diarrhea. The glycosides present in the plant are thought to provide some basis for its nervine properties. Because of its high tannin content, caution should be exercised with large doses or prolonged use.

Dietary supplements

Magnesium. Since approximately 70% of patients with tension-type headaches exhibit muscle tightness and tenderness, it is possible that problems in magnesium metabolism, dietary intake, or both are linked to concomitant muscle tension and tension-type headache.[38] Platelet levels of ionized magnesium in patients with tension-type headaches have been found to be significantly lower than those in healthy controls.[39] Open trials have demonstrated that 1 g of intravenous magnesium sulfate can relieve the pain of migraine and chronic tension-type headaches.[40] A recent randomized study found intravenous administration of magnesium sulfate effective in completely or partially relieving pain in 56% of patients with acute headache in the emergency-department setting; however, prochlorperazine completely or partially relieved pain in 90% of patients in the same setting, with fewer side effects.[41]

Research in this area should be focused on oral administration of magnesium for both prevention and treatment of tension-type headache, given the fact that the supplement is readily available and inexpensive and has a reasonably good safety profile.

SAMe. S-adenosyl-L-methionine (SAMe; pronounced "sammy") is an amino acid that is manufactured in the brain from the amino acid methionine. SAMe is the most active methyl donor in the body. Supplementation with SAMe increases levels of serotonin, dopamine, and phosphatides and improves serotonin and dopamine receptor site binding.[42] Research indicates that SAMe is beneficial for those with depression and osteoarthritis. Although no studies address the efficacy of SAMe for patients with chronic headache, it may be beneficial given its effect on neurotransmitter levels.

Mind/body interventions. Over the past three decades, mind/body interventions (chiefly relaxation, biofeedback, and stress management) have become standard components of the management of migraine and tension-type headaches. Meta-analytic literature reviews of these interventions have consistently identified clinically significant reductions in recurrent headache. Across studies, these interventions have yielded reductions of approximately 35% to 50% in migraine and tension-type headaches. Although we have only recently begun to directly compare standard drug and nondrug treatments for headache, the available evidence suggests that the level of headache improvement with mind/body interventions rivals that obtained with widely used pharmacologic therapies in representative patient samples.[43]

Spinal manual therapy. Many people seek chiropractic care for the treatment of chronic tension-type headaches and many claim that it is helpful. A recent systematic review of eight randomized trials involving spinal manipulation for the treatment of headaches failed to find evidence of benefit. Three studies examined tension-type headaches, three migraine headaches, one "cervicogenic" headache, and one "spondylogenic" chronic headache. In two studies, patients undergoing spinal manipulation showed comparable improvement in migraine and tension headaches compared with the relief obtained through drug treatment; however, most of the trials had considerable methodologic limitations— primarily inadequate control for nonspecific (placebo) effects. The authors concluded, "Despite claims that spinal manipulation is an effective treatment for headache, the data available to date do not support such definitive conclusions. It is unclear to what extent the observed treatment effects can be explained by manipulation or by nonspecific factors (e.g., of personal attention, patient expectation). Whether manipulation produces any long-term changes in these conditions is also uncertain. Future studies should address these two crucial questions and overcome the methodological limitations of previous trials."[44]

Massage therapy.   Therapeutic massage is used by many patients to obtain relief from chronic pain. Two studies have demonstrated beneficial effects of massage in patients with chronic tension-type headaches.[45,46] A special form of massage, neuromuscular therapy, may be particularly beneficial in patients with pericervical muscle tenderness.

Trigger point therapy.   Trigger points are discrete focal hyperirritable points located in taut bands of fascia and skeletal muscle. Early work on trigger points and trigger point therapy was performed by Dr. Janet Travell, a private personal physician to President John F. Kennedy. Trigger points, which produce both localized and referred pain, are often found in patients with chronic musculoskeletal pain. Trigger points may also manifest as tension headache, temporomandibular joint pain, and low back pain. Palpation of a hypersensitive bundle or nodule of muscle fiber of harder-than-normal consistency is the physical finding typically associated with a trigger point. Palpation of the trigger point elicits pain directly over the affected area, causes radiation of pain toward a zone of reference and a local twitch response, or both. Various modalities such as the "spray and stretch" technique, ultrasonography, manipulative therapy, and injection are used to deactivate trigger points. Trigger point injection has been shown to be one of the most effective treatment modalities to deactivate trigger points and provide prompt relief of symptoms.[47]

Trigger point injection therapy is often used in chronic myofascial pain syndromes.[48] Researchers have demonstrated that a 1:3 mixture of 1% lidocaine with water causes less pain on injection and is more effective than unaltered 1% lidocaine in treating chronic myofascial pain syndromes.[49] Lidocaine and mepivacaine are suitable local anesthetics, and a water-diluted concentration of 0.2% to 0.25% is considered most effective.[50]

References

1. Rasmussen BK, Jensen R, Schroll M, et al: Epidemiology of headache in a general population: a prevalence study, *J Clin Epidemiol* 44:1147-1157, 1991.
2. Rasmussen BK, Jensen R, Olesen J: Impact of headache on sickness absence and utilisation of medical services: a Danish population study, *J Epidemiol Community Health* 46:443-446, 1992.
3. Jensen R, Bendtsen L, Olesen J: Muscular factors are of importance in tension-type headache, *Headache* 38:10-17, 1998.
4. Sakai F, Ebihara S, Akiyama M, et al: Pericranial muscle hardness in tension-type headache, *Brain* 118:523-531, 1995.
5. Vandenheede M, Schoenen J: Central mechanisms in tension-type headaches, *Curr Pain Headache Rep* 6:392-400, October 2002.

6. Woolf CJ, Doubell TP: The pathophysiology of chronic pain—increased sensitivity to low threshold A beta-fibre inputs, *Curr Opin Neurobiol* 4:525-534, 1994.
7. Bendtsen L, Jensen R, Olesen J: Qualitatively altered nociception in chronic myofascial pain, *Pain* 65:259-264, 1996.
8. Meller ST, Gebhart GF: Nitric oxide (NO) and nociceptive processing in the spinal cord, *Pain* 52:127-136, 1993.
9. Haley JE, Dickenson AH, Schachter M: Electrophysiological evidence for a role of nitric oxide in prolonged chemical nociception in the rat, *Neuropharmacology* 31:251-258, 1992.
10. Mao J, Price DD, Zhu J, et al: The inhibition of nitric oxide–activated poly(ADP-ribose) synthetase attenuates trans-synaptic alteration of spinal cord dorsal horn neurons and neuropathic pain in the rat, *Pain* 72:355-366, 1997.
11. Ashina M, Lassen LH, Bendtsen L, et al: Inhibition of nitric oxide synthase has an analgesic effect in chronic pain, *Lancet* 353:287-289, 1999.
12. Ashina M, Bendtsen L, Jensen R, et al: Possible mechanisms of action of nitric oxide synthase inhibitors in chronic tension-type headache, *Brain* 122(pt 9):1629-1635, 1999.
13. Bendtsen L: Sensitization: its role in primary headache, *Curr Opin Invest Drug* 3:449-453, 2002.
14. Bendtsen L, Jensen R: Amitriptyline reduces myofascial tenderness in patients with chronic tension-type headache, *Cephalalgia* 20:603-610, 2002.
15. Sarchielli P, Alberti A, Floridi A, et al: L-Arginine/nitric oxide pathway in chronic tension-type headache: relation with serotonin content and secretion and glutamate content, *J Neurol Sci* 198(1-2):9-15, 2002.
16. Masdeu JC, Drayer BP, Anderson RE, et al: Atraumatic isolated headache—when to image. American College of Radiology appropriateness criteria, *Radiology* 215(suppl):487-493, 2000.
17. Headache Classification Committee of the International Headache Society: Classification and diagnostic criteria for headache disorders, cranial neuralgias and facial pain, *Cephalalgia* 8(suppl 7):29-34, 1988.
18. Schachtel BP, Furey SA, Thoden WR: Nonprescription ibuprofen and acetaminophen in the treatment of tension-type headache, *J Clin Pharmacol* 36:1120-1125, 1996.
19. Millea PJ, Brodie JJ: Tension-type headache, *Am Fam Phys* 66:797-804, 2002.
20. Holroyd KA: Behavioral and psychologic aspects of the pathophysiology and management of tension-type headache, *Curr Pain Headache Rep* 6:401-407, 2002.
21. Mathew NT, Bendtsen L: Prophylactic pharmacotherapy of tension-type headache. In Olesen J, Tfelt-Hansen P, Welch KM, editors: *The Headaches*, ed 2, Philadelphia, 2000, Lippincott, Williams & Wilkins, pp 667-673.
22. Moller HJ, Glaser K, Leverkus F, et al: Double-blind, multicenter comparative study of sertraline versus amitriptyline in outpatients with major depression, *Pharmacopsychiatry* 33:206-212, 2000.
23. Gobel H, Hamouz V, Hansen C, et al: Chronic tension-type headache: amitriptyline reduces clinical headache duration and experimental pain sensitivity but does not alter pericranial muscle activity readings, *Pain* 59:241-249, 1994.
24. Langemark M, Olesen J: Sulpiride and paroxetine in the treatment of chronic tension-type headache: an explanatory double-blind trial, *Headache* 34:20-24, 1994.
25. Oguzhanoglu A, Sahiner T, Kurt T, et al: Use of amitriptyline and fluoxetine in prophylaxis of migraine and tension-type headaches, *Cephalalgia* 9:531-532, 1999.
26. Gallagher RM, Verma S: Managing pain and comorbid depression: a public health challenge, *Semin Clin Neuropsychiatry* 4:203-220, 1999.
27. Adelman LC, Adelman JU, Von Seggern R, et al: Venlafaxine extended release (XR) for the prophylaxis of migraine and tension-type headache: a retrospective study in a clinical setting, *Headache* 40:572-580, 2000.
28. Stone E: On the success of the bark of the willow in the cure of agues, *Phil Trans* 195-200, 1763.
29. Chrubasik S, Kunzel O, Model A, et al: Treatment of low back pain with a herbal or synthetic anti-rheumatic: a randomized controlled study. Willow bark extract for low back pain, *Rheumatology* 40:1388-1393, 2001.
30. Schmid B, Ludtke R, Selbmann HK, et al: Efficacy and tolerability of a standardized willow bark extract in patients with osteoarthritis: randomized placebo-controlled, double blind clinical trial, *Phytother Res* 15:344-350, 2001.

31. Marz RW, Kemper F: Willow bark extract—effects and effectiveness. Status of current knowledge regarding pharmacology, toxicology and clinical aspects. *Wien Med Wochenschr* 152 (15-16):354-359, 2002.
32. Krivoy N, Pavlotzky E, Chrubasik S, et al: Effect of salicis cortex extract on human platelet aggregation. *Planta Med* 67:209-212, 2001.
33. Wichtl M, Bisset N: *Herbal drugs and phytopharmaceuticals: a handbook for practice on a scientific basis,* Stuttgart, Germany, 1994, Medpharm Scientific Publishers.
34. Hardy M, Kirk-Smith MD, Stretch DD: Replacement of drug treatment for insomnia by ambient odour, *Lancet* 346:701, 1995 [letter].
35. Gobel H, Fresenius J, Heinze A, et al: Effectiveness of Oleum menthae piperitae and paracetamol in therapy of headache of the tension type, *Nervenarzt* 67:672-681, 1996.
36. Andreatini R, Sartori VA, Seabra ML, et al: Effect of valepotriates (valerian extract) in generalized anxiety disorder: a randomized placebo-controlled pilot study, *Phytother Res* 16:650-654, 2002.
37. Wheatley D: Stress-induced insomnia treated with kava and valerian: singly and in combination, *Hum Psychopharmacol* 16:353-356, 2001.
38. Altura BM, Altura BT: Tension headaches and muscle tension: is there a role for magnesium? *Med Hypotheses* 57:705-713, 2001.
39. Mishima K, Takeshima T, Shimomura T, et al: Platelet ionized magnesium, cyclic AMP, and cyclic GMP levels in migraine and tension-type headache, *Headache* 37:561-564, 1997.
40. Mauskop A, Altura BT, Cracco RQ, et al: Intravenous magnesium sulfate rapidly alleviates headaches of various types, *Headache* 36:154-160, 1996.
41. Ginder S, Oatman B, Pollack M: A prospective study of i.v. magnesium and i.v. prochlorperazine in the treatment of headaches, *J Emerg Med* 18:311-315, 2000.
42. Baldessarini RJ: Neuropharmacy of S-adenosyl methionine, *Am J Med* 83:95-103, 1983.
43. Penzien DB, Rains JC, Andrasik F: Behavioral management of recurrent headache: three decades of experience and empiricism, *Appl Psychophysiol Biofeedback* 27:163-181, 2002.
44. Astin JA, Ernst E: The effectiveness of spinal manipulation for the treatment of headache disorders: a systematic review of randomized clinical trials, *Cephalalgia* 22:617-623, 2002.
45. Quinn C, Chandler C, Moraska A: Massage therapy and frequency of chronic tension headaches, *Am J Public Health* 92:1657-1661, 2002.
46. Puustjarvi K, Airaksinen O, Pontinen PJ: The effects of massage in patients with chronic tension headache, *Acupunct Electrother Res* 15:159-162, 1990.
47. Alvarez DJ, Rockwell PG: Trigger points: diagnosis and management, *Am Fam Phys* 65:653-660, 2002.
48. Criscuolo CM: Interventional approaches to the management of myofascial pain syndrome, *Curr Pain Headache Rep* 5:407-411, 2001.
49. Iwama H, Akama Y: The superiority of water-diluted 0.25% to neat 1% lidocaine for trigger-point injections in myofascial pain syndrome: a prospective, randomized, double-blinded trial, *Anesth Analg* 91:408-409, 2000.
50. Iwama H, Ohmori S, Kaneko T, et al: Water-diluted local anesthetic for trigger-point injection in chronic myofascial pain syndrome: evaluation of types of local anesthetic and concentrations in water, *Reg Anesth Pain Med* 26:333-336, 2001.

Migraine Headaches

Migraine is a common, painful headache disorder that affects at least 10% of the general population. Migraine is more common in women than in men. The American Migraine Study II reported that 20.9 million women and 6.9 million men suffer from severe headaches.[1] Prevalence varies with age: Migraines typically begin in childhood or adolescence and are most prevalent in young and middle-aged adults; the incidence of migraine generally declines after the fifth decade of life.[2] In women, menstrual migraines begin at menarche, abate during pregnancy, and continue through menopause.[3] Roughly half of all individuals who experience migraines consult a physician, and migraines are correctly diagnosed in about 50% of these patients. The remaining patients are often prescribed ineffective therapies, with many relying on over-the-counter medications.[4] Chronic daily headache (CDH), which can be a consequence of poor migraine management, remains a significant cause of morbidity.[5]

CLASSIFICATION OF MIGRAINE HEADACHE

Migraine pain is typically described as throbbing, aching, stabbing, or burning. The pain is generally unilateral but may be bilateral, appearing suddenly and escalating rapidly. Head pain may last hours to days if not treated and may be accompanied by nausea, anorexia, abdominal discomfort, visual disturbances (e.g., flashing lights, spots), visual field defects (e.g., homonymous hemianopsia), fatigue, numbness, or tingling. The majority of patients report being fatigued or "wiped out" after a migraine.

Migraine headaches are classified on the basis of criteria established by the International Headache Society (IHS). The IHS diagnostic criteria for migraine without and with aura are outlined in Box 10-1.

Migraine without aura usually presents with one-sided, throbbing pain of moderate to severe intensity. Nausea and sensitivity to noise and light are generally reported, and episodes last as long as 72 hours. Most patients find that physical activity intensifies the pain.

Patients who have migraine with aura may experience visual auras (the most common symptom), parasthesias, paresis, and dysphasia. Auras are localized to the brainstem or cerebral cortex and may last as long as 60 minutes. An aura is typically followed by pain.

157

Box 10-1

Migraine headaches

MIGRAINE WITHOUT AURA

1. At least five attacks
2. Attack duration 4 to 72 hours
3. At least two of the following characteristics:
   - Unilateral location
   - Pulsating quality
   - Moderate or severe intensity (hinders daily activities)
   - Aggravated by routine physical activity
4. During headache, at least one of the following:
   - Nausea, with or without vomiting
   - Photophobia and phonophobia

MIGRAINE WITH AURA

1. At least two attacks satisfying all of the following characteristics:
   - One or more fully reversible aura symptoms
   - At least one aura symptom lasting 4 minutes, or two or more symptoms in succession
   - Aura less than 60 minutes; if more than one aura, duration increases proportionately
2. Headache onset follows aura within 60 minutes

In rare cases, an aura may be experienced without a subsequent headache, or it may be experienced concurrently with migraine pain.

PATHOGENESIS OF MIGRAINE

Migraine is a heterogeneous condition in which headaches vary in frequency, duration, symptom presentation, and degree of disability, both between patients and in the same patient between attacks. The cause of migraine has been hotly debated over the years: Is it vascular, muscular, biochemical, neuronal, or a combination thereof?

The vascular theory suggests that vasoconstriction is followed by vasodilation, aura, and finally, throbbing headache. Blood vessels in the cerebellum and meninges expand and contract at various rates, depending on blood-flow changes.[6] Small blood vessels are dramatically stretched during these spasms, resulting in throbbing pain. A limitation of this theory, however, is that these changes in blood flow are neither correlated with headache intensity nor exclusive to migraine.

Although it is well known that muscle tension and contraction occur in tension-type headaches, electromyographic studies demonstrate greater muscle contraction in the patient with migraine; hence the muscular theory.[7]

The biochemical theory, also known as the cervicotrigeminovascular hypothesis, holds that migraine headaches are triggered by a decrease in the level of serotonin in the brain.

Serotonin receptors on the trigeminal nerve inhibit the release of substance P. When the serotonin level decreases, the release of substance P is enhanced, thereby triggering vasodilation, local inflammation, and pain. It is thought that the trigeminal neurons spontaneously fire with the depolarization of the ophthalmic branch of this nerve. Substance P, a neurotransmitter, is then released, causing vasodilation and increased permeability. This leads to local inflammation and edema, which results in the unilateral frontal pain of a migraine. This models holds that neurogenic inflammation and vasoconstriction are the two major factors in the development of a migraine.

Menstrual Migraine

The precise definition of *menstrual migraine* remains a matter of controversy, and debate over what exactly constitutes the diagnosis continues.[8] The IHS does not distinguish menstrual migraine as a separate entity from migraine without aura.[9] However, most physicians and researchers agree that menstrual migraine is a migraine headache that occurs regularly each month but only between the second day before the menses and the end of menstruation. Menstrual migraine is believed to occur in approximately 14% of women. Menstrual migraine is thought to result from declining estrogen levels and interactions between estrogen and other biochemicals.[10] Estrogen and progesterone have potent effects on central serotonergic and opioid neurons, modulating both neuronal activity and receptor density. One hypothesis holds that the decrease in estrogen during the late luteal phase makes the blood vessels more susceptible to compounds associated with migraines such as serotonin, substance P, norepinephrine, dopamine, endorphins, prolactin, and progesterone.[11]

From 1971 through 1994, 32 articles on menstrual migraine were published; however, the definition of menstrual migraine varied among these studies with respect to the timing and type of attacks.[10] Researchers have investigated the effectiveness of extended-duration oral contraceptives to prevent fluctuations in estrogen. Although research clearly shows that only a few women experience relief with this regimen, women who experience menstrual migraines and are taking oral contraceptives may achieve a reduction in the number of attacks by changing to a low-dose monophasic oral contraceptive with an extended-duration regimen. Other treatments that have been studied include transdermal estrogen patches, which failed to show benefit[12,13]; two small open studies of tamoxifen, which showed benefit[14,15]; an open nonrandomized study with danazol, which showed benefit in women older than 40 years[16]; and leuprolide (with add-back hormone therapy) in an open study of 5 women, which indicated beneficial effects.[17] Frovatriptan, 5 mg twice daily on the first dosing day, followed by 2.5 mg twice daily for 5 more days, has been shown to prevent menstrual migraine in 50% of women, compared with 26% of women given placebo when the treatment was started 2 days before the anticipated start of menstrual migraines.[18] Naratriptan, 1 mg twice daily, taken 3 days before the anticipated start of the menstrual migraine and continued for 6 days, has also been found superior to placebo.[19]

TREATMENT

Once the diagnosis of migraine has been made, a thorough history of the illness must be gathered, including past treatments the patient has tried, frequency of headache, impact on quality of life, and the identification/elimination of any known triggers. A comprehensive headache treatment plan should include treatments for acute migraine attacks and long-term preventive therapy to reduce attack frequency, severity, and duration.

Studies demonstrate that acetaminophen, aspirin, ibuprofen, and an aspirin-acetaminophen-caffeine combination are more effective than placebo in reducing moderate or severe migraine pain to mild or no pain 2 hours after administration in patients who experience vomiting or severe disability with their migraines.[20]

Triptans are relatively safe and effective medications for the treatment of acute migraine. The differences among them are generally minor. Considerations in selecting a triptan include individual patient response/tolerance, characteristics of the patient's attacks, relief of associated symptoms, consistency of response, headache recurrence, delivery systems, and patient preference.[21]

In both well-controlled single-episode studies and long-term multiple-episode studies, sumatriptan nasal spray has been effective and well tolerated in the short-term treatment of migraine in children and adolescents. Except for its unpleasant taste, sumatriptan nasal spray has a tolerability profile similar to that of placebo in young patients.[22]

Lifestyle Modification

Many people who experience migraines can identify triggers for the headaches. One hundred patients who fulfilled the diagnostic criteria for migraine without aura were evaluated through the use of a personal interview. Stress was the most frequently cited trigger, causing migraine in 76% of patients. Stress was followed, in descending order of frequency, by sensory stimuli (75%), sleep deprivation (49%), hunger (48%), environmental factors (47%), food (46%), menses (39%), fatigue (35%), alcohol (28%), sleep excess (27%), caffeine (22%), physical exertion (20%), head trauma (20%), travel (4%), sexual activity (3%), medication (2%), neck movement (2%), smoking (1%), and the use of a low-profile pillow (1%).[23] A headache diary may help identify triggers, allowing practitioners and patients to develop a strategy for reducing the frequency of acute attacks.

Many factors can affect serotonin levels, including food allergies or sensitivities, certain drugs, fluctuating hormone levels, anxiety, and certain dietary deficiencies. As the serotonin level increases, the incidence of headaches usually decreases. The diminishing number of postsynaptic serotonin receptors that accompanies the normal aging process partly explains the reduction of migraine frequency that occurs with age.[24]

The list of foods, beverages, and additives that have been reported to trigger migraines includes cheese, chocolate, citrus fruits, hot dogs, monosodium glutamate, aspartame, fatty foods, ice cream, and alcoholic drinks (especially red wine and beer), as well as caffeine withdrawal. Tyramine, phenylethylamine, histamine, nitrites, and sulfites affect phases of the migraine process by influencing the release of serotonin and norepinephrine, causing vasoconstriction or vasodilation, or by directly stimulating the trigeminal ganglia, the brainstem, and cortical neuronal pathways.[25] Patients should be informed of the most common food triggers and asked to keep a diary of acute attacks and their relation to any identifiable trigger.

Because stress has been cited as the most common precipitating factor, practitioners must help patients explore ways of managing or coping with stressful situations. A considerable body of evidence indicates that several mind/body therapies are effective in the treatment of headaches in adults[26] and that psychological treatments—mainly relaxation and cognitive behavioral therapy—are effective in reducing the severity and frequency of chronic headache among children and adolescents.[27] Although cognitive behavioral therapy has a great deal to offer individuals who experience recurrent headaches, issues surrounding cost and access are considerable in some populations. Many communities now offer classes in yoga, tai chi, relaxation, and fitness, and books written for the consumer provide tips for managing stress. Practitioners would be wise to familiarize themselves with community resources and steer patients toward such self-care initiatives when possible.

Dietary Supplements

Magnesium. Research has been focused on the role of magnesium in the pathogenesis of migraine. A low magnesium level may cause brain hyperexcitability by opening calcium channels, leading to increased intracellular calcium levels, glutamate release, and extracellular potassium levels, which may in turn trigger the cortical spreading depression seen with migraine.[28] A randomized, double-blind, placebo-controlled study was conducted to assess the efficacy of magnesium sulfate in patients with migraine with and without aura. Sixty patients in each group were randomly assigned to receive 1 g of intravenous magnesium sulfate or 0.9% physiologic saline solution. Seven parameters of analgesic evaluation and an analog scale for the assessment of nausea, photophobia, and phonophobia were used. No statistically significant difference in pain relief or nausea was seen in the migraine-without-aura group between patients who received magnesium sulfate and those who were given placebo; however, the intensity of photophobia and phonophobia was significantly lower. The migraine-with-aura group patients given magnesium sulfate had a statistically significant improvement in pain and all associated symptoms compared with that of controls.[29] The findings of this study are consistent with those of a smaller trial involving 30 patients with acute migraine in which 1 g of intravenous magnesium was an effective treatment for the relief of pain and associated symptoms.[30]

The evidence for magnesium supplementation as a prophylactic agent is contradictory. A 12-week double-blind, placebo-controlled study of 81 patients, ranging in age from 18 to 65 years, with migraine (mean attack frequency 3.6 headaches per month) showed that 600 mg/day oral magnesium dicitrate (24 mmol/day) was superior to placebo in reducing the frequency of migraine attacks. During weeks 9 through 12, the attack frequency was reduced by 42% in the magnesium group and by 16% in the placebo group compared with baseline ($P < 0.05$). The number of days with migraine and drug consumption for symptomatic treatment per patient also decreased significantly in the magnesium group. Diarrhea (19%) and gastric irritation (5%) were reported in the active treatment group.[31]

This study is in contrast to a randomized, placebo-controlled study of 69 patients with two to six migraines per month without aura and a history of migraine of at least 2 years that studied magnesium as a prophylactic agent. A 4-week baseline period without medication was followed by 12 weeks of treatment with magnesium aspartate (10 mmol twice daily) or placebo. The primary efficacy end point was a reduction of at least 50% in intensity or duration of migraine attacks in hours at the end of the 12 weeks of treatment compared with baseline. Of the participants in the study, 35 had received magnesium and 34 had received placebo. The number of responders was 10 in each group. Magnesium demonstrated no advantage over placebo with regard to the number of migraine attacks or migraine days. With respect to tolerability and safety, 46% of patients in the magnesium group reported primarily mild adverse events (e.g., soft stool, diarrhea), in contrast to 24% of the placebo group. The study was discontinued before its completion because researchers were not able to identify any benefit of magnesium.[32] It is unclear whether benefit would have occurred had the trial been continued for the full 12 weeks; the other preventive study found a strongly statistically significant difference between magnesium and placebo during weeks 9 through 12. The two studies also differed with regard to dose (the first study used more than double the dose) and magnesium preparation.

Until larger research trials are conducted to more adequately determine efficacy, optimal dose, and dosage form, some practitioners feel that given the relative safety and low cost of magnesium, a trial of a magnesium salt at doses of 200 mg twice daily or 400 mg four times daily makes good sense.[33] Some preliminary data suggest that a low magnesium level is related to the development of menstrual migraine,[34] and a 3 month-trial may be warranted in this group as well.

Riboflavin (vitamin B$_2$). Riboflavin is a key player in energy metabolism. Some researchers have postulated that a low level of cellular energy plays a role in migraine pathogenesis.[35] Preliminary studies suggest that riboflavin holds some promise in the prevention of migraines.

The authors of an open pilot study monitored 49 patients with migraine (45 without aura, 4 with) who were treated with 400 mg of riboflavin in a single daily oral dose for at least 3 months. Twenty-three patients also received 75 mg of aspirin each day. Mean global improvement after therapy was 68%, with no difference between the two groups. With the exception of one patient in the riboflavin-plus-aspirin group who withdrew because of gastric intolerance, no drug-related side effects were reported.[36] This clinical trial was followed by a randomized, double-blind, placebo-controlled study of 55 patients with migraine.[37] Riboflavin (400 mg/day) was significantly superior to placebo in reducing attack frequency ($P = 0.005$) and headache days ($P = 0.012$). With regard to headache days, the proportion of patients who experienced at least 50% improvement (i.e., "responders") was 15% for those treated with placebo and 59% for those given riboflavin ($P = 0.002$). Three minor adverse events occurred, two in the riboflavin group (diarrhea and polyuria) and one in the placebo group (abdominal cramps). None were considered serious.

It is obvious that comparative trials should be conducted with riboflavin and other preventive therapies; however, because of its low cost and excellent safety profile, practitioners may wish to consider riboflavin as a prophylactic agent in patients with migraine.

Botanicals

Feverfew (Tanacetum parthenium). Feverfew is the most commonly used and recommended herb for the prevention of migraine. The species name, *parthenium*, is said to have been given by the Greeks after the herb was used to save the life of someone who had fallen from the Parthenon in ancient Greece,[38] although others believe it is a reference to the use of feverfew for the relief of menstrual cramps in young girls (*parthenos* is Greek for "virgin").[39] In addition to being used for a variety of female complaints, the herb was considered beneficial for the treatment of fever (hence its common name), headache, arthritis, and other inflammatory conditions. Most modern research has been directed toward the use of feverfew for migraine prophylaxis and the relief of arthritis.

A systematic review of randomized, placebo-controlled, double-blind trials of feverfew monopreparations for the prevention of migraine in human subjects was published in 2000. Two independent reviewers extracted data in a predefined, standardized fashion and evaluated the methodologic quality of the trials using the Jadad score. To assess safety issues, they also consulted major reference texts. Six trials met the inclusion criteria. Most favored feverfew over placebo for the prevention of migraine.[40]

The authors of a 2002 study that was not included in the aforementioned systematic review employed a feverfew extract manufactured with supercritical CO_2 in a randomized, double-blind, placebo-controlled trial of 147 patients with migraine; 24% ($n = 35$) did not complete the study, for various reasons.[41] A 4-week baseline period without migraine prophylaxis was followed by a 12-week phase of treatment with feverfew extract or placebo. Three doses—2.08 mg (0.17 mg parthenolide), 6.25 mg (0.5 mg parthenolide), and 18.75 mg (1.5 mg parthenolide)—were taken three times a day. The primary outcome measure was the total number of migraine attacks during the last 28 days (weeks 13 to 16). Secondary outcomes included the total and average duration of migraine attacks, the mean duration of a single attack, and additional assessment of overall migraine severity. At the conclusion of the trial, a global assessment of efficacy revealed a "clinically relevant" decrease in the number of migraine attacks in the 6.25-mg group, but only within the sub-group of 49 patients who had reported at least four attacks during the 4-week baseline period. Adverse events were similar in the two groups. This study suggests that feverfew is most appropriate for individuals who experience frequent attacks.

Feverfew probably contains many active ingredients that work through more than one mechanism. Although many authors list parthenolide, a sesquiterpene lactone, as the active constituent, it should be stated that at the time of this writing no principle for the purported efficacy of feverfew in migraine has been identified. Medicinal feverfew contains considerable amounts of parthenolide (0.2% to more than 1% of dry weight), which can make this substance a marker of herb quality but not a guarantee of efficacy.

A 1996 trial by deWeerdt et al that produced negative results[42] involved an ethanolic extract of feverfew containing appropriate levels of the marker compound parthenolide. (The dried pulverized leaf was used in the trials that showed a positive effect on migraine.) It has been suggested that the extract or its method of preparation caused the degradation of potentially active constituents. These researchers suggest that another compound, such as chrysanthenyl acetate, detected in significantly reduced amounts in the extract compared with dried whole-leaf material, may contribute to the antimigraine activity through its inhibitory effect on prostaglandins.[39] However, the mechanism by which fever-few purportedly prevents migraine is unclear at this time.

Experts suggest that because the active constituents are not established, preparations containing whole leaf, fresh or dried, should be used. Feverfew should also be stored in a cool, dry, dark environment to prevent the breakdown of key constituents.[43]

Dosage and preparation. An optimal dosage of feverfew for the prevention of migraine has not been established. Depending on the source, dosages range from 50 to 150 mg/day dried leaf to 2.5 fresh leaves/day taken with food. A randomized study involving CO_2 extracts (not currently available in the United States) showed that a dosage of 6.25 mg thrice daily is most effective. Herbalists in both the United States and United Kingdom often recommend feverfew tincture, usually in combination with other herbs. The one study conducted with an ethanol extract failed to reveal any benefit, and no trials involving combinations have been conducted at this time.

Side effects. Feverfew is generally contraindicated during pregnancy because of its purported emmenagogue activity. Long-term users have reported withdrawal syndrome after abrupt discontinuation of feverfew; symptoms include headache, abdominal pain, diarrhea, fatigue, and joint pain.[44] Mouth ulceration and gastric disturbance occur in a small number of patients.[45] Feverfew inhibits platelet aggregation[46]; however, a study of 10 patients who had taken feverfew for long periods (3.5 to 8 years) revealed that adenosine diphosphate (ADP) and thrombin-stimulated platelet aggregation were no different than those in controls, although serotonin-induced aggregation was reduced.[47] Allergic reactions are possible, especially in individuals who are sensitive to members of the Asteraceae family (e.g., ragweed, marigold, daisy).

Butterbur (Petasites hybridus). Butterbur, a hardy perennial, is found throughout Europe and in parts of Asia and North America. The common names, butterbur and butterdock, refer to the historical practice of wrapping butter in the plant's large leaves during warm weather. The herb was used for the treatment of plague and fever during the Middle Ages and gained popularity during the 17th century for the treatment of respiratory complaints.[48] Today, butterbur is used mainly to prevent migraine and as a remedy for coughs, colds, and allergies. Sesquiterpene esters in butterbur are believed to account for much of its pharmacologic activity. Petasins (petasin, isopetasin, and neopetasin) isolated from extracts of butterbur have been shown to inhibit leukotriene synthesis in leukocytes.[49] The antiinflammatory activity of butterbur may contribute to its purported prophylactic effect in migraine. Animal, in vitro data, and two clinical trials support the use of butterbur as prophylaxis in migraine.

A randomized, placebo-controlled, double-blind clinical study was carried out with a special CO_2 extract from the rhizome of *Petasites hybridus* (Petadolex; Weber & Weber International GmBH & Co. KG-USA, Windermere, Fla.). After a 4-week run-in phase, 60 patients (28 male, 32 female) received butterbur extract (100 mg/day) or placebo for 12 weeks. Outcome variables included frequency, intensity, and duration of migraine attacks, plus accompanying symptoms. Fifty-eight patients completed the trial. One dropped out because of a suspected pregnancy, and another was unwilling to complete the study but gave no reason for withdrawal; both dropouts were in the active-treatment group. After the fourth week of treatment, the Petadolex group had a significant reduction in the number of migraine attacks compared with the placebo group ($P < 0.05$). In the active group, migraine frequency was reduced from 3.4 to 1 by the end of the twelfth week. The placebo group experienced a mean decrease in the frequency of migraine from 2.9 at baseline to 2.6 by the end of the 12-week study. The mean attack frequency per month decreased from 3.4 at baseline to 1.8 after 3 months ($P = 0.0024$) in the active group and from 2.9 to 2.6 in the placebo group. The responder rate (improvement of migraine frequency $\geq 50\%$) was 45% in the verum group and 15% in the placebo group.[50] No adverse events were reported.[51]

The second study enrolled 202 migraine patients (ages 19 to 65 years) who were divided into three groups. Group 1 took 50 mg of butterbur extract twice a day, Group 2 took 75 mg of butterbur extract twice a day, and Group 3 took placebo twice daily for 3 months after completing a "run-in" month without any medication. The primary endpoint, frequency of migraine attacks per 4 weeks, was reduced by 38%, 44%, 58%, and 51% in patients treated with 150 mg/day of Petadolex after 1 (baseline), 2, 3, and

4 months, respectively. The 100-mg/day group had a reduction of 24%, 37%, 42%, and 40%, whereas the placebo group results were 19%, 26%, 26%, and 32%, respectively. Although the treatment differences between those taking 100 mg/day of petasites were not significant compared with placebo, those taking 150 mg/day had a significant reduction in migraine number and intensity over the treatment period compared with those who received the placebo ($P < 0.001$). Adverse events were evenly distributed among all three groups. The most frequently reported adverse event was burping, which was reported by approximately 20% of patients taking the herbal preparation.[52] Other studies suggest benefit in allergic rhinitis[53] and asthma.[54] Low amounts of toxic pyrrolizidine alkaloids, mainly senecionine and intergerrimine, are concentrated in the metabolically active parts of the rhizome. Pyrrolizidine alkaloids are also present in the flower stalks but are almost absent from the leaf buds, petioles, and leaf blades.[55] Pyrrolizidine alkaloid–free extracts are available in the marketplace and should be recommended over crude preparations. Petadolex, the product used in the clinical trials, is a CO_2 extract of the butterbur rhizome (concentrated at a ratio of 28:1 to 44:1) standardized to 15% petasin and isopetasin with pyrrolizidine alkaloids reduced to less than 0.08 ppm in the finished product, which represents the lower limit of detection. Adults and children older than 12 years take 50 mg of the extract two to three times per day.

Documentation of adverse events from 1976 to June 30, 2002, found a total of 75 reports of suspected adverse reactions from Germany and 18 spontaneous reports from other countries received by the manufacturer of Petadolex.[56] Eight adverse reports were determined to be "probably causally related" and 18 "possibly causally related" to ingestion of butterbur extract. One case of cholestatic hepatitis was diagnosed as a hypersensitivity reaction with a probable causal reaction to butterbur. Butterbur should not be used during pregnancy or lactation because of the lack of safety data.

Other Botanicals

Herbalists use a variety of botanicals in their approach to the treatment of migraines. Combination formulas are usually developed on the basis of an individual's clinical profile. Combination treatments for acute migraine headache often include willow bark (*Salix* spp), valerian (*Valeriana officinalis*), wood betony (*Stachys betonica* or *S. officinalis*), or Jamaican dogwood (*Piscidia erythrina*). Ginger (*Zingiber officinale*) is often used in traditional Asian medicine as an abortive agent in the treatment of migraine.[57] For prophylaxis, if stress is a strong factor in the presentation, as it frequently is, nervine tonics, such as oats (*Avena sativa*) or skullcap (*Scutellaria lateriflora*), would be added. Rosemary (*Rosmarinus officinalis*) may be included in migraine formulations, likely on the basis of its historical use for the treatment of headache. No research on combination formulas for the short-term relief of migraine or migraine prophylaxis has been published.

Massage and Manual Therapy

Many patients with headache, both migraine and chronic, report the use of massage or chiropractic manipulation as part of their health care approach. Satisfaction appears to be quite high among patients who use a combination of medication and manual therapy. Nine trials involving 683 patients were included in a recent review of the role of spinal manual therapy in the treatment of chronic headache.[58] Methodologic-quality (validity) scores ranged from 21 to 87 on a 100-point scale. Spinal manual therapy appeared to have a better effect than massage on cervicogenic headache. Before any firm conclusions can be drawn, however, further testing must be conducted in rigorous trials with sufficiently long follow-up periods.

Acupuncture

Preliminary research suggests that acupuncture is effective in the treatment of some types of headache pain.[59] However, interpretation of the literature on acupuncture for the treatment of headache is complicated by the fact that researchers often neglect to report important clinical details adequately and do not discuss the reliability, validity, and clinical significance of the outcome measures used in the trials.[60] No definitive recommendation can be made on the basis of the current literature with regard to the efficacy of acupuncture in the treatment of some common pain syndromes, including headache and neck and back pain.[61]

If the patient chooses to try acupuncture, she should see a licensed acupuncturist (acupuncture is licensed in most states and the District of Columbia) and understand that it may take 6 to 8 weeks for benefits to be noted.

References

1. Lipton RB, Stewart WF, Diamond S, et al: Prevalence and burden of migraine in the United States: data from the American migraine study II, *Headache* 41:646-657, 2001.
2. Breslau N, Rasmussen BK: The impact of migraine: epidemiology, risk factors, and co-morbidities, *Neurology* 56(suppl 1):4-12, 2001.
3. Kornstein SG, Parker AJ: Menstrual migraine: etiology, treatment, and relationship to premenstrual syndrome, *Curr Opin Obstet Gynecol* 9:154-159, 1997.
4. Edmeads J, Láinez JM, Brandes JL, et al: Potential of the Migraine Disability Assessment (MIDAS) questionnaire as a public health initiative and in clinical practice, *Neurology* 56 (suppl 1):S29-S34, 2001.
5. Silberstein SD, Lipton RB: Chronic daily headache, *Curr Opin Neurol* 13:277-283, 2001.
6. Marcus DA: Serotonin and its role in headache pathogenesis and treatment, *Clin J Pain* 9: 159-167, 1993.
7. Lichstein KL, Fisher SM, Eakin TL, et al: Psycho-physiological parameters of migraine and muscle-contraction headaches, *Headache* 31:27-34, 1991.
8. Loder E: Prophylaxis of menstrual migraine with triptans: problems and possibilities, *Neurology* 59:1677-1681, 2002.
9. Headache Classification Committee of the International Headache Society: Classification and diagnostic criteria for headache disorders, cranial neuralgias, and facial pain, *Cephalalgia* 8(suppl 7): 1-96, 1988.
10. MacGregor EA: Menstruation, sex hormones, and migraine, *Neuro Clin* 15:125-141, 1997.
11. Boyle CA: Management of menstrual migraine, *Neurology* 53(suppl 1):14-18, 1999.
12. Pfaffenrath V: Efficacy and safety of percutaneous estradiol versus placebo in menstrual migraine, *Cephalalgia* 13:168, 1993.
13. Smits MG, van der Meer YG, Pfeil JP, et al: Perimenstrual migraine: effect of Estraderm TTS and the value of contingent negative variation and exteroceptive temporalis muscle suppression test, *Headache* 34:103-106, 1993.
14. O'Dea JP, Davis EH: Tamoxifen in the treatment of menstrual migraine, *Neurology* 40:1470-1471, 1990.
15. Powles TJ: Prevention of migrainous headaches by tamoxifen [letter], *Lancet* 6:1344, 1986.

16. Lichten EM, Bennett RS, Whitty AJ, et al: Efficacy of danazol in the control of hormonal migraine, *J Reprod Med* 36:419-424, 1991.
17. Murray SC, Muse KN: Effective treatment of severe menstrual migraine headaches with gonadotropin-releasing hormone agonist and "add-back" therapy, *Fertil Steril* 67:390-393, 1997.
18. Silberstein SD, Elkind AH, Schreiber C: Frovatriptan, a selective 5HT1B/1D agonist, is effective for prophylaxis of menstrually associated migraine. In *Program and abstracts of the 55th Annual Scientific Meeting of the American Academy of Neurology*, Honolulu, Hawaii, March 29-April 5, 2003 (abstract S15.004).
19. Nett R, Manix LK, Landy S, et al: A randomised, double-blind, placebo-controlled, parallel group evaluation of oral naratriptan 1 mg twice daily as prophylactic treatment for menstrually-associated migraine. In *Program and abstracts of the 55th Annual Scientific Meeting of the American Academy of Neurology*, Honolulu, Hawaii, March 29-April 5, 2003 (abstract 15.006).
20. Wenzel RG, Sarvis CA, Krause ML: Over-the-counter drugs for acute migraine attacks: literature review and recommendations, *Pharmacotherapy* 4:494-505, 2003.
21. Gawel MJ, Worthington I, Maggisano A: A systematic review of the use of triptans in acute migraine, *Can J Neurol Sci* 28:30-41, 2001.
22. Hamalainen M, Jones M, Loftus J, et al: Sumatriptan nasal spray for migraine: a review of studies in patients aged 17 years and younger, *Int J Clin Pract* 56:704-709, 2002.
23. Ierusalimschy R, Moreira Filho PF: Precipitating factors of migraine attacks in patients with migraine without aura [in Portuguese], *Arq Neuropsiquiatr* 60:609-613, 2002.
24. Stewart WF, Lipton RB, Celentano DD, et al: Prevalence of migraine headache in the United States, *JAMA* 267:64-69, 1992.
25. Millichap JG, Yee MM: The diet factor in pediatric and adolescent migraine, *Pediatr Neurol* 28: 9-15, 2003.
26. Astin JA, Shapiro SL, Eisenberg DM, et al: Mind-body medicine: state of the science, implications for practice, *J Am Board Fam Pract* 16:131-147, 2003.
27. Eccleston C, Yorke L, Morley S, et al: Psychological therapies for the management of chronic and recurrent pain in children and adolescents, *Cochrane Database Syst Rev* 1:CD003968, 2003.
28. Tepper SJ, Rapoport A, Sheftell F: The pathophysiology of migraine, *Neurology* 7:279-286, 2001.
29. Bigal ME, Bordini CA, Tepper SJ, et al: Intravenous magnesium sulphate in the acute treatment of migraine without aura and migraine with aura: a randomized, double-blind, placebo-controlled study, *Cephalalgia* 22:345-353, 2002.
30. Demirkaya S, Vural O, Dora B, et al: Efficacy of intravenous magnesium sulfate in the treatment of acute migraine attacks, *Headache* 41:171-177, 2001.
31. Peikert A, Wilimzig C, Kohne-Volland R: Prophylaxis of migraine with oral magnesium: results from a prospective, multi-center, placebo-controlled and double-blind randomized study, *Cephalalgia* 16:257-263, 1996.
32. Pfaffenrath V, Wessely P, Meyer C, et al: Magnesium in the prophylaxis of migraine—a double-blind placebo-controlled study, *Cephalalgia* 16:436-440, 1996.
33. Bigal ME, Rapoport AM, Sheftell FD, et al: New migraine preventive options: an update with pathophysiological considerations, *Rev Hosp Clin* 57:293-298, 2002.
34. Mauskop A, Altura BT, Altura BM: Serum ionized magnesium levels and serum ionized calcium/ionized magnesium ratios in women with menstrual migraine, *Headache* 42:242-248, 2002.
35. Welch KM, Ramadan NM: Mitochondria, magnesium and migraine, *J Neurol Sci* 134:9-14, 1995.
36. Schoenen J, Lenaerts M, Bastings E: High-dose riboflavin as a prophylactic treatment of migraine: results of an open pilot study, *Cephalalgia* 14(5):328-329, 1994.
37. Schoenen J, Jacquy J, Lenaerts M: Effectiveness of high-dose riboflavin in migraine prophylaxis: a randomized controlled trial, *Neurology* 50:466-470, 1998.
38. Hobbs C: Feverfew. *Tanacetum parthenium*: a review. *HerbalGram* 20:26-35, 1989.
39. Blumenthal M: *The ABC clinical guide to herbs*, Austin, Texas, American Botanical Council, 2003, pp 138-142.
40. Ernst E, Pittler MH: The efficacy and safety of feverfew (*Tanacetum parthenium* L.): an update of a systematic review, *Public Health Nutr* 3(4A):509-514, 2004.

41. de Weerdt GJ, Bootsma HPR, Hendriks H: Herbal medicines in migraine prevention. Randomized, double blind, placebo-controlled crossover trial of a feverfew preparation, *Phytomedicine* 3:225-230, 1996.
42. Pfaffenrath V, Diner HC, Fisher M, et al: The efficacy and safety of *Tanacetum parthenium* (feverfew) in migraine prophylaxis—a double blind, multicentre, randomized placebo-controlled dose-response study, *Cephalagia* 22:523-532, 2002.
43. Heptinstall S, Awang D: Feverfew: a review of its history, its biological and medicinal properties, and the status of commercial preparations of the herb. In *ACS Symposium Series 691: Phytomedicines of Europe—chemistry and biological activity*, New York, 1998, American Chemical Society (distributed by Oxford University Press), pp 158-175.
44. Johnson ES, Kadam NP, Hylands DM, et al: Efficacy of feverfew as a prophylactic treatment of migraine, *BMJ* 291:569-573, 1985.
45. Bradley PR: *British Herbal Compendium, vol. 1*, Dorset, UK, British Herbal Medicine Association, 1992.
46. Heptinstall S, White A, Williamson L, et al: Extracts of feverfew inhibit granule secretion in blood platelets and polymorphonuclear leucocytes, *Lancet* 1:1071-1074, 1985.
47. Biggs MJ, Johnson ES, Persaud NP, et al: Platelet aggregation in patients using feverfew for migraine (letter). *Lancet* 2:776, 1982.
48. Mauskop A: *Petasites hybridus*: ancient medicinal plant is effective prophylactic treatment for migraine, *Townsend Lett* 202:104-106, 2002.
49. Thomet OA, Wiesmann UN, Schapowal A, et al: Role of petasin in the potential anti-inflammatory activity of a plant extract of *Petasites hybridus*, *Biochem Pharmacol* 15(61):1041-1047, 2001.
50. Diener HC, Rahlfs VW, Danesch U: The first placebo-controlled trial of a special butterbur root extract for the prevention of migraine: reanalysis of efficacy criteria, *Eur Neurol* 51:89-97, 2004.
51. Grossmann W, Schmidramsl H: An extract of *Petasites hybridus* is effective in the prophylaxis of migraine, *Int J Clin Pharmacol Ther* 38:430-435, 2000.
52. Lipton RB, Gobel H, Wilkes K, et al: Efficacy of Petasites 50 and 75 mg for prophylaxis of migraine: results of a randomised, double-blind, placebo-controlled study, *Neurology* 58(suppl 3):A472, 2002.
53. Thomet OA, Simon HU: Petasins in the treatment of allergic diseases: results of preclinical and clinical studies, *Int Arch Allergy Immunol* 129:108-112, 2002.
54. Danesch UC. *Petasites hybridus* (butterbur root) extract in the treatment of asthma—an open trial, *Altern Med Rev* 9:54-62, 2004.
55. Chizzola R, Ozelsberger B, Langer T: Variability in chemical constituents in *Petasites hybridus* from Austria, *Biochem Syst Ecol* 28:421-432, 2000.
56. Danesch U, Rittinghausen R: Safety of a patented special butterbur root extract for migraine prevention, *Headache* 43:76-78, 2003.
57. Mustafa T, Srivastava KC: Ginger (*Zingiber officinale*) in migraine headache, *J Ethnopharmacol* 29:267-273, 1990.
58. Bronfort G, Assendelft WJ, Evans R, et al: Efficacy of spinal manipulation for chronic headache: a systematic review, *J Manipulative Physiol Ther* 24:457-466, 2001.
59. Allais G, De Lorenzo C, Quirico PE, et al: Non-pharmacological approaches to chronic headaches: transcutaneous electrical nerve stimulation, laser therapy and acupuncture in transformed migraine treatment, *Neurol Sci* 24(suppl 2):S138-S142, 2003.
60. Elorriaga Claraco A, Hanna SE, Fargas-Babjak A: Reporting of clinical details in randomized controlled trials of acupuncture for the treatment of migraine/headaches and nausea/vomiting, *J Altern Complement Med* 9:151-159, 2003.
61. Rabinstein AA, Shulman LM: Acupuncture in clinical neurology, *Neurology* 9:137-148, 2003.

Depression

I n *Webster's Dictionary*, definitions for depression include "a psychoneurotic or psychotic disorder marked especially by sadness, inactivity, difficulty in thinking and concentration, a significant increase or decrease in appetite and time spent sleeping, feelings of dejection and hopelessness, and sometimes suicidal tendencies; a lowering of vitality or functional activity; and a state of feeling sad." Synonyms include sadness, the blues, dejection, being down in the dumps, gloom, heavyheartedness, melancholy, mournfulness, and unhappiness (Figure 11-1). It is part of the human condition to experience periods of sadness and dejection. Unhappiness with a situation can be a prime motivator for change. However, persistent and prolonged feelings of hopelessness and despair often require medical investigation and appropriate treatment.

Depression currently ranks fourth among the major causes of disability worldwide, after respiratory infections, perinatal conditions, and human immunodeficiency virus infection/acquired immunodeficiency syndrome.[1] In the United States, depression is the second greatest source of disability among women.[2] It is relatively straightforward to diagnose a mood disorder in someone who presents to the health care system complaining of being sad, down, or tired; the diagnosis is less clear when a patient reports only somatic symptoms. Although recurrent headache, back pain, stomachache, dizziness, chest pain, and fatigue occur in both depressive and physical illnesses, the possibility of depression is often overlooked. This may be due in part to medical curricula that generally teach medical students to rule out physical disorders before considering a mental disorder. A clinician should consider hypothyroidism, anemia, multiple sclerosis, and other conditions that can cause depression, but it is equally important that he or she consider the diagnosis of depression when an individual presents with chronic somatic symptoms. In many cultures, the reporting of somatic complaints by individuals with depression is common. An international study found that nearly 70% of patients with major depression reported only *physical* symptoms as the primary reason for consulting a physician.[3]

Because no definitive biologic marker for depression exists, no biochemical test exists to confirm the diagnosis of depression. The diagnosis is made after a thorough history and physical examination and, if necessary, appropriate laboratory tests to rule out other biochemical imbalances that can cause depressive symptoms (e.g., hypothyroidism).

169

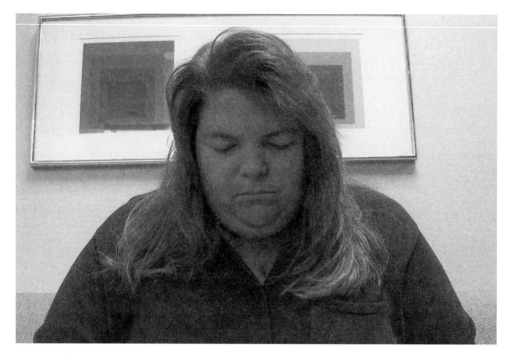

Figure **11-1** Persistent depression and feelings of despair can require medical treatment. *(From Freeman L: Mosby's complementary and alternative medicine: a research-based approach, St. Louis, 2004, Mosby.)*

DSM-IV Criteria for a Major Depressive Episode

A. Five or more of the following symptoms have been present during the same 2-week period and represent a change from previous functioning; at least one of the symptoms is depressed mood or loss of interest or pleasure. *Note: Do not include symptoms that are clearly caused by a general medical condition or mood-incongruent delusions or hallucinations.*

1. Depressed mood most of the day, nearly every day, as indicated by either subjective report (e.g., feels sad or empty) or observation made by others (e.g., appears tearful.)
2. Markedly diminished interest or pleasure in all, or almost all, activities most of the day, nearly every day.
3. Significant weight loss when not dieting or weight gain (e.g., a change of >5% of body weight in a month), or decrease or increase in appetite nearly every day.
4. Insomnia or hypersomnia nearly every day.

5. Psychomotor agitation or retardation nearly every day (observable by others, not merely subjective feelings of restlessness or being slowed down).
6. Fatigue or loss of energy nearly every day.
7. Feelings of worthlessness or excessive or inappropriate guilt (which may be delusional) nearly every day (not merely self-reproach or guilt about being sick).
8. Diminished ability to think or concentrate, or indecisiveness, nearly every day (either by subjective account or as observed by others).
9. Recurrent thoughts of death (not just fear of dying), recurrent suicidal ideation without a specific plan, or a suicide attempt or a specific plan for committing suicide.
B. Exclusion of other causes or symptoms
1. The symptoms cause clinically significant distress or impairment in social, occupational, or other important areas of function.
2. The symptoms are not a result of the direct physiologic effects of a substance (e.g., a drug of abuse or a medication) or general medical condition (e.g., hypothyroidism).
3. The symptoms are not better accounted for by bereavement.

MEDICAL CAUSES OF DEPRESSION

Prescription drugs: α-methyldopa, barbiturates, benzodiazepines, β-blockers, cholinergic drugs, corticosteroids, estrogens, levodopa, ranitidine, cimetidine, reserpine, progestins, and others.

- Endocrine/metabolic: hyperthyroidism, hypothyroidism, hyperadrenalism, hypercalcemia, hyponatremia, diabetes mellitus, lead poisoning, porphyria, uremia
- Neurologic: brain tumor, dementia, Huntington's disease, multiple sclerosis, Parkinson's disease, dominant-hemisphere stroke, syphilis, epilepsy, Wilson's disease
- Nutritional: pellagra; deficiency of vitamin B_{12}, vitamin B_6, pantothenic acid, or folate
- Miscellaneous: alcohol or cocaine abuse, systemic lupus erythematosus, mononucleosis, Lyme disease, hypoglycemia, solvent exposure

---

PATHOPHYSIOLOGY

The pathophysiology of depression remains poorly understood but appears to be a complex interplay of genetics, biochemistry, and developmental and social factors. Traumatic events in childhood such as physical or sexual abuse can increase the risk for depression in adulthood[4] and a recent stressful event often precedes a depressive episode in a vulnerable individual.[5] With advances in decoding the human genome, genetic polymorphisms and their role in depression are being explored. For many years, however, a substantial amount of research has been focused on the role of monoamine transmitters in mood disorders.

Although disturbances in norepinephrine and serotonin levels have been repeatedly demonstrated in models of depression, it remains unclear whether these disturbances are the cause of depression or an effect of it. Many biochemical abnormalities have been identified in individuals with depression, among them increased production and release of corticotropin-releasing factor (CRF), which results in abnormalities in hypothalamic pituitary adrenal axis activity. Disruption of glutamate, γ-aminobutyric acid (GABA), growth hormone, and thyroid hormone levels has also been demonstrated, as have abnormalities in secondary messenger systems such as cyclic adenosine monophosphate (AMP).[6] Activation of secondary messenger systems is important in the maintenance of healthy levels of neurotrophic factors, including brain-derived neurotrophic factor.[7] An increase in expression of brain-derived neurotrophic factor appears to facilitate both neuronal survival and neurogenesis. Some antidepressant medications may work through this proposed mechanism.

It may be far too simple to assume that depression is simply the result of disruption in monoamine transmitter levels. Treatment failure, in addition to nonadherence with therapy, may be due to our inability to accurately identify subgroups of patients with depression and to provide treatments specifically targeted to their unique neurobiologic characteristics.

TREATMENT

Psychotherapy

An article in the *Journal of the Medical American Association* reported that between 1987 and 1998, the number of Americans being treated for depression increased from 1.7 million to 6.3 million. The proportion of depressed people taking antidepressants increased from 37% to 75%, whereas the number undergoing psychotherapy decreased from 71% to 60%. This change is likely due in part to the improved availability of medications that are better tolerated by patients. The trend of medicating patients without psychotherapy is cause for concern but not altogether surprising in the era of managed care. In many cases primary-care providers are encouraged to prescribe antidepressant drugs but support for mental-health counseling is limited. Most experts are convinced, however, that the majority of patients do best with a combination of medication and psychotherapy. This is especially true in cases of chronic major depression, in which combined treatment has been found significantly superior to medication or psychotherapy alone.[8]

Prescription Medication

Several different classes of antidepressants have been shown to be effective in clinical trials. These include monoamine oxidase (MAO) inhibitors, tricyclic antidepressants (TCAs), selective serotonin-reuptake inhibitors (SSRIs), and novel agents including serotonin- and norepinephrine-reuptake inhibitors (SNRIs). Current treatments often produce only partial symptomatic improvement (response) rather than symptom resolution and optimal function (remission). Some new agents, including CRF antagonists, substance P antagonists, and antiglucocorticoids, hold promise in the refinement of treatment options, especially among subgroups of patients who do not fully respond to first-line treatments.[9]

Debate continues over the differences in efficacy and tolerability among the different classes of antidepressant drugs. A systematic review of 108 metaanalyses of antidepressant medications revealed the following: only small differences in efficacy exist between most new and old antidepressants (old being defined as those on the market before the 1980s); superior efficacy of SNRIs over SSRIs; slower onset of therapeutic action of fluoxetine compared to other SSRIs; superior general tolerability of SSRIs over TCAs; poorer tolerability of fluvoxamine than of other SSRIs in a within-group comparison; and no increase in the risk of suicidal acts or ideation with fluoxetine compared with TCAs (or placebo) in low-risk patients.[10]

Serotonin is a major player in mood, whereas norepinephrine is involved in drive and energy state. There is interaction between them in matters of appetite, sleep regulation, and anxiety. It is generally accepted that depletion of serotonin is related to depressive symptoms. A strong link also exists between stress and depression. Stress systems in the brain are, for the most part, mediated by norepinephrine transmission.

One hypothesis holds that dual-action antidepressant drugs such as venlafaxine and milnacipran are superior in efficacy to those that mainly affect the serotonergic pathway. Some research is available to support this hypothesis. A recent metaanalysis showed that venlafaxine had greater efficacy than SSRIs in the treatment of depression.[11] Venlafaxine is also being promoted as a treatment for menopausal flushing, especially in women who cannot or prefer not to take estrogen replacement therapy (ERT; see Chapter 6).

In addition to relieving the symptoms of depression, substances that modulate both the serotonin and norepinephrine (NE) pathways can be helpful to patients with pain. Both serotonin and NE neural circuits directly modulate the descending pathways and make up an integral part of the complex system that controls pain perception.[12] The TCAs have been shown clinically to reduce pain; however, their side effect profile often limits their use in general practice. The SNRIs may prove a useful tool in patients with chronic pain or the dual diagnosis of pain and depression. The authors of one study found that extended-release venlafaxine at a dosage of 150 to 220 mg/day was significantly better than placebo in relieving diabetic neuropathic pain by the third week of treatment.[13]

Estrogen Replacement Therapy

Many practitioners believe that ERT improves mood in perimenopausal and menopausal women, but current research neither validates nor disproves this assertion. Although neurobiological studies show promising antidepressant effects of estradiol on serotonergic, noradrenergic, cholinergic, dopaminergic, and GABA-ergic functions, no consistent findings of a correlation between any serum hormone level and the severity or presence of depressive symptoms have been reported. Most clinical trials have shown a modest effect on symptoms of depression; however, the methodologic limitations of the research do not permit generalization or recommendations.[14] Given concerns with long-term use of ERT (see Chapter 6), more definitive information is needed.

Integrative Approaches

Any truly integrative approach to the treatment of depression should include investigation of the patient's physical and emotional well-being, as well as a careful examination of lifestyle. Stress reduction is an important part of the wellness strategy for anyone with depression. Relaxation, meditation, yoga, prayer, and journal-keeping can all be effective tools in helping reduce stress and create a sense of empowerment in the patient. Research suggests that regular exercise improves mood.[15] The clinician should discuss and encourage healthy dietary habits, including a reduction in the consumption of caffeinated beverages, especially if the patient is feeling anxious or not sleeping well, and the limitation of alcohol-containing beverages to one per day.

Supplements and Botanicals

Omega-3 fatty acids. A growing body of evidence demonstrates the many health benefits of fish oil. Intervention trials in human subjects show that omega-3 fatty acids may have positive effects in the treatment of various psychiatric disorders.[16] The findings of epidemiologic surveys indicate that populations consuming large amounts of fish have lower rates of depression than do members of groups that consume small amounts.[17] Research indicates that individuals with major depression have marked depletions in omega-3 fatty acids (especially docosahexaenoic acid [DHA]) in erythrocyte phospholipids compared with controls.[18] Arachidonic acid and DHA account for roughly half of total brain phospholipids, substances necessary for the proper function of the nerve-cell membranes and second messenger systems believed to play a role in depression and other mood disorders.

Although epidemiologic and basic-science studies suggest that long-chain fatty acids are beneficial for individuals prone to or experiencing depression, well-controlled clinical trials are needed. To date, only two double-blind studies have been completed. Four weeks of supplementation with 2 g/day of eicosapentaenoic acid ethyl ester (E-EPA) enhanced the antidepressant effects of conventional drug therapy in a double-blind, placebo-controlled study of 20 patients with recurrent unipolar depressive disorder treated with maintenance antidepressant therapy. The 24-item Hamilton Rating Scale for Depression (HAM-D) was administered at baseline and weekly thereafter. The average HAM-D baseline score was 18 or less. By the end of the study, E-EPA–treated patients showed a mean reduction of 12.4 points, compared with a mean reduction of 1.6 points among patients receiving a placebo. The researchers were unsure whether E-EPA augments the effect of the antidepressant therapy by way of the secondary messenger system or whether it exerts an independent antidepressant effect.[19] A 12-week randomized, double-blind, placebo-controlled study of 60 patients with persistent depression who were taking conventional antidepressant drugs found that 1 g/day of E-EPA improved depression scores more than did placebo. Higher doses of 2 g/day or 4 g/day did not lead to further improvement.[20]

Given the relatively inexpensive cost of omega-3 fatty-acid capsules, the other health benefits of omega-3, and the very low side-effect profile, patients with depression may wish to add fish to the diet twice a week or supplement the diet with omega-3 capsules. Quality control of fish-oil capsules has been a concern as fish can accumulate toxins such as mercury, dioxins, and polychlorinated biphenyls. Neither the Food and Drug Administration (FDA) nor any other federal or state agency tests fish oil supplements for quality before sale. Consumer Labs tested 20 fish oil products and found that none contained any detectable level of mercury; however, six of the 20 products failed to pass review because they contained inadequate amounts of DHA ranging from just 50% to 83% of the amounts stated on the labels.[21] Although the optimal dose has not yet been determined, most authorities recommend 1 to 3 g/day of omega-3 fatty acids.

SAMe. S-adenosyl-L-methionine (SAMe), derived from the sulfur-containing amino acid methionine and adenosine triphosphate (ATP), is a natural substance that plays an important role in many of the body's biochemical processes. SAMe is the most important methyl donor in transmethylation reactions occurring in the central nervous system. Serum and cerebrospinal-fluid levels of SAMe are reported to be low in some patients with depression.

The Agency for Healthcare Research and Quality published a review of the evidence on SAMe in the treatment of depression, osteoarthritis, and liver disease. Of 39 studies considered, 28 were included in a metaanalysis of the efficacy of SAMe in reducing symptoms of depression.[22] Reviewers found that SAMe was superior to placebo. Compared with treatment with conventional antidepressant drugs, SAMe was not associated with a statistically significant difference in outcome.

This dietary supplement must be taken as an enteric-coated tablet in the morning, before breakfast. The dosage used to treat depression generally ranges from 400 to 1200 mg/day. The patient should be instructed to start with 400 mg/day for 5 days and then increase the dosage by 200 mg/day every 3 to 5 days as needed. The main side effects are gastrointestinal upset, nausea, agitation, and insomnia. Taking the supplement with food will reduce the incidence of gastrointestinal complaints. Agitation and insomnia are often dosage-related. SAMe is contraindicated in patients with bipolar disorder as it can induce mania.

St. John's wort (Hypericum perforatum). St. John's wort is the most heavily studied botanicals for depression. Its use as a mood-elevating substance may date back 2000 years or more. *H. perforatum,* meaning "over an apparition," is the botanical name given by the ancient physician Dioscorides (70 CE). The name was apparently chosen because the plant was believed to protect the user from evil or wandering spirits. It is quite possible that early users of St. John's wort found that the herb "lifted" the spirits (or eased depression). Early Christians, noting the red oil glands on the plant's leaves, claimed that they represented the blood spilled by John the Baptist during his beheading and gave the herb its common name, St. John's wort. Others say the common name is derived from the fact that the herb blooms on St. John's Day (Figure 11-2).

A 1996 metaanalysis of St. John's wort in the *British Medical Journal*[23] revealed that St. John's wort is more effective than placebo in the treatment of mild to moderate depression. This review helped focus attention on this herb in the United States, and sales quickly increased. Sales remained high until 1998-1999, when reports of herb-drug interactions began to be reported in the media. By the spring of 2002, results from 34 controlled double-blind trials of *Hypericum* extracts in some 3000 patients, mostly with mild to moderate depression, had been published.[24]

The most recent Cochrane review found 27 trials with a total of 2291 patients that met inclusion criteria for a metaanalysis. Seventeen trials with 1168 patients were placebo-controlled (16 trials involved monopreparations and one involved St. John's wort plus four other herbs), and 10 trials (eight single preparations and two combinations of St. John's wort and valerian) with 1123 patients compared *Hypericum* with other antidepressant or sedative drugs. Most trials lasted 4 to 6 weeks, and the diagnosis in most participants was "neurotic depression" or "mild to moderate severe depressive disorder." The authors concluded, "There is evidence that extracts of Hypericum are more effective than placebo for the short-term treatment of mild to moderately severe depressive disorders. The current evidence is inadequate to establish whether *Hypericum* is as effective as other antidepressants. Further studies comparing *Hypericum* with standard antidepressants in well defined groups of patients over longer observation periods, investigating long-term side effects, and comparing different extracts and doses are needed."[25]

Another meta-analysis of 22 randomized, controlled trials showed St. John's wort to be significantly more effective than placebo (relative risk 1.98) and not significantly different

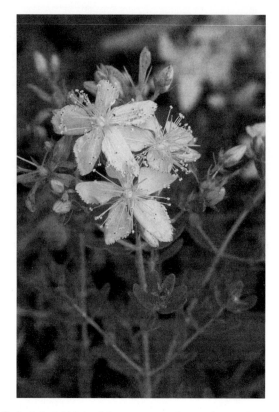

Figure 11-2 St. John's Wort *(Hypericum perforatum)*. *(Courtesy Martin Wall Botanical Services.)*

in efficacy from other antidepressant agents (relative risk 1.0). Adverse effects occurred more frequently with standard antidepressants than with St. John's wort.[26] At the time of this writing, on the basis of the existing data, it appears that St. John's wort is superior to placebo in the treatment of mild to moderately severe depression. Equivalency, or superiority, to conventional antidepressants has not been adequately addressed, although the Whiskey metaanalysis suggests that St. John's wort is not significantly different from prescription medication.

The vast majority of studies have demonstrated that St. John's wort extract is superior to placebo in the treatment of depression, with the notable exception of two studies published in the *Journal of the Medical Association*. The first of these trials was published in 2001. A randomized, double-blind, placebo-controlled clinical trial was conducted in 200 patients with major depression and a baseline HAM-D score of at least 20. After a 1-week single-blind run-in of placebo, participants were randomized to receive either 900 mg/day St. John's wort extract (0.3% hypericin) or placebo for 4 weeks. The dose could be increased to 1200 mg/day for the remainder of the 8-week study if treatment response was inadequte. Response rates in the intention-to-treat analysis were not significantly different between the two groups: 26.5% for St. John's wort and 18.6% for placebo. The number of participants achieving remission of symptoms was significantly higher with St. John's wort than with placebo ($P = 0.02$), but the rates were low in the full intention-to-treat analysis (14.3% and 4.9%, respectively). The authors conclude, "These results do not support significant antidepressant or antianxiety effects for St. John's wort when contrasted with placebo in a clinical sample of depressed patients."[27] The study was challenged for its lack of a historical active, study population of severely depressed patients and its very low placebo response, an uncommon finding in antidepressant trials, where placebo response is generally 25% to 30%.

The National Institutes of Health–sponsored study is the longest and most rigorous study of St. John's wort conducted so far.[28] Three hundred forty moderately to severely depressed patients were randomly assigned to receive St. John's wort extract, placebo, or sertraline for 8 weeks. On the basis of clinical response, the daily dose of St. John's wort extract could range from 900 to 1500 mg and sertraline from 50 to 100 mg. Patients who demonstrated a response at week 8 could continue their blinded treatment for an additional 18 weeks. The two primary outcomes were change in the HAM-D between baseline and 8 weeks and the rates of full response (as determined by changes in HAM-D and Clinical Global Impressions scores). With regard to change in the HAM-D score, neither sertraline nor St. John's wort extract was statistically different from placebo. Full response occurred in 31.9% of the placebo-treated patients, compared with 23.9% of the St. John's wort extract–treated patients ($P = 0.21$) and 24.8% of the sertraline-treated patients ($P = 0.26$). Neither sertraline nor St. John's wort extract performed as well as placebo with regard to this primary outcome. Sertraline was better than placebo on the Clinical Global Impressions improvement scale ($P = 0.02$), which was used as a secondary measure in this study.

The media reports, based on the findings of this trial, that St. John's wort is ineffective in the treatment of major depressive disorder, do not provide an entirely accurate picture. In studies of antidepressants, the tested drug often fails to do better than placebo. This is a result of both the high subjectivity of the scales used and the typically large placebo response. A review of clinical-trial data from the nine antidepressants approved by the FDA between 1985 and 2000 included 10,030 patients with depression who participated in 52 antidepressant clinical trials evaluating 93 treatment arms. The researchers found that fewer than half (48%, 45 of 93) of the antidepressant-treatment arms showed superiority to placebo.[29] To avoid a false-negative result (type II error), antidepressant trials would have to involve 300 or more patients per arm; otherwise, more sensitive research designs must be developed.[30] The appropriate conclusion from this trial is that it was not sensitive enough to detect the effectiveness of either sertraline or St. John's wort extract or that this was primarily a group of "nonresponders."

Mechanism of action.   The mechanism behind the antidepressant effects of St. John's wort is not well understood. Originally it was thought that the flowering tops inhibited monoamine oxidase (MAO), the enzyme responsible for the degradation of the neurotransmitters norepinephrine and serotonin. However, research has shown that inhibition of MAO does not occur in vivo. The antidepressant activity of St. John's wort may be mediated by serotonergic (5-HT), noradrenergic, and dopaminergic systems,[31,32] as well as by GABA and glutamate amino-acid neurotransmitters.[33]

Difficulties in determining the mechanism of effect may be a result of the duration of administration. Studies in rats and cats have demonstrated that short-term treatment with

St. John's wort does little to alter the neurochemistry of the brain.[34] In cats, St. John's wort extract and hypericin significantly decreased levels of corticotropin-releasing hormone messenger RNA by 16% to 22% in the hypothalamus and serotonin 5-HT(1A) receptor messenger RNA by 11% to 17% in the hippocampus at 8 weeks but not at 2 weeks.[35]

Recent in vitro research suggests that the herb has an antagonist effect at the CRF(1) receptor. Abnormalities in the hypothalamic-pituitary-adrenal axis have been noted in many patients with depression. These abnormalities are believed to be caused, in part, by increased CRF activity. Pseudohypericin is a selective CRF antagonist, hypericin was shown to be a competitive antagonist for CRF, and hyperforin is a noncompetitive antagonist for CRF and calcitonin.[36] This finding is consistent with animal research indicating decreased levels of corticotropin-releasing hormone and normalized activity of the hypothalamic-pituitary-adrenal axis with St. John's wort administration.[35]

Other researchers have demonstrated increased production and release of aspartate, glutamate, serine, glycine, and GABA by hyperforin by way of facilitation of entry of sodium into the neuron, leading to the release of calcium from intracellular stores.[37] Other scientists have demonstrated inhibition of glutamate and GABA uptake by hyperforin as well.[38]

The question of which constituent, or constituents account for the antidepressant activity of St. John's wort, is being hotly debated. Biologically active constituents may include hyperforin and adhyperforin, hypericin and pseudohypericin, flavonoids, xanthones, oligomerics, procyanidines, and amino acids.[39] "Standardizing" the herb to achieve maximal beneficial effect is a matter of difficulty, as multiple constituents within the herb account for the plant's therapeutic effects.

Contraindications, adverse effects, and herb-drug interactions. Systematic reviews have verified that St. John's wort has fewer side effects than prescription antidepressants: 26% for St. John's wort and 45% for standard antidepressants.[25] A review of adverse events in patients taking St. John's wort from 1991 to 1999, involving approximately 8 million people, documented 95 reports of adverse events.[40] Side effects, which are generally mild, include headache, gastrointestinal upset, fatigue, sedation, restlessness, dizziness, and skin reactions. Coordination, concentration, and attentiveness (necessary for the safe operation of motor vehicles and machinery) were not impaired in 32 patients with depression taking 900 mg/day of St. John's wort extract for 4 weeks in a double-blind, placebo-controlled study.[41] St. John's wort does not appear to potentiate or modify the effects of alcohol.[42]

Pruritus was experienced by 2% of patients taking St. John's wort for depression.[43] Phototoxicity is rare but may occur in light-skinned individuals prone to sunburn. A randomized, placebo-controlled trial showed that fair-skinned subjects who sunburned easily had a "slight reduction in the minimum-tanning dose."[44] Phototoxicity appears to be caused by hypericin, pseudohypericin, and naphthodianthrones, which produce singlet oxygen and free radicals on exposure to light.

Numerous drug interactions have been reported in the literature. In a preclinical study, the administration of St. John's wort extract to rats for 14 days resulted in a 3.8-fold increase of intestinal P-glycoprotein/Mdr1 expression and a 2.5-fold increase in hepatic CYP3A4 expression (as detected on Western-blot analysis).[45] A study of hyperforin showed that this constituent is a potent ligand for the pregnane X receptor, an orphan nuclear receptor that regulates expression of the cytochrome P-450 (CYP) 3A4 monooxygenase. Treatment of primary human hepatocytes with hypericum extracts or hyperforin resulted in a marked induction of CYP3A4 expression.[46] Researchers have reported in vivo and in vitro CYP 2C9, 2D6, and 3A4 inhibition[47]; however, a 3-day study in human subjects failed to demonstrate a similar significant effect on drugs metabolized by CYP 2D6 or 3A4 enzymes.[48] It appears that St. John's wort inhibits CYP 3A4 acutely and then induces this enzyme with repeated administration, which helps explain the negative 3 day study.[49]

REPORTED HERB-DRUG INTERACTIONS

Anticoagulants: Reduction in International Normalized Ratio in seven patients whose condition was previously stable while they were taking warfarin suggests induction of cytochrome P-450 2C9,[1] although this finding could also be due to induction of P-glycoprotein.

Cyclosporine: A significant decrease in cyclosporine levels was observed in 30 kidney-transplant recipients taking St. John's wort. Cyclosporine levels increased markedly after the herb was discontinued.[2] The authors of one recent article reviewed 11 case reports and two case series involving decreased blood levels of cyclosporine, and several cases of transplant rejection, associated with the use of St. John's wort.[3] In addition to induction of CYP3A4, cyclosporine levels may be affected by the induction of the drug pump P-glycoprotein.[4]

Digoxin: A 25% decrease in digoxin in the area under the curve occurred in a 10-day placebo-controlled trial. The interaction with digoxin suggests induction of the drug transporter P-glycoprotein.[5]

Medications for the treatment of human immunodeficiency virus infection (HIV): The oral clearance of nevirapine was significantly increased in five HIV-positive patients treated concurrently with St. John's wort.[6] Reduced serum levels of indinavir were noted in an open trial of healthy volunteers.[7]

Nifedipine: An open study in human subjects showed reduced midazolam concentrations, possibly a result of the induction of CYP3A4.[8]

Oral contraceptives: Three months' administration of St. John's wort extract (300 mg three times daily; preparation unspecified) was associated with increased clearance of norethindrone and breakthrough bleeding in 7 of 12 female volunteers in a study of the effects of St. John's wort on a combination oral contraceptive (ethinylestradiol/norethindrone).[9] At the time of this writing, other trials to confirm these results are under way.

SSRIs: There are several reports of older patients developing confusion, agitation, confusion, nausea, vomiting and headache after adding St. John's wort to their SSRI therapy.[10]

Statins: Fourteen days' consumption of St. John's wort (300 mg three times daily) reduced the plasma simvastatin level after a single dose of simvastatin (10 mg), but had no effect on plasma pravastatin levels after a single dose of pravastatin (20 mg), in a double-blind, placebo-controlled, crossover study of 16 healthy men.[11]

TCAs: A 14-day open study of 12 depressed patients showed a significant reduction in amitriptyline concentration when 900 mg/day of St. John's wort was taken concurrently,[12] most likely as a result of the induction of CYP3A4.

References

1. Kaminsky LS, Zhang ZY: Human P450 metabolism of warfarin, *Pharmacol Ther* 73:6774, 1997.
2. Breidenbach T, Kliem V, Burg M, et al: Profound drop of cyclosporin A whole blood trough levels caused by St. John's wort (*Hypericum perforatum*) [letter], *Transplantation* 69:2229-2230, 2000.
3. Ernst E: St. John's wort supplements endanger the success of organ transplantation, *Arch Surg* 137:316-319, 2002.
4. Cott JM: Herb-drug interactions, *CNS Spectrum* 6:827-832, 2001.
5. Johne A, Brockmoller J, Bauer S, et al: *Interaction of St. John's Wort extract with digoxin*, Berlin, June 10-12, 1999, Jahreskongress fur Klinische Pharmakologie.
6. de Maat MM, Hoetelmans RM, Mathot RA, et al: Drug interaction between St. John's wort and nevirapine, *AIDS* 15:420-421, 2001.
7. Piscitelli SC, Burstein AH, Chaitt D, et al: Indinavir concentrations and St. John's wort, *Lancet* 355:547-548, 2000.
8. Smith M, Lin KM, Zheng YP: PIII-89 an open trial of nifedipine-herb interactions: nifedipine with St. John's wort, ginseng or ginkgo biloba, *Clin Pharmacol Ther* 69:P86, 2001.
9. Gorski JC, Hamman MA, Wang Z, et al: *The effect of St. John's wort on the efficacy of oral contraception* [abstract MPI-80]. Atlanta, Georgia, March 27-27, 2002, American Society for Clinical Pharmacology and Therapeutics Annual Meeting.
10. Hammerness P, Basch E, Ulbricht C, et al: St. John's wort: a systematic review of adverse effects and drug interactions for the consultation psychiatrist, *Psychosomatics* 44:271-282, 2003.
11. Fujimura A, Sugimoto K, Ohmori M, et al: *Different effects of St. John's wort on the pharmacokinetics of simvastatin and pravastatin* [abstract TPII-81], Atlanta, Georgia, March 24-27, 2002, American Society for Clinical Pharmacology and Therapeutics Annual Meeting.
12. Johne A, Schmider J, Brockmöller J, et al: Decreased plasma levels of amitriptyline and its metabolites on co-medication with an extract from St. John's wort (*Hypericum perforatum*), *J Clin Psychopharmacol* 22:46-54, 2002.

Dose and preparation.   The recommended dosage of standardized extracts of St. John's wort generally ranges from 900 to 1500 mg/day. Yet no current scientific consensus has been reached as to which constituent(s) to standardize and at what level. Many herbalists recommend the flowering tops in tincture (1:5 in 25%-40% alcohol), alone or combined with other herbs, at a dosage of 3 to 5 mL thrice daily.

Ginkgo (Ginkgo biloba).   Standardized extracts of ginkgo have been intensely studied in Europe for more than 30 years. The main foci of research have been cerebrovascular disease, dementia, and peripheral vascular disease. In 1994, the German government approved a standardized form of leaf extract (EGb761) for the treatment of dementia. The standardized extract contains 22% to 27% flavonoids and 5% to 7% terpene lactones. The psychological and physiologic benefits of ginkgo are thought to be a result of its primary action of regulating neurotransmitters and exerting neuroprotective effects on the brain, protecting against or retarding nerve-cell degeneration.[50]

Ginkgo is recognized by the German Commission E and the World Health Organization as a symptomatic treatment for disturbed performance in organic brain syndrome with the following principal characteristics: memory deficits, disturbances in concentration, depressive emotional condition, dizziness, tinnitus, and headache. Ginkgo may be helpful in alleviating depressive symptoms in individuals with dementia syndromes. Despite these endorsements, however, the authors of a recent review of *G. biloba* for the treatment of cognitive impairment and dementia concluded that although ginkgo appears to be safe, a large trial involving modern methodology to estimate the extent and possible mechanism of any treatment effect(s) is needed, given the methodologic limitations of the clinical trials.[51]

Older individuals with treatment-resistant depression may benefit from the addition of ginkgo to their treatment regimens. A double-blind, placebo-controlled study of 40 patients (age range 51-78 years) with persistent depression despite treatment with antidepressant medication revealed that 240 mg/day of a standardized extract of ginkgo (EGb761) improved depressive symptoms better than did placebo.[52] It is unclear whether ginkgo has direct antidepressant effects, whether it augments the effects of conventional medications, or whether it mainly improves symptoms such as deficits in sleep and cognition. Insomnia and cognitive impairment are frequent complaints of patients taking conventional antidepressant medications. An open, nonrandomized pilot study of 16 patients treated with a trimipramine monotherapy (200 mg) showed that individuals given an adjunct dose of 240 mg/day of a standardized extract of ginkgo (LI1370) experienced increased sleep efficiency and decreased incidence of nighttime wakening.[53]

Animal studies have demonstrated that ginkgo may reduce the activity of cortisol-releasing hormone, which is related to depressive mood and behavior, particularly sleep and cognition.[54] Other animal research has demonstrated an increased number of serotonin-binding sites, which may improve mood and alleviate depressive symptoms.[55] In light of the complexity of the biochemical changes involved in depression, it may be that ginkgo improves specific symptoms in particular subgroups of patients. More research, however, is needed in both the clinical and basic science arenas before it can be predicted who might benefit from this therapy.

The German Commission E lists occasional gastrointestinal upset, headache, and allergic skin reactions as side effects of ginkgo and deems the herb contraindicated in individuals with hypersensitivity to ginkgo preparations. Ten cases of hemorrhage have been reported with use of ginkgo, a small number given the millions of doses taken over the years. Although the true risk of gingko's interaction with warfarin or antiplatelet agents is not known,[56] it is probably best to recommend that patients taking anticoagulant medications avoid ginkgo until more conclusive research has been conducted in this area. A recent randomized, double-blind, placebo-controlled study of 32 young healthy male volunteers failed to show any alteration of platelet function or coagulation when the volunteers were given 120, 240, or 480 mg/day of EGb761 for 14 days.[57] The dosage generally used in clinical trials is 120 to 240 mg/day of standardized extract.

Ginseng (Panax ginseng).   Ginseng is often reported to improve an individual's sense of well-being and has a long history of use as a "tonic" herb. Three ginseng species are commonly used in herbal medicine. *P. ginseng* grows in China and Korea and is typically referred to as Asian ginseng, *P. quinquefolius* (American ginseng) is indigenous to the United States and Canada, and *P. notoginseng* grows in southern Asia. Siberian ginseng (*Eleutherococcus senticosus*) does not belong to the genus *Panax*, and although it is also purported to have tonic effects, most experts now refer to the herb as eleuthero in an attempt to avoid confusion.

Clinical trials of the effectiveness of ginseng in the treatment of depression and other mood disorders are rare. Two studies of quality of life with a multivitamin and ginseng yielded contradictory results. An 8-week placebo-controlled study involving the administration of a commercial ginseng-multivitamin/multimineral preparation to 60 patients admitted to the geriatric unit of a hospital found no differences between the two groups with regard to duration of stay, activities of daily living, cognitive function, or somatic symptoms.[58] However, this vitamin provided only 40 mg/day of a standardized ginseng extract (G115), whereas the typical dose is generally 100 to 200 mg/day. A double-blind study of a multivitamin complex supplemented with ginseng compared with a multivitamin complex without ginseng in 625 patients complaining of stress or fatigue found significant improvement in the quality-of-life index at 4 months in those receiving ginseng.[59]

Two studies have been conducted in menopausal women to investigate the herb's purported estrogenic activity. A randomized, double-blind, placebo-controlled study of *P. ginseng* in 384 women with menopausal symptoms failed to note a reduction in vasomotor symptoms. However, the application of a validated tool for the evaluation of mood and well-being yielded *P* values of less than 0.05 for depression, well-being, and health subscales in favor of ginseng compared with placebo.[60] This finding is consistent with the results of a small open study showing that 30 days' treatment with 6 g/day of Korean red ginseng improved symptoms of fatigue, insomnia, and depression in women with menopausal symptoms.[61] These results are intriguing because women experienced an improved sense of well-being and less depression despite continued vasomotor symptoms.

The pharmacologic activity of ginseng is not completely understood, although corticosteroid-like actions and hypoglycemic activity have been documented.[62] Researchers have found that ginseng has a favorable effect on stress models.[65]

American ginseng has been shown to exert GABA-ergic activity in animal studies,[66] and research on Vietnamese ginseng (*P. vietnamensis*) suggests interaction of GABA-A receptor and CRF.[65]

Adverse effects, which are rare, generally occur only with high doses or prolonged use. They include sleeplessness, nervousness, early-morning diarrhea, and hypertony.[66] Three incidents of hormonelike effects in older women have been reported.[67] However, it is important to note that most of these case reports failed to accurately identify the product as ginseng, and it is well known that ginseng has historically been replaced and adulterated with less expensive herbs. The *British Herbal Compendium* states that the use of ginseng is contraindicated during pregnancy, but the German Commission E and the American Herbal Products Association do not. No fetal abnormalities have been noted in rats or rabbits given 40 mg/kg of a standardized extract on days 1 through 15 of pregnancy. No teratogenic

POTENTIAL DRUG-GINSENG INTERACTIONS

Diabetic agents: Hypoglycemic effects have been documented with ginseng.[1] Patients with diabetes should monitor their blood sugar and adjust medications.
Stimulants: Some authors suggest that large amounts of caffeinated beverages (or other stimulants) should be avoided by individuals taking ginseng.[1]
MAO inhibitors: An isolated case report suggests that the combination of ginseng tea and phenelzine induces headache, insomnia, and tremor.[1] In another case, a woman taking phenelzine experienced what may have been a manic reaction to the
Continued

POTENTIAL DRUG-GINSENG INTERACTIONS—CONT'D

combination of ginseng and bee pollen.[1] Neither of these case reports includes appropriate identification of the herb involved. In the 1980s it was not uncommon for ginseng to be replaced or adulterated with other substances, including ephedra.[1] Although interaction is possible, it is difficult to form any definitive conclusion from these two case reports.

Anticoagulant/antiplatelet agents: Ginsenoside Rg2 inhibits platelet aggregation,[1] whereas ginsenoside Rg3 inhibits the activity of platelet-activating factor in vitro.[1] In one case report of a patient taking warfarin, a decreased International Normalized Ratio is discussed[1]; however, animal studies have failed to show interaction between ginseng and warfarin when single or multiple doses of ginseng are concomitantly administered.[1] Until this issue is further clarified, practitioners should monitor patients taking anticoagulant medications and ginseng.

---

effects were observed in two generations of rats fed as much as 2700 mg of ginseng extract per day.[62]

Given the extensive historical use of this herb, more basic-science and clinical research are justified to determine what value ginseng offers individuals living with unrelenting stress and mood disorders.

Valerian (**Valeriana officinalis**).   Valerian has been used as a sedative and sleep aid since the time of Hippocrates. Valerian is listed officially in the pharmacopoeias of many countries, including Austria, France, Great Britain, Hungary, Russia, and Switzerland.[68] Although numerous species of valerian exist, the one most commonly researched and used in the herbal supplement industry is *V. officinalis*. In vitro and animal research has confirmed that constituents in the root have GABAergic activity.[69-71] Two clinical trials have been conducted on a combination of valerian and St. John's wort for the treatment of depression. The combination was found to be equivalent or superior to the TCAs amitriptyline and desipramine when given for 6 weeks.[25]

References

1. *Mental health: new understanding, new hope,* Geneva, Switzerland, 2001, World Health Organization.
2. Michaud CM, Murray CJ, Bloom BR: Burden of disease: implications for future research, *JAMA* 285:535-539, 2001.
3. Simon GE, VonKorff M, Piccinelli M, et al: An international study of the relation between somatic symptoms and depression, *N Engl J Med* 341:1329-1335, 1999.
4. Heim C, Nemeroff CB: The role of childhood trauma in the neurobiology of mood and anxiety disorders: preclinical and clinical studies, *Biol Psychiatr* 49:1023-1039, 2001.
5. Kendler KS: Major depression and the environment: a psychiatric genetic perspective, *Pharmacopsychiatry* 31:5-9, 1998.
6. Vaidya VA, Duman RS: Depression: emerging insights from neurobiology. *Br Med Bull* 57:61-79, 2001.
7. Duman RS, Heninger GR, Nestler EJ: A molecular and cellular theory of depression, *Arch Gen Psychiatr* 54:597-606, 1997.
8. Arnow BA, Constantino MJ: Effectiveness of psychotherapy and combination treatment for chronic depression, *J Clin Psychol* 59:893-905, 2003.

9. Farvolden P, Kennedy S, Lam R: Recent developments in the psychobiology and pharmacotherapy of depression: optimising existing treatments and novel approaches for the future, *Expert Opin Invest Drug* 12:65-86, 2003.

10. Anderson IM: Meta-analytical studies on new antidepressants, *Br Med Bull* 57:161-178, 2001.

11. Smith D, Dempster C, Glanville J, et al: Efficacy and tolerability of venlafaxine compared with selective serotonin reuptake inhibitors and other antidepressants: a meta-analysis, *Br J Psychiatr* 180:396-404, 2002.

12. Jessell TM, Kelly DK: Pain and analgesia. In Kandell ER, Schwartz JH, Jessell TM, editors: *Principles of neural science*, ed 3. Norwalk, Conn, 1991, Appleton & Lange.

13. Kunz NR, Goli V, Entsuah R, et al: Diabetic neuropathic pain management with venlafaxine extended release, *Eur Neuropsychopharmacol* 10:S389, 2000.

14. Stoppe G, Doren M: Critical appraisal of effects of estrogen replacement therapy on symptoms of depressed mood, *Arch Women Mental Health* 5:39-47, 2002.

15. Ernst E, Rand JI, Stevinson C: Complementary therapies for depression: an overview, *Arch Gen Psychiatr* 55:1026-1032, 1998.

16. Haag M: Essential fatty acids and the brain, *Can J Psychiatr* 48:195-203, 2003.

17. Hibbeln JR: Fish consumption and major depression, *Lancet* 351:1213, 1998.

18. Mischoulon D, Fava M: Docosahexanoic acid and omega-3 fatty acids in depression, *Psychiatr Clin North Am* 23:785-794, 2000.

19. Nemets B, Stahl Z, Belmaker RH: Addition of omega-3 fatty acid to maintenance medication treatment for recurrent unipolar depressive disorder. *Am J Psychiatr* 159:477-479, 2002.

20. Peet M, Horrobin DF: A dose-ranging study of the effects of ethyl-eicosapentaenoate in patients with ongoing depression despite apparently adequate treatment with standard drugs, *Arch Gen Psychiatr* 59:913-919, 2002.

21. Fish oil omega-3, Consumberlabs.com. Last accessed July 27, 2003.

22. *S-adenosyl-L-methionine for treatment of depression, osteoarthritis, and liver disease: summary, evidence report/technology assessment number 64*, AHRQ publication no. 02-E033, Rockville, Maryland, August 2002, Agency for Healthcare Research and Quality.

23. Linde K, Ramirez G, Mulrow CD, et al: St. John's wort for depression: an overview and meta-analysis of randomised clinical trials, *BMJ* 313:253-258, 1996.

24. Schulz V: Clinical trials with hypericum extracts in patients with depression: results, comparisons, conclusions for therapy with antidepressant drugs, *Phytomedicine* 9:468-474, 2002.

25. Linde K, Mulrow CD: St. John's wort for depression. *Cochrane Database Syst Rev* (2): CD000448, 2002.

26. Whiskey E, Werneke U, Taylor D: A systematic review and meta-analysis of *Hypericum perforatum* in depression: a comprehensive clinical review, *Int Clin Psychopharmacol* 16:239-252, 2001.

27. Shelton RC, Keller MB, Gelenberg A, et al: Effectiveness of St. John's wort in major depression: a randomized controlled trial, *JAMA* 285:1978-1986, 2001.

28. Hypericum Depression Trial Study Group: Effect of *Hypericum perforatum* (St. John's wort) in major depressive disorder: a randomized controlled trial, *JAMA* 287:1807-1814, 2002.

29. Khan A, Khan S, Brown WA: Are placebo controls necessary to test new antidepressants and anxiolytics? *Int J Neuropsychopharmacol* 5:193-197, 2002.

30. Thase ME: Comparing the methods used to compare antidepressants, *Psychopharmacol Bull* 36(suppl 1):1-17, 2002.

31. Di Matteo V, Di Giovanni G, Di Mascio M, et al: Effect of acute administration of *Hypericum perforatum*–CO_2 extract on dopamine and serotonin release in the rat central nervous system, *Pharmacopsychiatry* 33:14-18, 2000.

32. Chatterjee SS, Bhattacharya SK, Singer A, et al: Hyperforin inhibits synaptosomal uptake of neurotransmitters in vitro and shows antidepressant activity in vivo, *Pharmazie* 53:9, 1998.

33. Nathan PJ: *Hypericum perforatum* (St. John's wort): a non-selective reuptake inhibitor? A review of the recent advances in its pharmacology, *J Psychopharmacol* 15:47-54, 2001.

34. Butterweck V, Bockers T, Korte B, et al: Long-term effects of St. John's wort and hypericin on monoamine levels in rat hypothalamus and hippocampus. *Brain Res* 930(1-2):21-29, 2002.

35. Butterweck V, Winterhoff H, Herkenham M: St. John's wort, hypericin, and imipramine: a comparative analysis of mRNA levels in brain areas involved in HPA axis control following short-term and long-term administration in normal and stressed rats, *Mol Psychiatr* 6:547-564, 2001.

36. Simmen U, Bobirnac I, Ullmer C, et al: Antagonist effect of pseudohypericin at CRF(1) receptors, *Eur J Pharmacol* 458:251-256, 2003.
37. Marsh WL, Davies JA: The involvement of sodium and calcium ions in the release of amino acid neurotransmitters from mouse cortical slices elicited by hyperforin, *Life Sci* 71:2645-2655, October 18, 2002.
38. Muller WE, Singer A, Wonnemann M: Hyperforin: antidepressant activity by a novel mechanism of action. *Pharmacopsychiatry* 34(suppl 1):S98-S102, 2001.
39. Nahrstedt A, Butterweck V: Biologically active and other chemical constituents of the herb of *Hypericum perforatum* L. *Pharmacopsychiatry* 30(suppl 2):129-134, 1997.
40. Schulz V: Incidence and clinical relevance of the interactions and side effects of Hypericum preparations, *Phytomedicine* 8:152-160, 2001.
41. Schmidt U: Evaluation of reaction time under antidepressive therapy with Hypericum preparation LI 160, *Nervenheilkunde* 10:311-312, 1991.
42. Schmidt U, Harrer G, Kuhn U, et al: Interaction of hypericum extract with alcohol. Placebo controlled study with 32 volunteers. *Nervenheilkunde* 12:314-319, 1993.
43. Wheatley D: Hypericum extract: potential in the treatment of depression, *CNS Drugs* 9:431-440, 1998.
44. Brockmoller J, et al: Hypericin and pseudohypericin: pharmacokinetics and effects of photosensitivity in humans, *Pharmacopsychiatry* 30(suppl 2):94-101, 1997.
45. Durr D, Stieger B, Kullak-Ublick GA, et al: St. John's Wort induces intestinal P-glycoprotein, MDRI and intestinal and hepatic CYP3A4, *Clin Pharmacol Ther* 68:598-604, 2000.
46. Moore LB, Goodwin B, Jones SA, et al: St. John's wort induces hepatic drug metabolism through activation of the pregnane X receptor, *Proc Natl Acad Sci U S A* 97:7500-2c, June 20, 2000.
47. Obach RS: Inhibition of human cytochrome P450 enzymes by constituents of St. John's wort, an herbal preparation used in the treatment of depression, *J Pharmacol Exp Ther* 294:88-95, 2000.
48. Markowitz JS, DeVane CL, Boulton DW, et al: Effect of St. John's wort (*Hypericum perforatum*) on cytochrome P-450 2D6 and 3A4 activity in healthy volunteers, *Life Sci* 66:L133-L139, 2000.
49. Cott JM: Herb-drug interactions, *CNS Spectrum* 6:827-832, 2001.
50. EGb 761: ginkgo biloba extract, Ginkor, *Drugs R D* 4:188-193, 2003.
51. Birks J, Grimley Evans J, et al: *Ginkgo biloba* for cognitive impairment and dementia (Cochrane Review). In *The Cochrane Library*, issue 4, Oxford, UK, 2002.
52. Schubert H, Halama P: Depressive episode primarily unresponsive to therapy in elderly patients: efficacy of *Ginkgo biloba* (Egb 761) in combination with antidepressants, *Geriatr Forschung* 3:45-53, 1993.
53. Hemmeter U, Annen B, Bischof R, et al: Polysomnographic effects of adjuvant ginkgo biloba therapy in patients with major depression medicated with trimipramine, *Pharmacopsychiatry* 34:50-59, 2001.
54. Marcilhac A, Dakine N, Bourhim N, et al: Effect of chronic administration of *Ginkgo biloba* extract or Ginkgolide on the hypothalamic-pituitary-adrenal axis in the rat. *Life Sci* 62:2329-2340, 1998.
55. Huguet F: Decreased cerebral 5-HT1a receptors during aging: reversal by *Ginkgo biloba* extract (Egb 761), *J Pharm Pharmacol* 46:316-318, 1994.
56. Vaes LP, Chyka PA: Interactions of warfarin with garlic, ginger, ginkgo, or ginseng: nature of the evidence, *Ann Pharmacother* 34:1478-1482, 2000.
57. Sollier CBD, Caplain H, Drouet L: No alteration in platelet function or coagulation induced by Egb761 in a controlled study, *Clin Lab Haem* 25:251-253, 2003.
58. Thommessen B, Laake K: No identifiable effect of ginseng (Gericomplex) as an adjuvant in the treatment of geriatric patients, *Aging Clin Exp Res* 8:417-420, 1996.
59. Fugh-Berman A, Cott JM: Dietary supplements and natural products as psychotherapeutic agents, *Psychosom Med* 61:712-728, 1999.
60. Wiklund IK, Mattsson LA, Lindgren R, et al: Effects of a standardized ginseng extract on quality of life and physiological parameters in symptomatic postmenopausal women: a double-blind, placebo-controlled trial. Swedish Alternative Medicine Group, *Int J Clin Pharmacol Res* 19:89-99, 1999.
61. Tode T, Kikuchi Y, Hirata J, et al: Effect of Korean red ginseng on psychological functions in patients with severe climacteric syndromes, *Int J Gynaecol Obstet* 67:169-174, 1999.

62. Newall CA, Anderson LA, Phillipson JD: *Herbal medicines: a guide for health-care professionals*, London, 1996, Pharmaceutical Press.
63. Kim DH, Moon YS, Jung JS, et al: Effects of ginseng saponin administered intraperitoneally on the hypothalamo-pituitary-adrenal axis in mice, *Neurosci Lett* 343:62-66, 2003.
64. Yuan CS, Attele AS, Wu JA, et al: Modulation of American ginseng on brainstem GABAergic effects in rats, *J Ethnopharmacol* 62:215-222, 1998.
65. Huong NT, Matsumoto K, Watanabe H: The antistress effect of majonoside-R2, a major saponin component of Vietnamese ginseng: neuronal mechanisms of action, *Methods Find Exp Clin Pharmacol* 20:65-76, 1998.
66. Deleted in proof.
67. McGuffin M, Hobbs C, Upton R, et al: 1997.
68. Blumenthal M, Goldberg A, Brinckmann J: *Herbal medicine: expanded Commission E monographs*, Newton, Massachusetts, 2000, Integrative Medicine Communications, pp 394-397.
69. Ortiz JG, Nieves-Natal J, Chavez P: Effects of *Valeriana officinalis* extracts on [³H]flunitrazepam binding, synaptosomal [³H]GABA uptake, and hippocampal [³H]GABA release, *Neurochem Res* 24:1373-1378, 1999.
70. Cavadas C, Araujo I, Cotrim MD, et al: In vitro study on the interaction of *Valeriana officinalis* L. extracts and their amino acids on GABAA receptor in rat brain, *Arzneimittelforschung* 45:753-755, 1995.
71. Santos MS, Ferreira F, Cunha AP, et al: An aqueous extract of valerian influences the transport of GABA in synaptosomes, *Planta Med* 60:278-279, 1994.

CHAPTER

12

Insomnia

Insomnia is a term used to describe the chronic inability to sleep at times when sleep is normally expected to occur. Insomnia may consist of difficulty falling asleep or difficulty remaining asleep. The most common sleep disorder, insomnia reportedly affects at least 60 million Americans.[1] Of people who see primary care physicians, an estimated 69% have had insomnia, but this figure is considered low because only one third of those with insomnia speak to their physicians about the problem,[2] as many believe it is not a legitimate health problem.

Primary insomnia is generally the result of a combination of psychological and social factors. Secondary insomnia is caused by a disease process, underlying medical disorder, or external cause, such as the use of medications or an excessive amount of alcohol. Restless legs syndrome, *anxietas tibiarum,* is one medical condition that can impair an individual's ability to fall asleep. A person with restless legs syndrome complains of an uneasy feeling—usually relieved by movement—in the legs after lying down. Excessive fatigue can cause this condition, but it may also be an early sign of peripheral neuropathy.

Insomnia is more common in women than in men.[3] During menopause, women may experience sleep problems as a result of hot flashes, night sweats, or psychological stressors.[4] A longitudinal study in which women were monitored over a 3-year period, as they moved from perimenopause to menopause, revealed significant increases in the incidence and severity of sleep disturbances.[5] Women taking hormone replacement therapy experienced far less severe instances of these sleep disturbances, suggesting that therapies that reduce unpleasant symptoms such as hot flashes and night sweats may also improve sleep.

Patients often have difficulty quantifying the amount of time they actually sleep. Scientists have conducted research on patients with insomnia to determine whether patients could reliably detect whether they were asleep or awake by comparing diaries against polysomnograph readings.[6] Researchers found that insomniacs have a reduced ability to discriminate sleeping from waking and that they are prone to misclassify a sleeping episode as one in which they were awake. It appears that some insomniacs greatly overestimate the extent and duration of their insomnia.

TREATMENT OPTIONS

Chronic stress and insomnia can lead to many unhealthy daytime behaviors that further aggravate both problems; thus integrative treatment is probably the best approach. When people are tired, they often consume more caffeine and high-sugar, high-fat foods in an attempt to feel more energetic. Individuals are also less likely to exercise because they feel "too tired." Insomnia decreases the ability to concentrate and focus, causing job and school performance to suffer. More alarming, it may increase the risk for heart disease and obesity. The findings of studies published in leading medical journals suggest that sleep loss increases hunger and affects the body's metabolism, making it more difficult to maintain or lose weight. The National Sleep Foundation reports that roughly 100,000 car accidents per year are the result of drowsiness and estimates the direct and indirect annual costs of sleep disorders to the U.S. economy at $100 billion.

Lifestyle and Diet

A healthy diet is important to everyone, especially anyone who does not feel adequately rested. The B vitamins are important in improving the quality and quantity of sleep. Vitamin B_6 is involved in the synthesis of serotonin, a neurotransmitter used by the brain

---

SIMPLE TIPS FOR GETTING TO SLEEP

- Establish a regular sleep-wake schedule. A good way to begin is by getting up at the same time every morning, no matter what time you go to sleep. Yes, this means weekends, too!
- Create a pleasant place in which to rest. Purchase high-quality cotton sheets and a cozy comforter. Try soft music, candles, flowers—whatever makes you feel relaxed. Keep a fan or small water feature in your bedroom to block out nighttime noise.
- Darken your bedroom at bedtime. Light affects the brain hormones in charge of your sleep cycle. Even a small amount of light can disrupt sleep. Use window treatments to darken the room or wear a sleep mask to bed.
- The bed should be used only for sleeping and making love, not for working, studying, or watching TV.
- Don't consume any caffeine after 4 PM.
- Try drinking a strong cup of chamomile tea in the evening. Pour 1 cup of boiling water over two or three teabags, then steep the tea for 5 minutes. Sip slowly about 45 minutes before bedtime.
- Eat a light meal, preferably one containing some carbohydrates, in the evening.
- Consume no more than one serving of alcohol per day. Excessive amounts of alcohol disrupt sleep. Don't drink within 2 hours of bedtime.
- To reduce muscle tension, try a relaxation technique, such as meditation, yoga, or soaking in a warm bath.
- Regular exercise helps improve sleep and mood, but make sure to finish your workout at least 3 hours before bedtime.

---

to regulate sleep. Vitamin B_6 deficiency can lead to insomnia, depression, and increased irritability, all of which are reversible when adequate levels of the vitamin are supplied. Restless legs syndrome has been linked to abnormalities in iron stores in adults and adolescents.[7] Sleep specialists recommend evaluation of iron status, including serum iron, total iron-binding capacity, and ferritin levels, in any patient with chronic insomnia of unexplained origin, even when anemia is mild or absent. A high-magnesium diet seems to provide the highest-quality sleep time with the fewest nighttime awakenings.

A patient with insomnia should be advised to avoid caffeinated beverages. Any consumption of coffee, tea, or soda should be limited to early in the day and kept to a minimum. Coffee consumption causes a decrease in the total amount and quality of sleep, as well as an increase in the amount of time it takes to fall asleep. Researchers have also found that consumption of caffeine decreases the level of 6-sulfoxymelatonin, the main metabolite of melatonin in urine.[8]

Over-the-Counter Medications

A survey of adults ages 18 to 45 years revealed that self-medication for insomnia is relatively common.[9] Thirteen percent of respondents reported using alcohol, 10% reported using over-the-counter (OTC) medications, and 5% reported using prescription drugs. The main ingredients of most OTC insomnia remedies are the antihistamines diphenhydramine hydrochloride and doxylamine succinate. Diphenhydramine should be taken at bedtime, whereas doxylamine products should be taken half an hour before bedtime. During this 30-minute interval, the individual should not drive or perform any activity requiring vigilance.[10]

Although OTC antihistamines are effective and relatively safe for the treatment of insomnia, the U.S. Food and Drug Administration requires that manufacturers warn patients not to take the drugs if they are younger than 12 years or have a breathing problem (e.g., emphysema or chronic bronchitis), glaucoma, enlarged prostate or if they are pregnant or breastfeeding. The labels of these antihistamines carry a required caution to patients to stop use and consult a physician if sleeplessness lasts for more than 2 weeks. The labeling also advises individuals against taking the drugs with alcohol and encourages them to check with a health care provider before using them at the same time as sedatives or tranquilizers.[10]

Melatonin

Melatonin (*N*-acetyl-5-methoxytryptamine), a neurohormone produced in the pineal gland, is involved in the regulation of the sleep-wake cycle. Melatonin is normally secreted during darkness in response to the release of norepinephrine from retinal photoreceptors. Levels begin to rise at nightfall, with peak serum concentrations typically occurring between 2 and 4 AM in adults. Individuals with impaired melatonin production or secretion may experience chronic disturbances in the onset and duration of sleep. In these patients, exogenous melatonin may be beneficial to help regulate the sleep-wake cycle.[11]

Although most consider melatonin a dietary supplement, in 1993 the Food and Drug Administration classified it as an orphan drug for the entrainment of circadian rhythm in blind people (the absence of light cues results in disturbances of sleep and sleep-related neuroendocrine patterns). In a double-blind crossover study, 12 totally blind individuals received 5 mg of oral melatonin or placebo 1 hour before bedtime, starting at 11 PM. This dose of melatonin increased total sleep time and reduced time spent awake ($P < 0.05$) while normalizing pituitary-adrenal activity.[12]

In addition to improving the sleep-wake cycle in blind people, melatonin has been shown to be remarkably effective in preventing or reducing jet lag. Cochrane reviewers state that "it should be recommended to adult travelers flying across five or more time zones, particularly in an easterly direction, and especially if they have experienced jet lag on previous journeys. Travelers crossing 2-4 time zones can also use it if need be."[13]

Melatonin is often given to children and adolescents with severe neurodevelopmental disabilities. Turk et al conducted a literature review and concluded that melatonin is a potentially useful and safe adjunct to psychological and social approaches to the treatment of severe sleep disturbances in these children.[14] Melatonin is sometimes recommended for children with attention deficit/hyperactivity disorder, but whether it is beneficial in this group is less clear. The National Sleep Foundation notes that melatonin may be useful in teenagers who are unable to fall asleep during the early nighttime hours and consequently experience problems awakening the next morning.[15]

Oral melatonin therapy appears to be well tolerated. No adverse effects have been noted in most clinical trials and case series. Headache, excessive sedation, and transient depression have been reported with dosages greater than 8 mg/day. The typical dose of melatonin is 3 mg/day. The effect of melatonin in people with epilepsy is not completely understood. In a 1998 study published in the *Lancet,* melatonin administration to six children with underlying seizure disorders produced a worsening of seizures in three.[16] Melatonin may also interact with warfarin; patients should be monitored if taking these substances concurrently.[13]

Botanical Remedies

Valerian **(Valeriana officinalis).**   Valerian is a common ingredient in products sold as mild relaxants and the relief of nervous tension and insomnia (Figure 12-1). The genus *Valeriana* includes more than 250 species, but *V. officinalis,* in root and rhizome form, is the species most often used in the United States and Europe. The herb is sold as a single ingredient but is more commonly found in combination products. Valerian has been used medicinally since at least the time of ancient Greece and Rome; in the second century AD, Galen recommended valerian as a treatment for insomnia. During World War II, valerian was used in England to relieve the stress of air raids.[17] The German Commission E endorses the use of valerian for restlessness and sleeping disorders caused by nervous conditions. The World Health Organization lists the following uses for valerian: mild sedative, sleep-promoting agent, milder alternative to or possible substitute for stronger sedatives (e.g., benzodiazepines), and treatment for nervous excitation and sleep disturbances induced by anxiety.[18] The European Scientific Cooperative on Phytotherapy lists the following therapeutic indications for valerian: tenseness, restlessness, and irritability accompanied by difficulty falling asleep. Valerian root, root powder, and root extract are official (with legally recognized standards of identity, strength, quality, purity, packaging, and labeling) in the *United States Pharmacopoeia* (25th edition).[19]

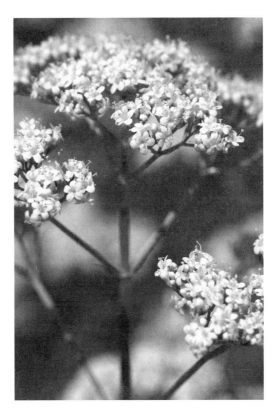

Figure **12-1** Valerian *(Valeriana officinalis). (Courtesy Martin Wall Botanical Services.)*

Although valerian is recognized in many countries as a traditional medicine to aid sleep and reduce nervousness and herbalists strongly believe in its beneficial effects, clinical trials have yielded conflicting results. In a systematic review, nine randomized, placebo-controlled, double-blind clinical trials of valerian and sleep disorders were identified and evaluated for evidence of efficacy of valerian as a treatment for insomnia.[20] Three of the nine trials earned the highest rating (5 on a scale of 1 to 5), although the reviewers concluded overall that the evidence supporting the efficacy of valerian in the treatment of insomnia is inconclusive and that more rigorous trials are necessary. The following text provides a quick review of the three best studies cited in the review, all of which yielded positive findings.

In a 1982 study by Leathwood et al, 128 volunteers were randomly assigned to take one of the three preparations three times in random order on nine consecutive nights. The study preparations included a 400-mg dose of an aqueous extract of valerian, a combination preparation containing 60 mg of valerian and 30 mg of hops, and a placebo.[21] Each participant filled out a questionnaire on the morning after each treatment. Compared with the placebo, the valerian extract resulted in a statistically significant subjective improvement in the time required to fall asleep, quality of sleep, and the number of nighttime awakenings. The combination preparation did not produce a statistically significant improvement in any of these three measures, although this would not be unexpected given the low levels of both valerian and hops in the product. Although the study scored high rating for its design, it had two major drawbacks: a participant-withdrawal rate of 22.9% and, more important, the fact that volunteers were not screened for insomnia, meaning that some participants had trouble sleeping but others did not.

In another study, Leathwood et al compared 450- and 900-mg dosages of valerian aqueous extract to placebo in eight patients with mild insomnia. Patients were randomly assigned to receive one of the three test samples each night, Monday through Thursday, for 3 weeks. Results were based on nighttime motion as measured with the use of activity meters worn on the wrist and responses to questionnaires about sleep quality, latency, depth, and morning sleepiness that were completed the morning after each treatment. The 450-mg dosage of valerian extract reduced sleep latency from 16 to 9 minutes; no statistically significant shortening of sleep latency was observed with the 900-mg dose. The time required to fall asleep was shortened by 7 minutes and was therefore a statistically significant result, but this finding may not be clinically significant. The 900-mg sample increased the patients' perception of sleep improvement, but participants noted increased sleepiness the next morning.[22]

A more recent study, published by Vorbach et al in 1996, also received a rating of 5 from the review team. This is the only one of the three studies in which the sustained use of valerian extract over an extended period was examined. One hundred twenty-one individuals with documented nonorganic insomnia received either 600 mg of a standardized extract of dried valerian root (LI 156, Sedonium; Lichtwer Pharma AG, Berlin, Germany; each tablet contains 300 mg of extract of valerian with a drug/extract ratio of 5:1) or placebo for 28 days.[23] Three different questionnaires were provided to participants; one evaluated the therapeutic effect on days 14 and 28, one evaluated change in sleep patterns on day 28, and one evaluated change in sleep quality and well-being on days 0, 14, and 28. After 28 days, the group receiving the valerian extract showed a decrease in insomnia symptoms, compared with the placebo group, on all questionnaires. The differences in improvement between valerian and placebo increased between the assessments conducted on days 14 and 28. The findings of this study are consistent with my own clinical experience that individuals with insomnia experience better results with valerian when they take it every night for an extended period, usually 4 to 6 weeks. Patients often tell me that occasional use of valerian to relieve sleeplessness has hit-or-miss results.

Not included in the review was a double-blind, randomized study by Ziegler et al comparing the effects of a 6-week course of 600 mg/day standardized valerian extract (LI 156 Sedonium) or 10 mg/day of oxazepam in 202 patients ages 18 to 73 years with nonorganic insomnia. Changes in sleep quality were assessed with the use of Sleep Questionnaire B (CIPS [Collegium Internationale Psychiatrie Scalarum] 1996), which revealed that 600 mg of valerian extract was at least as efficacious as treatment with 10 mg of oxazepam. Both treatments markedly increased sleep quality compared with baseline ($P < 0.01$). Other Sleep Questionnaire B subscales (e.g., feeling of refreshment after sleep, dream recall, duration of sleep) showed similar effects for the two treatments. The Clinical Global Impressions scale and Global Assessment of Efficacy by investigator and patient showed similar effects of the two treatments. Adverse events occurred in 29 patients (28.4%) receiving valerian extract LI 156 and in 36 patients (36.0%) taking oxazepam; all were rated as mild to moderate. No serious adverse drug reactions were reported in either group. Most patients assessed their treatment as very good (82.8% in the valerian group, 73.4% in the oxazepam group).[24]

The aforementioned studies were all conducted with the use of monopreparations of valerian, although most consumers likely purchase combination products. Three double-blind, placebo-controlled studies showed that the combination of valerian and lemon balm (*Melissa officinalis*), an herb with documented anxiolytic activity, was effective in improving sleep quality among individuals with insomnia. Combinations of valerian, hops, and lemon balm yielded similarly positive effects.[25] Although most practitioners associate the use of valerian with sleep and, to a lesser extent, anxiety, two clinical trials of a combination of valerian and St. John's wort for the treatment of depression have been conducted. The combination was equivalent or superior to the tricyclic antidepressants amitriptyline and desipramine when given for a period of 6 weeks.[26] It is unclear whether the antidepressant effect was primarily the result of St. John's wort or whether synergism exists between the two herbs.

Controversy over the active constituents of valerian continues. Most research has been focused on two main groups of substances: the volatile oil fraction and the valepotriates. Three cyclopentane sesquiterpenoids (valerenic acid, acetoxyvalerenic acid, and valeranal) are present only in *V. officinalis,* distinguishing it from other species of the genus.[18] The volatile oil fraction is responsible for only part of the sedative effect; likewise, the valepotriates do not account for all the sedative activity of the plant extract.[27] The isolation of 6-methylapigenin, a flavone derivative that acts as a ligand for the benzodiazepine-binding site of the $GABA_A$ receptor[28]; and 2S(–)-7-rhamnoglucosyl-hesperetin, a flavanone glycoside with sedative and sleep-enhancing properties from both *V. wallachii* and *V. officinalis,* continues to expand our understanding of the complex biochemistry of this genus.

Valerian's mechanism of action is poorly understood. Compounds in valerian have been shown to have a direct effect on the amygdaloid body of the brain, and valerenic acid has been shown to inhibit enzyme-induced breakdown of γ-aminobutyric acid (GABA) in the brain, resulting in sedation.[29] The valepotriates act as prodrugs, which are transformed into homobaldrinal, a compound found to reduce the spontaneous motility of mice, and a lignan, hydroxypinoresinol, which has been shown to bind to benzodiazepine receptors.[29] The proprietary valerian extract LI 156 has been found to act on the melatonin receptor in a dose-dependent manner in vitro.[30]

Valerian is generally quite safe when taken appropriately. The crude herb is usually taken in a dosage of 2 or 3 g, equivalent to 10-15 mL of tincture (1:5 strength), approximately 1 hour before bedtime. Standardized extracts are also widely available and should be taken as directed on the label. Valerian may need to be taken for several weeks for its maximal effect to be achieved. The World Health Organization notes that the use of valerian is contraindicated during pregnancy and lactation due to lack of studies in this area.

Passionflower (**Passiflora incarnata**).   Passionflower has traditionally been used by South American Indians as a mild sedative. The herb exported to Europe in 1569 by Spanish explorers returning from Peru, who named the plant for its appearance, which evokes Christ's Passion, with five anthers resembling the stigmata and a fringelike crown resembling a crown of thorns. Passionflower is a popular herb in the United States and Europe, where it is used in the management of anxiety, insomnia, epilepsy, and morphine addiction. *P. incarnata* is official in the pharmacopoeias of many countries, including Great Britain, the United States, India, France, Egypt, Germany, and Switzerland.[31] The

German Commission E endorses the use of passionflower for the treatment of nervous restlessness. It is generally used in combination with other sedative herbs such as valerian, lemon balm, and hops (*Humulus lupulus*).

In recent studies, a methanol extract of the leaves of *P. incarnata* was shown in animal studies to have anxiolytic,[32] antitussive,[33] and aphrodisiac properties.[34] A trisubstituted benzoflavone moiety isolated from the methanol extract was found to counter dependence on and the development of tolerance to, morphine, cannabinoids, nicotine, and ethanol in mice at a dosage range of 10 to 50 mg/kg.[35] Sedative and anxiolytic effects have also been documented with aqueous and hydroethanolic extracts of passionflower in mice.[36]

The pharmacologically active constituents of passionflower are not precisely known, but current thinking holds that the flavonoids play a significant role. Flavonoids (up to 2.5% content in the plant) include vitexin, isovitexin, coumarin, apigenin, umbeliferone, and maltol. Harmala alkaloids, including harmaline and harmine, have been reported and are believed to contribute to the plant's sedative activity but may be present in subtherapeutic quantities. The stability of flavonoids in passionflower tinctures (60% vol/vol) is roughly 6 months,[37] calling into question the efficacy of these products shelved for many years.

Human clinical research with passionflower herb is lacking. However, given what is known of its biochemistry, as well as its widespread use, modern research is warranted. Passionflower appears to be relatively safe when used appropriately. Pregnancy is not listed as a contraindication to the use of passionflower by the German Commission E, the *British Herbal Compendium*, or the American Herbal Products Association. The herb may potentiate the sedative effects of benzodiazepines, although this is a theoretical interaction and not based on actual case reports. The dosage listed in the German Commission E monograph is 4 to 8 g/day in tea or equivalent preparations. This is far greater than what is generally available in OTC dietary supplements in the United States.

Skullcap (Scutellaria lateriflora). Skullcap, also known as mad dog weed, has traditionally been used as a sedative and to treat various nervous disorders such as anxiety. It is often found in combination formulas with valerian, hops, lemon balm, and passionflower. Animal studies suggest that the formula indeed has some anxiolytic activity.[38] The 70% ethanol extract of *S. lateriflora* is characterized chemically by the presence of flavonoids; the predominant ones are baicalin, lateriflorin, dihydrobaicalin, and baicalein.[39] These compounds may play a role in anxiolytic activity; baicalin and baicalein are known to bind to the benzodiazepine site of the GABA-A receptor, GABA being the primary inhibitory neurotransmitter.[38] Levels of these compounds are even higher in a related species, *Scutellaria baicalensis*.

One author has reported that large amounts of skullcap can cause giddiness, stupor, confusion, and seizures.[40] Liver damage and acute hepatitis following the use of herbal preparations that purportedly contained skullcap (*Scutellaria* spp) and valerian have been reported.[41] It is believed that the adverse effects were actually the result of substitution of germander (*Teucrium* spp), an herb known to have hepatotoxic effects, for skullcap.[42] The substitution or adulteration of *S. lateriflora* with *Teucrium canadense* and *T. chamaedrys* is well known. Analytical methods have been developed[39] to prevent this occurrence in the marketplace; however, manufacturers are not mandated to perform the tests.

CASE REPORT OF LIVER TOXICITY

In July 2002, a 56-year-old woman who had been previously well, apart from a history of benign monoclonal gammopathy (IgG 24 g/L; normal range 6.9–15.4 g/L), presented to her local physician with a 2-week history of fatigue, nausea, and increasing jaundice. She had no risk factors for viral hepatitis and no history of liver disease, and her alcohol consumption was minimal. During the preceding 3 months she had been taking a herbal supplement, prescribed and provided by a naturopath, for anxiety (Kava 1800 Plus, one tablet three times daily; labeled as containing kavalactones 60 mg, *P. incarnata* 50 mg and *S. lateriflora* 100 mg; Eagle Pharmaceuticals, Castle Hill, New South Wales, Australia). She had also been taking some vitamin and mineral supplements but was taking no other medications. Examination on presentation to the hospital revealed the patient to be deeply jaundiced but without the stigmata of chronic liver disease. The results of screening for recognized causes of acute liver failure were negative. The findings of assays for the hepatitis A, B, and C viruses; Epstein-Barr virus; and cytomegalovirus were all negative. Serum copper and ceruloplasmin levels were normal, and Kayser-Fleischer rings were not present. Antinuclear antibodies were detected at a titer of 1:160, but anti–smooth muscle antibodies were not detected. No acetaminophen was detected in the blood. An abdominal ultrasound revealed a small liver with normal flow in the hepatic arteries, hepatic veins, and portal veins. The paraprotein level had remained stable over the previous 12 months. A repeat bone-marrow biopsy did not suggest the presence of multiple myeloma. The patient underwent liver transplantation 17 days after being admitted to the hospital, but she died of progressive blood loss, hypotension, and circulatory failure. Subsequent analysis of the supplement she had taken revealed that it contained kava and *P. incarnata*, as labeled, and a third, as yet unidentified compound. Although the label listed *S. lateriflora* as an ingredient, none was identified in the product.[43] Although most reviewers have focused on the potential role of kava in this case of hepatotoxicity, the presence of an "unidentified" compound in the product prompts questioning as to whether this could be another case of replacement of *Scutellaria* with *Teucrium*. This case certainly highlights the need for superior quality control to avoid intentional or accidental substitution of toxic plant material in a product.

Hops (Humulus lupulus).   Beer brewers originally used hops as a preservative: Beer brewed with the herb could be stored longer before being sold, and the bitter flavor imparted by the hops became popular with beer drinkers. Hops were also widely used as a traditional medicine for insomnia and nervousness. Hops-filled pillows were extremely popular in England during the 17th through the 19th centuries. Such pillows purportedly brought sleep to King George III of England and Abraham Lincoln, both of whom had insomnia. Eberle wrote in an 1824 American medical text "everyone knows the effects of hop pillow in procuring sleep."[44] In traditional Chinese medicine, hops are used to treat insomnia, restlessness, dyspepsia, intestinal cramps, and lack of appetite. The German

Commission E endorses the use of hops for the treatment of mood disturbances such as restlessness and anxiety and for the relief of sleep disturbances. The European Scientific Cooperative on Phytotherapy lists hops as a remedy for tenseness, restlessness, and difficulty falling asleep.

Despite the long, rich history of hops as a sedative, virtually no human clinical trials have been conducted to study hops as a single therapy. Animal studies indicate that hops have sedative, hypnotic, anticonvulsant, and antinociceptive properties.[45] Findings from several small, methodologically weak clinical trials of products containing both valerian and hops show that the combination is useful in promoting sleep. Preliminary pharmacologic tests suggest that the soporific activity of hops can be explained by its content of 2-methyl-3-butene-2-ol in the volatile fraction.[46] Only trace amounts of this constituent are present in the fresh hops, but its concentration has been shown to continuously increase after they have been dried, reaching maximal levels (approximately 0.15%) within 2 years of hops' storage at room temperature, as a result of the degradation of the soft resin compounds humulone and lupulone.[47]

In addition to the inclusion of hops in dietary supplements intended for sleep and relaxation, the herb is being heavily promoted for its phytoestrogen content. Hops can now be found in numerous products designed to ease symptoms of menopause symptoms and for "breast enhancement." A novel phytoestrogen, 8-prenylnaringenin, has been identified in hops. This substance is strongly competitive with 17-estradiol for binding to both the α- and β-estrogen receptors.[48]

The estrogenic activity of this compound has been shown to be greater than that of established phytoestrogens such as coumestrol, genistein, and daidzein in vitro.[49] The presence of 8-prenylnaringenin in hops may provide an explanation for anecdotal accounts of menstrual disturbances in female hops workers.[50] However, levels of this substance are very low in beer. Researchers have concluded that the human health hazard of beer drinking originating from activity on the estrogen receptor-α is negligible.[51]

Hops appear to be relatively safe when used appropriately. Theoretically, hops may potentiate the sedative effects of barbiturates[45] because of the herb's effects on the central nervous system. Dosage varies among texts and practitioners. Traditionally, 0.5 g of dried herb as an infusion or 1 or 2 mL of tincture (1:5, 60% ethanol) is taken two or three times a day. Although this practice is not common, some products are standardized to provide 5.2% bitter acids, 4% flavonoids, or both per dose.

Lemon balm **(Melissa officinalis).**   Islamic physicians referred to lemon balm as the "gladdening" herb during the Middle Ages, likely referring to its mood-lifting effects. Herbalists often use the fresh or dried aerial parts, gathered just before flowering, to ease depression, reduce anxiety, promote rest, and improve mood. The German Commission E endorses the use of lemon balm for the treatment of "insomnia of nervous origin."

Data from in vitro, animal, and human studies confirm that the herb possesses sedative activity. Freeze-dried hydroalcoholic extract of lemon balm was shown to exert sedative activity in mice even at relatively low dosages; higher dosages exerted analgesic activity.[52] A randomized, double-blind, placebo-controlled study showed that a 300-mg dosage of lemon balm extract increased self-reported "calmness," and a dosage of 900 mg significantly reduced "alertness" in 20 young, healthy undergraduate volunteers (mean age 19.2 years, range 18 to 22 years).[53] Participants were administered single doses of lemon balm or placebo on 5 different study days. The study days were separated by 7-day washout periods. On the first study day, participants underwent a battery of cognitive tests but did not receive treatment. On the next 4 study days, participants were randomly assigned to receive either placebo or 300, 600, or 900 mg of lemon balm extract. Tests included immediate and delayed word recall, simple reaction time, a digit vigilance task, choice reaction time, spatial working memory, numeric working memory, delayed word recognition, delayed picture recognition, and serial subtraction tasks. The scores were collapsed into four global outcome factors, namely accuracy and speed of attention and accuracy and speed of memory. Interestingly, this study showed the lowest dose of lemon balm had the most beneficial effect on mood and did not reduce memory performance, whereas the highest dose used in this study (900 mg) was detrimental overall to cognitive function.[54] The product used in the study contains the dried leaves of *M. officinalis* extracted to exhaustion in a 30:70 methanol/water mixture.

Lemon balm is often combined with other herbs that possess nervine properties. Indeed, the German monograph on lemon balm notes that combining lemon balm with other sedative and carminative drugs may be advantageous. The findings of several studies have demonstrated the sedative activity of valerian/lemon balm combinations.[55-57] Herbalists often combine lemon balm with other herbs to treat individuals with anxiety, nervousness, or insomnia.

Lemon balm is quite safe when used appropriately. Some concerns have been raised with regard to its effects on thyroid function on the basis of in vitro studies showing that freeze-dried aqueous extracts of lemon balm were able to block the binding of bovine thyroid-stimulating hormone (TSH) and Graves' autoantibodies to human thyroid membranes.[58] Some practitioners recommend testing thyroid function 6 to 8 weeks after the start of therapy with lemon balm in patients taking thyroid medication, although no cases of interaction have been reported. To prepare an infusion, steep 1.5 to 2.5 g of lemon-balm leaf in 1 cup of water for 5 to 10 minutes (1 tsp of herb equals roughly 1 g). This preparation is generally taken two or three times a day or 30 minutes before bed. The dosage for tincture (1:5) is generally 3 to 5 mL, twice or thrice daily.

California poppy (Eschscholzia californica). California poppy was tradition medicine of the indigenous peoples of what is now the state of California. It is still widely used by rural populations for its analgesic and sedative properties. Animal studies have verified its sedative and anxiolytic activities.[59] A hydroethanolic extract of the herb has been shown to demonstrate an affinity for the benzodiazepine receptor; the sedative and anxiolytic effects of the herb were suppressed by flumazenil, a benzodiazepine-receptor antagonist. Peripheral analgesic effects have also been noted in mice.[60] No human clinical trials have been published, to my knowledge. The famed herbalist Michael Moore sums up the folk use of California poppy nicely: "Like so many of the family, a mild sedative and analgesic, suitable even for children. A rounded teaspoon of the chopped plant as tea. Excess quantities can cause a slight residual hangover the next morning. [Note to would-be "Opium Eaters": the tea is functional, not fun."[61]

References

1. Katz DA, McHorney CA: The relationship between insomnia and health-related quality of life in patients with chronic illness, *J Fam Pract* 51:229-235, 2002.
2. Epstein DR, Bootzin RR: Insomnia, *Nurs Clin North Am* 37:611-631, 2002.
3. Shaver JL: Women and sleep. *Nurs Clin North Am* 37:707-718, 2002.
4. Moline ML, Broch L, Zak R, et al: Sleep in women across the life cycle from adulthood through menopause, *Sleep Med Rev* 7:155-177, 2003.

5. Shaver JL, Zenk SN: Sleep disturbances in menopause, *J Women Health Gend Based Med* 9: 109-118, 2000.
6. Mercer JD, Bootzin RR, Lack LC: Insomniacs' perception of wake instead of sleep, *Sleep* 25:564-571, 2002.
7. Kryger MH, Otake K, Foerster J: Low body stores of iron and restless legs syndrome: a correctable cause of insomnia in adolescents and teenagers, *Sleep Med* 3:127-132, 2002.
8. Shilo L, Sabbah H, Hadari R, et al: The effects of coffee consumption on sleep and melatonin secretion, *Sleep Med* 3:271-273, 2002.
9. Johnson EO, Roehrs T, Roth T, et al: Epidemiology of alcohol and medication as aids to sleep in early adulthood, *Sleep* 21:178-186, 1998.
10. Pray JJ, Pray WS: The role of the pharmacist in treating insomnia, *US Pharmacist* 8(7), 2003. Available online at Medscape.
11. Jan JE, Freeman RD, Fast DK: Melatonin treatment of sleep-wake cycle disorders in children and adolescents, *Dev Med Child Neurol* 41:491-500, 1999.
12. Fischer S, Smolnik R, Herms M, et al: Melatonin acutely improves the neuroendocrine architecture of sleep in blind individuals, *J Clin Endocrinol Metab* 88:5315-5320, 2003.
13. Herxheimer A, Petrie KJ: Melatonin for the prevention and treatment of jet lag (Cochrane review). In *The Cochrane Library*, issue 2. Oxford, UK, 2003, Update Software.
14. Turk J: Melatonin supplementation for severe and intractable sleep disturbance in young people with genetically determined developmental disabilities: short review and commentary, *J Med Genet* 40:793-796, 2003.
15. Goldberg JR: Melatonin: the facts. Available at: www.sleepfoundation.org/publications/melatoninthefact.html#2. Accessed March 2003.
16. Sheldon SH: Pro-convulsant effects of oral melatonin in neurologically disabled children, *Lancet* 351:1254, 1998.
17. Grieve M: Valerian. In: *A modern herbal*, New York, 1974, Hafner Press, pp 824-830.
18. "Valeriane radix," *WHO Monographs on Selected Medicinal Plants*, vol 1, Geneva, Switzerland, 1999, World Health Organization, pp 267-276.
19. *United States Pharmacopeia/National Formulary*, Rockville, MD, 2001, The United States Pharmacopeial Convention.
20. Stevinson C, Ernst E: Valerian for insomnia: a systematic review of randomized clinical trials, *Sleep Med* 1:91-99, 2000.
21. Leathwood PD, Chauffard F, Heck E, et al: Aqueous extract of valerian root (*Valeriana officinalis* L.) improves sleep quality in man, *Pharmacol Biochem Behav* 17:65-71, 1982.
22. Leathwood PD, Chauffard F: Aqueous extract of valerian reduces latency to fall asleep in man, *Planta Medica* 2:144-148, 1985.
23. Vorbach EU, Gortelmeyer R, Bruning J: Treatment of insomnia: effectiveness and tolerance of a valerian extract [in German], *Psychopharmakotherapie* 3:109-115, 1996.
24. Ziegler G, Ploch M, Miettinen-Baumann A, et al: Efficacy and tolerability of valerian extract LI 156 compared with oxazepam in the treatment of non-organic insomnia—a randomized, double-blind, comparative clinical study, *Eur J Med Res* 7:480-486, 2002.
25. Blumenthal M: *The ABC Clinical Guide to Herbs*, Austin, Texas, 2003, American Botanical Council, pp 351-364.
26. Linde K, Mulrow CD: St John's wort for depression (Cochrane Review). In *The Cochrane Library*, Issue 1, 2004, Chichester, UK: John Wiley & Sons.
27. Carlini EA: Plants and the central nervous system, *Pharmacol Biochem Behav* 75:501-512, 2003.
28. Wasowski C, Marder M, Viola H, et al: Isolation and identification of 6-methylapigenin, a competitive ligand for the brain GABA$_A$ receptors, from *Valeriana wallichii* D.C. *Planta Med* 68:934-936, 2002.
29. Houghton PJ: The scientific basis for the reputed activity of valerian. *J Pharm Pharmacol* 51: 505-512, 1999.
30. Fauteck JD, Pietz B, Winterhoff H, et al: Interaction of *Valeriana officinalis* with melatonin receptors: a possible explanation of its biological action [abstract]. In: *Second International Congress on Phytomedicine*, Munich, Germany, September 11-14, 1996.

31. Dhawan K, Kumar S, Sharma A: Anti-anxiety studies on extracts of *Passiflora incarnata* Linneaus, *J Ethnopharmacol* 78:165-170, 2001.
32. Dhawan K, Kumar S, Sharma A: Comparative anxiolytic activity profile of various preparations of *Passiflora incarnata* Linneaus: a comment on medicinal plants' standardization, *J Altern Complement Med* 8:283-291, 2002.
33. Dhawan K, Sharma A: Antitussive activity of the methanol extract of *Passiflora incarnata* leaves, *Fitoterapia* 73:397-399, 2002.
34. Dhawan K, Kumar S, Sharma A: Aphrodisiac activity of methanol extract of leaves of *Passiflora incarnata* Linn in mice, *Phytother Res* 17:401-403, 2003.
35. Dhawan K, Dhawan S, Chhabra S: Attenuation of benzodiazepine dependence in mice by a tri-substituted benzoflavone moiety of *Passiflora incarnata* Linneaus: a non–habit forming anxiolytic, *J Pharm Pharm Sci* 6:215-222, 2003.
36. Soulimani R, Younos C, Jarmouni S, et al: Behavioural effects of *Passiflora incarnata* L. and its indole alkaloid and flavonoid derivatives and maltol in the mouse, *J Ethnopharmacol* 57:11-20, 1997.
37. Bilia AR, Bergonzi MC, Gallori S, et al: Stability of the constituents of Calendula, milk-thistle and passionflower tinctures by LC-DAD and LC-MS, *J Pharm Biomed Anal* 30(3):613-624, October 2002.
38. Awad R, Arnason JT, Trudeau V, et al: Phytochemical and biological analysis of skullcap (*Scutellaria lateriflora* L.): a medicinal plant with anxiolytic properties, *Phytomedicine* 10:640-649, 2003.
39. Gafner S, Bergeron C, Batcha LL, et al: Analysis of *Scutellaria lateriflora* and its adulterants *Teucrium canadense* and *Teucrium chamaedrys* by LC-UV/MS, TLC, and digital photomicroscopy, *J AOAC Int* 86:453-460, 2003.
40. Newall CA, Anderson LA, Phillipson JD: *Herbal medicines: a guide for health-care professionals*, London, UK, 1996, Pharmaceutical Press.
41. MacGregor FB, Abernethy VE, Dahabra S, et al: Hepatotoxicity of herbal remedies, *Br Med J* 299:1156-1157, 1989.
42. Perez Alvarez J, Saez-Royuela F, Gento Pena E, et al: Acute hepatitis due to ingestion of *Teucrium chamaedrys* infusions, *Gastroenterol Hepatol* 24:240-243, 2001.
43. Gow PJ, Connelly NJ, Hill RL, et al: Fatal fulminant hepatic failure induced by a natural therapy containing kava, *Med J Aust* 178:442-443, 2003.
44. Eberle J: *A treatise of the materia medica and therapeutics*, Baltimore, Maryland, 1824, Mcctccr.
45. Lee KM, Jung JS, Song DK, et al: Effects of *Humulus lupulus* extract on the central nervous system in mice, *Planta Med* 59(suppl):A691, 1993.
46. Hänsel R, Wohlfart R, Coper H: Sedative-hypnotic compounds in the exhalation of hops, II, *Z Naturforsch [C]* 35:1096-1097, 1980.
47. Hänsel R, Wohlfart R, Schmidt H: The sedative-hypnotic principle of hops. 3. Communication: contents of 2-methyl-3-butene-2-ol in hops and hop preparations, *Planta Med* 45:224-228, 1982.
48. Milligan SR, Kalita JC, Pocock V, et al: The endocrine activities of 8-prenylnaringenin and related hop (*Humulus lupulus* L.) flavonoids, *J Clin Endocrinol Metab* 85:4912-4915, 2000.
49. Milligan S, Kalita J, Pocock V, et al: Oestrogenic activity of the hop phyto-oestrogen 8-prenyl-naringenin, *Reproduction* 123:235-242, 2002.
50. Milligan SR, Kalita JC, Heyerick A, et al: Identification of a potent phytoestrogen in hops (*Humulus lupulus* L.) and beer, *J Clin Endocrinol Metab* 84:2249-2252, 1999.
51. Promberger A, Dornstauder E, Fruhwirth C, et al: Determination of estrogenic activity in beer by biological and chemical means, *J Agric Food Chem* 49:633-640, 2001.
52. Soulimani R, Fleurentin J, Mortier F, et al: Neurotropic action of the hydroalcoholic extract of *Melissa officinalis* in the mouse, *Planta Med* 57:105-109, 1991.
53. Kennedy DO, Scholey AB, Tildesley NT, et al: Modulation of mood and cognitive performance following acute administration of *Melissa officinalis* (lemon balm), *Pharmacol Biochem Behav* 72:953-964, 2002.
54. Pharmaton Natural Health Products, Pharmaton SA, Lugano, Switzerland.

55. Cerny A, Schmid K: Tolerability and efficacy of valerian/lemon balm in healthy volunteers: a double-blind, placebo-controlled, multicentre study, *Fitoterapia* 70:221-228, 1999.
56. Dressing H, Riemann D: Insomnia: are valerian/melissa combinations of equal value to benzodiazepine? *Therapiewoche* 42:726-736, 1992.
57. Dressing H, Kohler S, Muller W: Improvement in sleep quality with a high dose valerian-melissa preparation, *Psychopharmacotherapie* 3:123-130, 1996.
58. Auf'mkolk M, Ingbar JC, Kubota K, et al: Extracts and auto-oxidized constituents of certain plants inhibit the receptor-binding and the biological activity of Graves' immunoglobulins, *Endocrinology* 116:1687-1693, 1985.
59. Rolland A, Fleurentin J, Lanhers MC, et al: Behavioural effects of the American traditional plant *Eschscholzia californica*: sedative and anxiolytic properties, *Planta Med* 57:212-216, 1991.
60. Rolland A, Fleurentin J, Lanhers MC, et al: Neurophysiological effects of an extract of *Eschscholzia californica* Cham. (Papaveraceae), *Phytother Res* 15:377-381, 2001.
61. Moore M: *Medicinal plants of the mountain West*, Santa Fe, New Mexico, 1979, Museum of New Mexico Press, pp 49-50.

CHAPTER

13

Cognitive Disorders and Dementia

Alzheimer's disease (AD), first described in 1907, is defined as progressive loss of mental function and memory accompanied by a decline in cognitive function. More than 4 million Americans are afflicted with the condition. Related health care costs exceed $100 billion per year, according to the Alzheimer's Association. Millions more are afflicted worldwide. AD is classified as a primary degenerative dementia, with senile onset occurring after age 65 and presenile onset taking place before age 65. The incidence of dementia may be as high as 10% among people older than 65 years and 40% among individuals older than 80.

Cognitive impairment is thought to be associated with the degeneration of cholinergic neurons. AD involves disturbances in the amygdala, hippocampus, cerebral cortex, and basal forebrain. The main structural changes are neuronal loss, cortical atrophy, and the presence of neurofibrillary tangles and plaques. Tangles are twisted fibers caused by changes in a protein called tau. Plaques are dense, sticky substances comprising accumulations of a protein called β-amyloid. The β-amyloid plaques reside in the spaces between the billions of neurons in the brain and the neurofibrillary tangles clumped together inside the neurons. Plaques and tangles block the normal transport of electrical messages between neurons that enable us to think, remember, talk, and move. Neuronal structures deteriorate, which in turn affects the transport of neurotransmitters and alters receptor activity in specific areas of the brain. As AD progresses, nerve cells die, the brain shrinks, and the ability to function deteriorates.[1] Reduced cerebral blood flow has also been noted in subjects with AD. It appears that the more severe the reduction in blood flow, the more severe the dementia.

Specific changes in brain neurotransmitter levels occur in patients with AD. Levels of the enzyme choline acetyltransferase (ChAt) are reduced, as are muscarinic receptors types 1 and 2 (M_1 and M_2) and presynaptic nicotinic receptors in the cerebral cortex. The M_2 receptor, when bound, inhibits adenylate cyclase, causing the release and synthesis of acetylcholine. The activated nicotinic receptor facilitates the release of acetylcholine from the neuron. As a result, neuronal transmission in the brain is diminished because of reduced levels of acetylcholine, a neurotransmitter important in memory and cognitive function.

The locus ceruleus consists primarily of adrenergic nuclei that play a pivotal role in the processing of information and tolerance of stress and anxiety. Subjects with AD often experience neuronal loss in the locus ceruleus accompanied by an increase in the activity of monoamine oxidase, the enzyme responsible for the degradation of noradrenergic and dopaminergic neurotransmitters. Serotonin levels also are reduced in AD. The raphe system contains serotonergic nuclei that become overrun with neurofibrillary tangles.

Diagnosis

AD occurs gradually, starting with mild memory loss, changes in personality and behavior, and a decline in cognition. It progresses to loss of speech and movement, then total incapacitation and eventually death. It is normal for memory to decline and for the ability to absorb complex information to slow as we age, but AD is not a part of normal aging. The impact on both the individual and his or her family is devastating.

IDENTIFYING ALZHEIMER'S DISEASE

A patient with AD often presents with the following difficulties:

- Learning and retaining new information. The individual is more repetitive; has trouble remembering recent conversations, events, or appointments; and frequently misplaces objects.
- Handling complex tasks: The individual with AD has trouble following a complex train of thought or performing tasks that require many steps (e.g., balancing a checkbook, cooking a meal).
- Reasoning ability: The individual is unable to respond with a reasonable plan to problems at work or home, such as knowing what to do if the house is cold; shows uncharacteristic disregard for rules of social conduct and behavior.
- Spatial ability and orientation: An individual with AD has trouble driving, organizing objects around the house, or finding his or her way around familiar places.
- Language: The individual experiences increasing difficulty in finding the words to express himself or herself.
- Behavior: The individual appears more passive and less responsive, is more irritable or suspicious than usual, and misinterprets visual or auditory stimuli.

A thorough history and physical examination, laboratory studies (including assessments of folate and vitamin B_{12} levels; liver, thyroid, and kidney function; complete blood-cell count; a screen for advanced syphilis (Venereal Disease Research Laboratory [VDRL] slide test) and human immunodeficiency virus testing; and imaging studies such as magnetic resonance imaging (MRI) and computed tomography are conducted as necessary. The diagnosis of AD is made only after other causes of dementia have been ruled out. This diagnosis of exclusion is performed so that a potentially treatable problem (e.g., hypothyroidism, depression) is not missed and also because, at this time, the diagnosis of AD can only be conclusively made at autopsy.

New research may change this, however. Researchers have found that a radioactive compound known as FDDNP has a special affinity for the neurofibrillary tangles and β-amyloid plaques found in the brains of AD patients. The compound was first tested in vitro, then in animals, and finally in a small number of patients. If the accuracy of this test can be confirmed in larger studies, the test will become an invaluable tool for the early diagnosis of AD, enabling earlier initiation of treatment.

INTEGRATIVE TREATMENT STRATEGIES

Cognitive Stimulation

Some studies have shown that participation in mentally stimulating activities (e.g., reading, doing crossword puzzles, going to social events) may be associated with a reduced risk of AD. Stimulating activity, either mentally or socially oriented, may protect against dementia, indicating that both social interaction and intellectual stimulation may be important for preservation of mental function in the elderly.[2] Researchers speculate that repetition improves certain cognitive skills, making them less susceptible to brain damage.[1]

In a study funded by the National Institutes on Aging and published in the *Journal of the American Medical Association* in 2002, frequent cognitive activity in elderly people was found to reduce the risk of AD by almost 50%. The study included 801 Catholic nuns, priests, and brothers (at least 65 years old) without dementia, recruited from 40 religious organizations across the United States. Researchers documented the frequency of cognitive activity at baseline using a 5-point scale (e.g., doing crossword puzzles, reading books and newspapers, going to museums). Cognitive function (e.g., memory, language, attention, spatial ability) and physical activity were also documented. After 4.5 years of follow-up, researchers found that frequency of cognitive activity was inversely related to the risk of AD. After controlling for age, sex, and education, the investigators found that each one-point increase in cognitive activity was associated with a 33% reduction in risk for AD, and slowed the decline in cognitive function by 47%, working memory by 60%, and that of perceptual speed by 30%.[3]

Acetylcholinesterase Inhibitors

The cholinergic hypothesis has provided the rationale for our current pharmacotherapy for AD. Among the possible strategies for enhancing brain cholinergic activity, acetyl-cholinesterase inhibitors (AChEIs) have been studied most extensively. Cholinesterase inhibitors increase the amount of acetylcholine present in the neuronal synaptic cleft by inhibiting the enzyme responsible for the hydrolysis of acetylcholine, thus improving neuronal transmission. At the time of this writing, the U.S. Food and Drug Administration has approved four prescription drugs for people with mild to moderate AD: tacrine (Cognex), donepezil (Aricept), rivastigmine (Exelon), and galantamine (Reminyl).[4]

CURRENT DRUG THERAPY FOR ALZHEIMER'S DISEASE

Although many practitioners consider the drugs now available for the treatment of AD to be equivalently effective, with similar side-effect profiles, a systematic review by the Cochrane group revealed the following:

- No convincing evidence indicates that tacrine is a useful treatment for the symptoms of AD.[4]
- Rivastigmine appears to be beneficial for subjects with mild to moderate AD.[5] Improvements were noted in cognitive function, ability to carry out activities of daily living, and severity of dementia with daily dosages of 6 to 12 mg compared with placebo. Adverse events were consistent with the cholinergic actions of the drug.
- In patients with mild or moderate AD who were treated for 12, 24, or 52 weeks, donepezil produced modest improvements in cognitive function.[6] No improvements were seen with regard to patient-assessed quality-of-life, and data on other important outcomes are not available.
- Positive effects of galantamine were found in trials lasting 3, 5, and 6 months. Improvements with dosages greater than 8 mg/day were, for the most part, consistently statistically significant.[7]

Although these drugs offer hope for individuals with AD, the relatively short duration of action, frequent side effects, and dose-dependent hepatotoxicity have made the search for better-tolerated medications and treatments desirable.

Statins and Cholesterol Management

Accumulation of β-amyloid is associated with AD, and medicines that inhibit this peptide have been researched as a potential treatment. Recent evidence suggests that 3-hydroxy-3-methylglutaryl coenzyme A (HMG-CoA) reductase inhibitors, commonly known as statins, can inhibit β-amyloid production. In vitro and animal data show that a reduction in cholesterol reduces the production of β-amyloid, and in human subjects lovastatin, however, some has been shown to reduce blood peptide levels by as much as 40%.[8] Some researchers question whether blood levels of β-amyloid adequately correspond to levels found in the brain or signify the progression of AD. Two retrospective epidemiological studies have linked statin use with a reduction in risk for AD of 40% to 79%.[9] One study showed that individuals ages 50 years and older who were prescribed statins had a substantially decreased risk of dementia, independent of the presence or absence of untreated hyperlipidemia, or exposure to nonstatin lipid-lowering agents.[10] However, a prospective study of 4740 individuals older than age of 65 found that although statin use was associated with a reduced prevalence of dementia, statins had no statistically significant effect on the incidence of AD.[11] (Incidence is the number of *new* occurrences of a condition in a population over a given period.) This study also raised the issue of equal efficacy among statins and questioned the necessity of a drug to cross the blood-brain barrier. Atorvastatin, which does not penetrate the blood-brain barrier, was actually shown to offer a greater risk-reducing effect than statins that do enter into the brain.

At this time, evidence is insufficient to recommend statins as a means of reducing the risk of AD. However, a growing body of biologic, epidemiologic, and clinical evidence indicates that decreasing the serum cholesterol level may retard the pathogenesis of AD.[12] Rigorous research is needed to determine what role, if any, is played by statins in the prevention and treatment of AD.

Antiinflammatory Medications

People who take large doses of nonsteroidal antiinflammatory drugs (NSAIDs), commonly used to relieve joint pain, have been shown to have a reduced likelihood of developing AD in some studies.

A systematic review and metaanalysis of nine studies of NSAID use among adults ages 55 and older showed that NSAIDs offer some protection against the development of AD.[13] The authors note, however, that the optimal dosage, duration of use, and ratios of risk to benefit are unknown. A 12-month study of 351 patients with mild to moderate AD given rofecoxib (25 mg) once daily, naproxen sodium (220 mg) twice daily, or placebo failed to show any slowing of cognitive decline among the members of the treatment groups compared with subjects taking placebo. Results of secondary analyses showed no consistent benefit of either treatment. Fatigue, dizziness, hypertension, and more serious adverse events were more common in the active treatment groups.[14]

None of the studies performed to date with antiinflammatory drugs is definitive. The Alzheimer's Disease Anti-Inflammatory Prevention Trial was launched in 2001 to test the effectiveness of some NSAIDs in preventing AD. The study, comprising more than 2500 healthy participants ages 70 and older, is sponsored by the National Institute on Aging and is scheduled to run 5 to 7 years.[15]

Micronutrients

Folate and reduction of homocysteine. Folate is essential to the healthy development of the central nervous system. Recently it has been found that folate deficiency is associated with high blood levels of the amino acid homocysteine. Folate deficiency can occur because of insufficient folate in the diet, inefficient absorption, or altered metabolic use related to genetic variations. High blood levels of homocysteine have been linked to increased risk for arterial disease and dementia.

A prospective, observational study monitored 1092 patients (mean age 76 years), free of dementia at the time of enrollment, for approximately 8 years. Participants' homocysteine levels were measured near the beginning of the study (1979-1982) and again between 1986 and 1990. At the end of the study, it was found that dementia had developed in 111 participants. AD was thought to be the cause in 83 cases. This study found that patients with the highest levels of homocysteine were roughly twice as likely to experience dementia, compared with those with the lowest levels. The correlation between homocysteine level and dementia was present even after age, sex, blood levels of vitamins, and the presence of lipoprotein E genotype were accounted for. In fact, each 5 μmol/L increase in homocysteine concentration was associated with a 40% increased risk for AD.[16]

But does a reduction in homocysteine level prevent AD or slow its progression? A review by the Cochrane group showed no beneficial effect of 750 µg/day folic acid on measures of cognition or mood in older healthy women and no benefit on measures of cognition or mood among patients with mild to moderate cognitive decline and different forms of dementia receiving 2 mg/day folate.[17] The reviewers noted that one trial reported a significant decline, compared with patients taking placebo, in two cognitive-function tasks performed by dementia patients who had received high doses of folic acid (10 mg/day) for unspecified periods. Although no benefit was seen, folic acid plus vitamin B_{12} was effective in reducing the serum homocysteine concentration, and the treatment was well tolerated. Limitations of the currently available research include short duration of studies, which ranged from 5 to 12 weeks and may not have been long enough to see a treatment effect.

Given the comparatively low cost of vitamin supplements, it makes sense to study the possible relationship between high serum homocysteine levels and dementia. The National Institute on Aging is funding an 18-month clinical trial designed to test whether reduction of homocysteine levels with high-dose vitamin supplements can slow the rate of cognitive decline in people with AD. Although these vitamin supplements are relatively safe, folic acid given to people with undiagnosed vitamin B_{12} deficiency may cause neurologic damage. Vitamin B_{12} deficiency produces an anemia identical to that seen in folate deficiency but also causes irreversible damage to the central and peripheral nervous systems.[18] Folic acid corrects the anemia associated with vitamin B_{12} deficiency and so delays diagnosis but does not prevent progression to neurologic damage. For this reason, folic-acid supplementation should be accompanied by the simultaneous administration of vitamin B_{12}.

Antioxidants. Antioxidants help neutralize the free radicals produced through normal metabolism, helping prevent damage to important cell components. As people age, free radicals become increasingly prevalent, and many researchers believe that it is the inability to buffer against the effects of this oxidative stress that leads to age-related neuronal decline.[19]

If antioxidants reduce the damaging effects of free radicals that occur with aging, and if memory decline is related to oxidative neuronal destruction, perhaps antioxidants can help slow memory decline and improve memory.[20] Though frank vitamin deficiency is uncommon in the United States, suboptimal vitamin status is prevalent and puts aged individuals at high risk for such diseases as cardiovascular disease, dementia, and osteoporosis.[21]

Although researchers have revealed an association between high dietary antioxidant intake and decreased risk for AD,[22,23] clinical trials have failed to show a significant benefit in patients with AD.[20] Some researchers postulate that by the time clinical symptoms of AD appear, a large proportion of neuronal cells may have already been destroyed and, therefore, intervention with antioxidants represents a case of too little, too late.[24] Some experts note other potential flaws with clinical trials, citing a lack of design specificity to test a particular antioxidant, short duration of treatment and inappropriate choice of "time window" (for efficacy to be achieved, the antioxidant must be given during the time available between the damaging event and irreversible cell loss), the synthetic or natural source of antioxidant used, and the absence of evaluation of markers of oxidative stress as intermediate end points.[24]

Many unexplored issues warrant research. Because antioxidants work as a system, their effectiveness depends on adequate levels of other vitamins and minerals. Also, intake of an antioxidant may not directly translate to its serum level. Therefore, to find reliable benefits, researchers may need to be sensitive to levels of other micronutrients, as well as the serum level of the target antioxidant, not just the amount being supplemented.[25] Until more definitive answers are available, it would seem to be a common sense practice for most adults to take a daily multivitamin that provides adequate levels of antioxidants and other nutrients as part of a healthy diet and lifestyle.

Herbal Remedies

Ginkgo **(Ginkgo biloba).**   *Ginkgo biloba* extract (GBE) is one of the most heavily researched of all herbal remedies, and the most heavily researched herb for the treatment of dementia (Figure 13-1). A standardized extract of ginkgo leaf is widely prescribed by health care providers in Germany and France for relief of age-related conditions, peripheral vascular disorders, and dementia. The German Commission E has endorsed the use of gingko for the "symptomatic treatment of disturbed performance in organic brain syndrome within the regimen of a therapeutic concept in cases of demential syndromes with the following principal symptoms: memory deficits, disturbances in concentration, depressive emotional condition, dizziness, tinnitus and headache. The primary target groups are

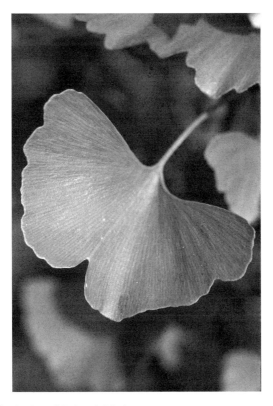

Figure 13-1 Ginkgo (*Ginkgo biloba*). (*Courtesy Martin Wall Botanical Services.*)

dementia syndromes, including primary degenerative dementia, vascular dementia and mixed forms of both."[26]

Several mechanisms of action have been proposed for ginkgo: increased blood supply through vasodilation, reduction of blood viscosity, modification of neurotransmitter systems, and reduction of oxygen free radicals.[27] The ginkgolides are thought to be primarily responsible for the inhibition of platelet-activating factor and inhibition of 3'4'-cyclic guanosine monophosphate phosphodiesterase.[28] The findings of in vitro and animal research indicate that the flavonoid fraction increases serotonin release and uptake, inhibits age-related reduction of muscarinic receptors and α-adrenoreceptors, stimulates choline uptake in the hippocampus, inhibits nitric oxide formation, and acts as a free-radical scavenger.[29] There is little question that the actions of ginkgo are complex and multifaceted, but the question remains: How much of these in vitro data and animal research, often involving exceedingly high doses of extract administered parenterally, are applicable to the typical oral dose used in human beings?

Although the precise mechanism(s) of action has not been clearly elucidated, the preponderance of evidence suggests that ginkgo plays a beneficial role in patients with early dementia. The Cochrane group conducted a systematic review of the research addressing the safety and efficacy of ginkgo in the treatment of cognitive impairment and dementia. They concluded, "*Ginkgo biloba* appears to be safe in use with no excess side effects compared with placebo. Many of the early trials used unsatisfactory methods, were small, and we cannot exclude publication bias. Overall, there is promising evidence of improvement in cognition and function associated with ginkgo. However, three more recent trials show inconsistent results. There is need for a large trial using modern methodology and permitting an intention-to-treat analysis to provide robust estimates of the size and mechanism of any treatment effects."[30]

The best trial to date, by Le Bars et al, was a randomized, double-blind, placebo-controlled, parallel-group, multicenter 52-week study of 309 patients with mild to severe AD or multiinfarct dementia who received either 120 mg/day of EGb 761 (standardized extract of ginkgo) or placebo.[31] The authors found ginkgo safe, and although the changes were modest, they were objectively measured on the Alzheimer's Disease Assessment Scale–Cognitive subscale and were of sufficient magnitude to be recognized by the caregivers in the Geriatric Evaluation by Relative's Rating Instrument. Le Bars has since published a retrospective analysis of this study showing that a treatment effect favorable to EGb could be observed with respect to cognitive performance ($P = 0.02$) and social function ($P = 0.001$). However, the relative changes from baseline that were measured at the end point depended heavily on the severity of dementia at baseline. Improvement was observed among patients with very mild to mild cognitive impairment, whereas in more severe dementia, the mean EGb effect was more in terms of stabilization or slowing down of worsening compared with the greater deterioration observed with placebo.[32]

Although gingko is widely accepted in Europe as a treatment for cognitive decline, skepticism continues among researchers and health care providers in the United States. Even the Cochrane reviewers, in their somewhat positive assessment, noted that many of the studies were of poor quality and that larger trials have provided conflicting data. Perhaps more definitive information will appear in the near future. The National Center for Complementary and Alternative Medicine at the National Institutes of Health is sponsoring two trials on ginkgo. The first is a randomized, double-blind 5-year study of 3000 healthy men and women, at least 75 years old, who will receive either 240 mg/day of GBE or placebo. The primary end point is dementia, specifically AD; secondary end points include the incidence of vascular disease, changes in cognitive-function scores over time, total mortality, and changes in functional status. The diagnosis of dementia will be based on neuropsychological testing, neurologic examination findings, MRI, functional measurements, and review by a central adjudication committee; the diagnosis will be classified on the basis of the *Diagnostic and Statistical Manual of Mental Disorders IV* and the joint task of the National Institute of Neurological and Communicative Disorders and Stroke and the Alzheimer's Disease and Related Disorders Association (NINCDS/ADRDA) criteria.[33] The second study is a randomized, placebo-controlled, double-blind 42-month study of the effects of standardized GBE on the prevention or delay of cognitive decline in people aged 85 years and older. This population offers an excellent opportunity to assess the effect of GBE as a primary prevention because of its members' particularly high risk for mild cognitive impairment. Approximately 200 elder cognitively healthy subjects will be enrolled and monitored for mild cognitive impairment. This study is important for determining whether GBE has a disease-modifying effect on the brain distinct from a symptomatic effect. The magnitude of biologic effect of the treatment will be assessed with the use of volumetric quantitative MRI and peripheral markers of oxidation status will assess the possible antioxidant effects of GBE.[33]

Ginkgo remains one of the most popular dietary supplements in the United States with total ginkgo sales in 2001 estimated at $180 million by the *Nutrition Business Journal*. A tremendous range of products containing a variety of dosages is available in a dizzying array of formulations, making it difficult for consumers to know which one to select. How these products compare to the concentrated phytopharmaceuticals used in clinical trials is open to debate. Thirty of the 33 studies reviewed by the Cochrane group were conducted using two proprietary ginkgo products manufactured in Germany. The leading extract used in 21 studies, EGb 761, is made by the W. Schwabe Pharmaceutical company and sold in the United States under the names Ginkoba and Ginkgold. The product used in the other 8 trials was LI 1370, made by Lichtwer Pharma and sold in the US as Ginkai.

The ginkgo used in most studies for the treatment of AD was a standardized extract (24% ginkgoflavones, 6% terpenes) at a dosage of 40 to 80 mg thrice daily. For subjects with early signs of dementia, a dose of 240 mg/day should probably be considered optimal at this time.

Ginkgo appears to be relatively safe when used appropriately. The German Commission E lists occasional gastrointestinal upset, headache, and allergic skin reactions as side effects of ginkgo and is contraindicated in subjects with hypersensitivity to ginkgo preparations. Reports of subarachnoid hemorrhage[34] and subdural hematoma[35] have been noted with the use of ginkgo alone. Several herb-drug interactions have also been reported. Spontaneous ocular hyphema was noted in a patient taking ginkgo and aspirin,[36] intracerebral hemorrhage was seen when ginkgo was taken with warfarin for 2 months,[37] bilateral subdural hematoma occurred in a 33-year-old woman who had been taking 120 mg/day ginkgo for 2 years,[38] and a subarachnoid hemorrhage occurred in a 61-year-old man with mildly prolonged bleeding time who had been taking 120 to 160 mg/day ginkgo for 6 months.[34] An additive effect on platelet inhibition was noted in normal rats and those in which thrombosis had been induced when they were given a combination of ticlopidine (50 mg/kg per day) and EGb 761 (40 mg/kg day). Bleeding time was prolonged by 150%[39] but this study involved a ginkgo dose much higher than the currently recommended therapeutic dose.

A prospective, double-blind, randomized, placebo-controlled study was carried out in 32 young, healthy male volunteers as a means of evaluating the effect of three dosages of EGb 761 (120, 240, and 480 mg/day) on hemostasis, coagulation, and fibrinolysis. After 14 days' administration, ginkgo did not induce any significant modification of bleeding time, platelet function, or coagulation at any dosage when compared with placebo.[40] Bleeding risk is probably quite low in otherwise healthy individuals who take ginkgo. However, whether there is a herb-drug interaction in patients who are using ginkgo and taking warfarin or antiplatelet agents is unclear.

Ginseng **(Panax ginseng).**   Ginseng has long been used to maintain physical vitality in the Far East, particularly in Korea and China. The genus name, *Panax*, means "cure-all" in Greek. Ginseng has been cultivated since 11 BC and honored as a medicinal agent for at least 50 centuries.[41] Other members of the genus include *P. quinquefolius* (American ginseng), *P. notoginseng*, and *P. japonicus*. Though commonly referred to as Siberian ginseng and used for similar purposes, *Eleutherococcus senticosus* is not a member of the genus *Panax* and is more appropriately referred to as eleuthero to prevent confusion. Asian ginseng is one of the most economically important medicinal herbs in world trade; in the United States, ginseng ranks second in total sales in food, drug, and mass-market retail stores, with sales in 2000 totaling $62.5 million.[42]

Ginseng is considered a general tonic and adaptogen used to enhance mental and physical energy. It has been approved by the German Commission E as a tonic for invigoration and fortification in times of fatigue and debility, in cases of declining capacity for work and concentration, and during convalescence.[26] An extensive pool of animal data exploring the effects of ginseng on the cardiovascular system, central nervous system, endocrine system, metabolism, and immune system has been compiled. Although widely popular, a review of the research to date finds an equivocal nature of evidence in both animal and human studies for most of the conditions for which the herb is taken.[43] Many of the studies suffer from such methodologic flaws such as inadequate sample size and lack of double-blind control. Although animal data demonstrate the cognition-enhancing effects of ginseng, the evidence of such effects after long-term administration is scarce in human subjects, especially those with dementia. A small study was conducted with a combination of *P. ginseng* and *P. notoginseng* in 25 patients with mild to moderate stroke-induced vascular dementia[44] and another 25 patients who took almitrine-raubasine (Duxil), a drug believed to improve oxygen delivery to the brain. Results showed that participants taking the herbal extract demonstrated greater improvement in overall memory than did those taking Duxil.

Does synergism result when ginkgo is combined with ginseng? The authors of a study published in 2000 tested a combination ginseng/ginkgo preparation in healthy adults ranging from 38 to 66 years of age who had no sign of memory-impairing disease.[45] Participants were randomly assigned to receive the herbal combination or placebo for 12 weeks. Memory testing was conducted before treatment, during the treatment period, and 2 weeks after the discontinuation of treatment. The memory tests assessed spatial and numeric working memory, immediate and delayed word recall, and word and picture recognition. Testing was repeated four times throughout each memory-test day, with the first test at 7:30 AM and the last at 2:30 PM. Across testing times, parallel versions of the tests were administered. After 4 weeks of treatment, the ginkgo/ginseng group showed significantly more improvement on the memory tests than did the placebo group. This improvement was still present 2 weeks after the discontinuation of treatment. When testing was conducted at 7:30 AM, little or no difference was detected with regard to memory improvement between the ginkgo/ginseng and placebo groups. By contrast, testing conducted at 2:30 PM produced consistent memory benefits that extended 2 weeks past the conclusion of treatment in the ginkgo/ginseng group. In some cases the benefits were remarkable, with the ginkgo/ginseng group showing a 63% improvement at week 14 over baseline for delayed word recall, compared with a 6% decrease in the placebo group.

The following is an excerpt from a comprehensive review by Kennedy et al. on ginseng and its effects on cognition and mood[46]:

> The evidence reviewed above from in vitro, in vivo, and animal behavioral studies suggests that ginseng and its component ginsenosides can modulate a number of physiological mechanisms and may improve indices of stress, fatigue, and learning in rodents. This review has concentrated on behavior-relevant indices. However, it is interesting to note that most of this research has been undertaken in regions of the world with indigenous *Panax* cultivation and a long history of usage. By contrast, the human behavioral studies, which have produced equivocal results, have been largely undertaken in Western areas of the world to which the *Panax* genus is a relative newcomer to the armory of the behavioral pharmacopoeia. This interesting dichotomy suggests two distinct philosophical approaches. In the case of the former, the research would seem to be driven by a curiosity as to the mechanisms underlying what is taken to be the known efficacy of a traditional medication; and in the case of the latter, the impetus is a desire to 'prove' the putative effects in humans of a potentially beneficial herb. Unfortunately, whilst these two approaches are mutually beneficial in the long run, the literature pertaining to the chronic effects of ginseng in humans is riddled with so many methodological inadequacies that the question of efficacy remains open.

Ginseng products are often sold as "white" or "red". White ginseng is raw; red ginseng has been steamed. Most studies have involved extracts standardized to contain 4% ginsenosides. Doses used in trials have ranged from 100 to 400 mg/day of standardized extract. High-quality crude root can also be used. The dosage is generally 3 to 6 g/day or its equivalent in tincture or fluid extract. Ginseng has a long history of adulteration, and care should be taken to ensure a quality product. Adverse effects, which are rare and generally occur only with high dosages or prolonged use, include sleeplessness, nervousness, early-morning diarrhea, and hypertony.[47] Three incidents of hormonelike effects in older women have been reported, although the estrogenic activity of ginseng remains controversial.

Red ginseng is said to be more stimulating than raw ginseng, and herbalists often contraindicate its use in people with hypertension. However, little evidence supports this caution. The authors of a recent study observed that heated ginseng was superior to raw ginseng in inducing endothelium-dependent relaxation.[49] A prospective, randomized, double-blind, placebo-controlled study of 30 healthy adults randomly assigned to receive 28 days of 200 mg of *P. ginseng* extract or placebo showed that ginseng *reduced* diastolic blood pressure from 75 ± 5 mm Hg at baseline to 70 ± 6 mm Hg at the same time point ($P = 0.02$).[50]

Huperzia (Huperzia serrata).   Huperzine A is a plant-based alkaloid found in the Chinese club moss *H. serrata,* also known as *Lycopodium serrata.* The plant, traditionally called *qian ceng ta,* meaning "thousand-laid pagodas,"[51] has been used for centuries in Asian medicine to treat fever, inflammation, and mental disorders. Chinese club moss contains triterpenoids and various alkaloids, including lycodoline, lycoclavine, serratinine, and huperzines.[52] Alkaloids represent 0.2% of the total content. Most researchers have focused on one alkaloid, huperzine A, which has been found to reverse or attenuate cognitive deficits in animal models and reduce neuronal cell death caused by an excess of glutamate, making it a substance of interest not only in AD but also in human immunodeficiency virus–associated dementia and Parkinson's disease.

Huperzine A acts as a potent, highly specific, and reversible AchEI that readily crosses the blood-brain barrier.[52] The findings of several studies conducted in China, where huperzine A is approved for the symptomatic treatment of AD, indicate that it has beneficial effects in older people with AD. In the following paragraphs I discuss two of the larger randomized, placebo-controlled studies; however, both were of short duration and neither involved a dosage greater than 400 µg/day.

A randomized, double-blind, placebo-controlled study of 103 patients with a diagnosis of AD based on *Diagnostic and Statistical Manual III-R* criteria was undertaken to evaluate the efficacy of huperzine A.[53] Patients were randomly assigned to receive 200 µg of oral huperzine A or placebo twice daily for 8 weeks. Their condition was evaluated with the the Wechsler Memory Scale, the Hasegawa Dementia Scale, the Mini-Mental State Examination, and the Activities of Daily Living Scale. Twenty-nine patients (58%) treated with huperzine A showed significant improvement in memory over baseline on all tests, compared with 19 (36%) of the placebo group. The incidence of diarrhea (10%), anorexia (10%), hyperactivity (10%), and nausea or vomiting (8%) was comparable to that seen with placebo. The authors detected no changes from baseline on the laboratory tests, but vital-signs assessment revealed clinically relevant bradycardia (a decrease in mean heart rate from 72 to 47 beats/min).

A 12-week multicenter, double-blind, randomized, placebo-controlled study was conducted in China among 202 patients (ages 50-80 years) with possible or probable AD.[54] Compared with patients receiving placebo, cognitive function (Mini-Mental State Examination, Alzheimer's Disease Assessment Scale (ADAS)–Cognitive Subscale), noncognitive function (mood and behavior ADAS–Noncognitive Subscale), and activities of daily living all demonstrated significant improvement by week 6, and particularly by week 12, among patients taking huperzine A. The dosage of huperzine A was titrated from an initial dosage of 100 µg taken orally with breakfast and dinner to 150 µg taken twice daily from week 2 to week 3 and, finally, to 200 µg taken twice daily from week 4 to week 12. The dose was adjusted on the basis of tolerance. The authors concluded that although huperzine A appears to be a safe and effective treatment for AD, these findings should be confirmed in larger and longer clinical trials, involving different dosage regimens.

In addition to AD, huperzine A may be protective on exposure to poisonous nerve agents. Anticholinergic agents have been a mainstay of prevention but are not without adverse effects. Huperzine A may prove an effective pretreatment against the irreversible AChEI soma nerve gas and other organophosphate poisons.[55] In a review, Lallement et al concluded that huperzine A is of value in the prophylaxis of organophosphate poisoning and it is relatively free of serious adverse effects in healthy subjects.

Huperzine A and *H. serrata* (club moss) are available in the United States as dietary supplements. They are marketed both for the treatment of dementia and as a memory-enhancing "smart" drug. Huperzine A appears to be fairly well tolerated when taken at the dosages used in clinical trials. High dosages of huperzine A could cause a cholinergic reaction, producing such side effects as sweating, nausea, vomiting, dizziness, cramps, and collapse. Studies of herb-drug interaction have shown that the activity and expression of liver cytochrome P450 (CYP450) isoenzymes are not affected in rats treated with pharmacologic doses of huperzine A but that higher doses may elicit a slight inductive response of CYP1A2.[56] In light of the results of basic-science, animal, and human clinical trials that are available at the time of this writing, rigorous clinical trials of longer duration should definitely be undertaken.

Muira puama (Ptychopetalum olacoides).   *Muira puama,* also called "potency wood," is a small tree that grows up to 5 m and is native to the Amazon rainforest. Two South American varieties—*P. olacoides* (found in Brazil, French Guiana, Guyana, and Suriname) and *P. uncinatum* (found only in Brazil)—are used interchangeably in South American herbal medicine. *P. olacoides* is generally preferred because it has a higher content of the active ingredient lupeol, a triterpene thought to significantly contribute to the plant's medicinal activity. A completely unrelated Brazilian tree, *Liriosma ovata,* also goes by the common name of *muira puama* and is often found in the marketplace instead of *P. olacoides.* The root and bark of *P. olacoides* have been used to treat a variety of conditions, including sexual impotence, hence the nickname potency wood; the herb is also used for muscle paralysis, menstrual disturbances, ataxia, and central nervous system disorders. It has been used topically for the relief of rheumatic pain. *Muira puama* has been official (monograph with standards) in the Brazilian pharmacopoeia since the 1950s. The herb is growing in popularity in the United States and is being marketed as both an aphrodisiac and, in some formulations, as a memory aid, although there is little scientific evidence to support either claim.

Research on the isolated constituent lupeol can be found in the scientific literature. In vitro studies confirm antiinflammatory activity by way of inhibition of prostaglandin synthesis,[57] and animal studies have demonstrated hepatoprotective[58] and anxiolytic activity.[59] The sparse research that has been conducted on the whole herb is mostly limited to animal studies. An ethanolic extract of *P. olacoides* was shown to improve long-term memory retrieval in adult mice in a dose-dependent fashion (significant improvement with 50 and 100 mg/kg), affecting neither memory consolidation nor task acquisition. The extract was found to inhibit AChE in vitro and in vivo. Neither the active compound(s) nor the mechanism(s) by which *muira puama* inhibits AchE is known at this time.[60]

Spanish sage (Salvia lavandulaefolia).   Sage has a long and respected history of use in herbal medicine. Different species (*S. officinalis, S. lavandulaefolia, S. miltiorrhiza*) have been used to treat a variety of health complaints, including depression and memory loss. Researchers have conducted preliminary studies of *S. lavandulaefolia* in the treatment of AD. This particular species of *Salvia* was chosen because it contains only trace amounts of thujone, a bicyclic monoterpene that possesses neurotoxic effects and, with prolonged use or high dosages, can cause renal damage, vertigo, vomiting, and convulsions. *S. lavandulaefolia* extracts and isolated constituents exhibit anticholinesterase activity in vitro and in vivo, as well as antioxidant, antiinflammatory, estrogenic, and central nervous system–depressant effects that may be relevant in the treatment of AD.[61] The essential oil inhibits AChE from human brain tissue, and individual monoterpenoid constituents inhibit the enzyme with varying degrees of potency. In vivo AChE inhibition of select brain tissue was achieved after oral administration of the essential oil to rats.[52]

Rosemary and sage are the most potent antioxidants of the commonly used spices. The antioxidant activity of sage polyphenols is mainly due to the presence of rosmarinic acid derivatives, whereas the flavonoids luteolin and apigenin exert comparatively weak to moderate activity.[62] Carvacrol and α-pinene are antiinflammatory components of the herb, and dose-dependent estrogenic activity has been demonstrated with the ethanolic extract of *S. lavandulaefolia*.[63]

A double blind, placebo-controlled study found that the administration of 50 µL/day of *S. lavandulaefolia* essential oil significantly improved immediate word recall in healthy participants.[64] In a 6-week open-label phase II pilot study of an *S. lavandulaefolia* essential oil administered orally to 11 patients with AD, statistically significant differences between baseline and results after 6 weeks' treatment included a reduction in neuropsychiatric symptoms and an improvement in attention.[52] Patients were given capsules containing 50 µL essential oil of *S. lavandulaefolia* plus 50 µL of sunflower oil (*Helianthus annuus*) as a carrier in the following manner: week 1, one capsule at 8 AM; week 2, one capsule at 8 AM and one at 7 PM; weeks 3 through 6, dosage as described above, with one additional capsule administered at 12:30 PM. None of the patients withdrew from the trial, and no patient experienced any adverse physical or neurologic effects. Blood samples taken at the end of the trial showed no statistically significant changes in any parameter in any patient. Blood pressure was measured weekly; two patients with a history of hypertension experienced an increase in blood pressure at 3 weeks, with the highest dosage. In one patient, diastolic pressure increased to 110 mm Hg and systolic pressure increased to 200 mm Hg. Inclusion of these data in the total analysis yielded a mean increase ($n = 11$) in diastolic blood pressure of 15.09 ($P = 0.025$) and a mean increase in systolic blood pressure of 6.19 ($P = 0.049$).

On the basis of the preliminary data, it appears that *S. lavandulaefolia* may offer some benefits for patients with AD. It may be worthwhile to study the herb extract in addition to the essential oil.

A larger, more rigorous study is needed to assess the tolerability and efficacy of the essential oil in patients with AD, especially those with existing hypertension.

Turmeric (Curcuma longa). Curcumin is one of the key ingredients in turmeric, a spice used worldwide as a seasoning and ingredient in curry. Numerous medicinal properties have been attributed to it, including antioxidant and antiinflammatory activity. Researchers at the University of California–Los Angeles showed that curcumin reduces inflammation caused by a buildup of β-amyloid. They postulated that it helps clear existing amyloid, reduces toxic compounds associated with chronic inflammation, and reverses oxidative damage.[65] Researchers injected amyloid proteins into the brains of aged mice in an attempt to mimic AD. Some mice were fed a diet high in curcumin, whereas others received a diet low in curcumin. Their brain tissue was later analyzed for inflammation, damage, and plaque formation. Both groups demonstrated a significant reduction in the buildup of amyloid proteins, the substance that causes inflammation and subsequent loss of memory. Studies of other antiinflammatory drugs have shown similar effects. Although considered preliminary, these findings suggest that turmeric is a healthy addition to the diet if one enjoys spicy food. More research is needed to determine the optimal dose when curcumin, or turmeric, is taken as a supplement.

Vinpocetine.   Vinpocetine is a *synthetic* ethyl ester of apovincamine, a vinca alkaloid obtained from the leaves of the lesser periwinkle (*Vinca minor*). Vinpocetine was developed in Hungary and has been used to treat patients with loss of memory and cognitive decline, although it has not been approved for the treatment of cognitive impairment by any regulatory body. It is available as a drug in Europe and is gaining popularity in the United States as a memory-enhancing dietary supplement.

Vinpocetine increases blood circulation and metabolism in the brain. Animal studies have shown that vinpocetine can reduce the loss of neurons caused by diminished blood flow. Thirty-four trials of vinpocetine have been conducted since 1976. Many of these were open, uncontrolled trials conducted before 1980. Vinpocetine was often administered parenterally in these studies. A Cochrane review revealed beneficial effects of vinpocetine at dosages of 30 and 60 mg/day compared with placebo, but the authors cautioned that the number of patients treated for 6 months or longer was small. They also noted that adverse effects were inconsistently reported, without regard for relationship to dose. The reviewers concluded, "While the basic science is interesting, the evidence for beneficial effect of vinpocetine on patients with dementia is inconclusive and does not support clinical use. The drug seems to have few adverse effects at the doses used in the studies. Large studies evaluating the use of vinpocetine for people suffering from well-defined types of cognitive impairment are needed to explore possible efficacy of this treatment."[66]

References

1. Bren L, Alzheimer's: searching for a cure, *FDA Consum* 37(July-August):19-25, 2003.
2. Wang HX, Karp A, Winblad B, et al: Late-life engagement in social and leisure activities is associated with a decreased risk of dementia: a longitudinal study from the Kungsholmen project, *Am J Epidemiol* 155:1081-1087, 2002.
3. Wilson RS, Mendes de Leon CF, Barnes LL, et al: Participation in cognitively stimulating activities and risk of incident Alzheimer disease, *JAMA* 287:742-748, 2002.
4. Qizilbash N, Birks J, Lopez Arrieta J, et al: Tacrine for Alzheimer's disease, *Cochrane Database Syst Rev* (3):CD000202, 2000.
5. Birks J, Grimley Evans J, Iakovidou V, et al: Rivastigmine for Alzheimer's disease, *Cochrane Database Syst Rev* (4):CD001191, 2000.
6. Birks JS, Melzer D, Beppu H: Donepezil for mild and moderate Alzheimer's disease, *Cochrane Database Syst Rev* (4):CD001190, 2000.
7. Olin J, Schneider L: Galantamine for Alzheimer's disease, *Cochrane Database Syst Rev* (4):CD001747, 2001.
8. Wolozin B: Cholesterol and Alzheimer's disease, *Biochem Soc Trans* 30:525-529, 2002.
9. Wolozin B, Kellman W, Ruosseau P, et al: Decreased prevalence of Alzheimer disease associated with 3-hydroxy-3-methylglutaryl coenzyme A reductase inhibitors, *Arch Neurol* 57:1439-1443, 2000.
10. Jick H, Zornberg GL, Jick SS, et al: Statins and the risk of dementia, *Lancet* 356:1627-1631, 2000.
11. Zandi P, Sparks DL, Khachaturian A, et al: Statins and dementia—does blood-brain barrier permeability matter? *Neurobiol Aging* 23(1S):S288, 2002.
12. Scott HD, Laake K: Statins for the prevention of Alzheimer's disease, *Cochrane Database Syst Rev* (4):CD003160, 2001.
13. Etminan M, Gill S, Samii A: Effect of non-steroidal anti-inflammatory drugs on risk of Alzheimer's disease: systematic review and meta-analysis of observational studies, *BMJ* 327:128-130, 2003.
14. Aisen PS, Schafer KA, Grundman M, et al: Effects of rofecoxib or naproxen vs placebo on Alzheimer disease progression: a randomized controlled trial, *JAMA* 289:2819-2826, 2003.

15. ADAPT Research Group, Martin BK, Meinert CL, Breitner JC: Double placebo design in a prevention trial for Alzheimer's disease, *Control Clin Trial* 23:93-99, 2002.
16. Seshadri S, Beiser A, Selhub J, et al: Plasma homocysteine as a risk factor for dementia and Alzheimer's disease, *N Engl J Med* 346:476-483, 2002.
17. Malouf M, Grimley EJ, Areosa SA: Folic acid with or without vitamin B_{12} for cognition and dementia, *Cochrane Database Syst Rev* (4):CD004514, 2003.
18. Malouf M, Grimley EJ, Areosa SA: Folic acid with or without vitamin B_{12} for cognition and dementia, *Cochrane Database Syst Rev* (4)CD004514, 2003.
19. Joseph JA, Shukitt-Hale B, Denisova NA, et al: Reversals of age-related declines in neuronal signal transduction, cognitive, and motor behavioral deficits with blueberry, spinach, or strawberry diet supplementation, *J Neurosci* 19:8114, 1999.
20. McDaniel MA, Maier SF, Einstein GO: "Brain-specific" nutrients: a memory cure? *Nutrition* 19:957-975, 2003.
21. Fairfield KM, Fletcher RH: Vitamins for chronic disease prevention in adults, *JAMA* 287:3116-3126, 2002.
22. Gonzalez-Gross M, Marcos A, Pietrzik K: Nutrition and cognitive impairment in the elderly, *Br J Nutr* 86:313-321, 2001.
23. Engelhart MJ, Geerlings MI, Ruitenberg A, et al: Dietary intake of antioxidants and risk of Alzheimer disease, *JAMA* 287:3223-3229, 2002.
24. Polidori MC: Antioxidant micronutrients in the prevention of age-related diseases, *J Postgrad Med* [serial online] 49:229-235, 2003. Accessed January 2, 2004.
25. Goodwin JS, Goodwin JM, Garry PJ: Association between nutritional status and cognitive functioning in a healthy elderly population, *JAMA* 249:2917, 1983.
26. Blumenthal M, Busse W, Goldberg A, et al, editors: *The Complete German Commission E monographs: therapeutic guide to herbal medicines,* Boston, 1998, Integrative Medicine Communications.
27. Nishida S, Satoh H: Comparative vasodilating actions among terpenoids and flavonoids contained in *Ginkgo biloba* extract, *Clin Chim Acta* 339:129-133, 2004.
28. *Folium ginkgo.* In: *WHO Monographs on selected medicinal plants,* vol 1, Geneva, Switzerland, 1999, World Health Organization, pp 154-167.
29. Blumenthal M: *The ABC clinical guide to herbs,* Austin, Texas, 2003, American Botanical Council, pp 185-200.
30. Birks J, Grimley Evans J, Van Dongen M: *Ginkgo biloba* for cognitive impairment and dementia (Cochrane review). In: *The Cochrane Library,* issue 4, Chichester, UK, 1993, John Wiley & Sons.
31. Le Bars PL, Katz MM, Berman N, et al: A placebo-controlled, double-blind, randomized trial of an extract of *Ginkgo biloba* for dementia. North American EGb Study Group, *JAMA* 278:1327-1332, 1997.
32. Le Bars PL, Velasco FM, Ferguson JM, et al: Influence of the severity of cognitive impairment on the effect of the *Ginkgo biloba* extract EGb 761 in Alzheimer's disease, *Neuropsychobiology* 45:19-26, 2002.
33. *Ginkgo biloba* Prevention Trial in Older Individuals. http://nccam.nih.gov. Accessed December 31, 2003.
34. Vale S: Subarachnoid hemorrhage associated with *Ginkgo biloba, Lancet* 352:36, 1998.
35. Gilbert GJ: *Ginkgo biloba, Neurology* 48:1137, 1997.
36. Rosenblatt M, Mindel J: Spontaneous hyphema associated with ingestion of *Ginkgo biloba* extract, *N Engl J Med* 336:1108, 1997.
37. Matthews MK: Association of *Ginkgo biloba* with intracerebral hemorrhage, *Neurology* 50:1933, 1998.
38. Rowin J, Lewis SL: Spontaneous bilateral subdural hematomas associated with chronic *Ginkgo biloba* ingestion, *Neurology* 46:1775-1765, 1996.
39. Kim YS, Pyo MK, Park KM, et al: Antiplatelet and antithrombotic effects of a combination of ticlopidine and *Ginkgo biloba* ext (Egb761), *Thromb Res* 91:33-38, 1998.
40. Bal Dit Sollier C, Caplain H, Drouet L: No alteration in platelet function or coagulation induced by Egb761 in a controlled study, *Clin Lab Haematol* 25:251-253, 2003.
41. Yun TK: *Panax ginseng*—a non–organ-specific cancer preventive? *Lancet Oncol* 2:49-55, 2001.

42. Blumenthal M: *The ABC clinical guide to herbs,* Austin, Texas, 2003, American Botanical Council, pp 213-225.
43. Bahrke MS, Morgan WR: Evaluation of the ergogenic properties of ginseng: an update, *Sports Med* 29:113-133, 2000.
44. Tian J, Adams R: Ginseng improves memory in dementia patients [presentation], American Stroke Association meeting, Phoenix, Arizona, Feb. 14, 2003.
45. Wesnes KA, Ward T, McGinty A, et al: The memory enhancing effects of a *Ginkgo biloba/Panax ginseng* combination in healthy middle-aged volunteers, *Psychopharmacology* 152:353, 2000.
46. Kennedy DO, Scholey AB: Ginseng: potential for the enhancement of cognitive performance and mood, *Pharmacol Biochem Behav* 75:687-700, 2003.
47. Wichtl M, Bisset NF, editors: *Herbal drugs and phytopharmaceuticals,* Stuttgart, Germany, 1994, Medpharm Scientific Publishers.
48. McGuffin M, Hobbs C, Upton R, et al, editors: *American Herbal Products Association's botanical safety handbook,* Boca Raton, FL, 1997, CRC Press.
49. Kim WY, Kim JM, Han SB, et al: Steaming of ginseng at high temperature enhances biological activity, *J Nat Prod* 63:1702-1704, 2000.
50. Caron MF, Hotsko AL, Robertson S, et al: Electrocardiographic and hemodynamic effects of *Panax ginseng, Ann Pharmacother* 36:758-763, 2002.
51. Pilotaz F, Masson P: Huperzine A: an acetylcholinesterase inhibitor with high pharmacological potential, *Ann Pharm Francaise* 57:363-373, 1999.
52. Zangara A: The psychopharmacology of huperzine A: an alkaloid with cognitive enhancing and neuroprotective properties of interest in the treatment of Alzheimer's disease, *Pharmacol Biochem Behav* 75:675-686, 2003.
53. Xu SS, Gao ZX, Weng Z, et al: Efficacy of tablet huperzine-A on memory, cognition, and behavior in Alzheimer's disease, *Acta Pharmacol Sinica* 16:391-395, 1995.
54. Zhang Z, Wang X, Chen Q, et al: Clinical efficacy and safety of huperzine alpha in treatment of mild to moderate Alzheimer disease: a placebo-controlled, double-blind, randomized trial, *Zhonghua Yi Xue Za Zhi* 82:941-944, 2002.
55. Lallement G, Baille V, Baubichon D, et al: Review of the value of huperzine as pretreatment of organophosphate poisoning. *Neurotoxicology* 23:1-5, 2002.
56. Ma XC, Wang HX, Xin J, et al: Effects of huperzine A on liver cytochrome P-450 in rats, *Acta Pharmacol Sinica* 24:831-835, 2003.
57. Fernandez MA, de las Heras B, Garcia MD, et al: New insights into the mechanism of action of the anti-inflammatory triterpene lupeol, *J Pharm Pharmacol* 53:1533-1539, 2001.
58. Sunitha S, Nagaraj M, Varalakshmi P: Hepatoprotective effect of lupeol and lupeol linoleate on tissue antioxidant defence system in cadmium-induced hepatotoxicity in rats, *Fitoterapia* 72:516-523, 2001.
59. da Silva AL, Bardini S, Nunes DS, et al: Anxiogenic properties of *Ptychopetalum olacoides* Benth. (Marapuama), *Phytother Res* 16:223-226, 2002.
60. Siqueira IR, Fochesatto C, da Silva AL, et al: *Ptychopetalum olacoides,* a traditional Amazonian "nerve tonic," possesses anticholinesterase activity, *Pharmacol Biochem Behav* 75:645-650, 2003.
61. Perry NS, Bollen C, Perry EK, et al: Salvia for dementia therapy: review of pharmacological activity and pilot tolerability clinical trial, *Pharmacol Biochem Behav* 75:651-659, 2003.
62. Lu Y, Foo LY: Antioxidant activities of polyphenols from sage (*Salvia officinalis*), *Food Chem* 75:197-202, 2001.
63. Perry NS, Houghton PJ, Sampson J, et al: In-vitro activity of *S. lavandulaefolia* (Spanish sage) relevant to treatment of Alzheimer's disease, *J Pharm Pharmacol* 53:1347-1356, 2001.
64. Tildesley NTJ, Kennedy DO, Perry EK, et al: *Salvia lavandulaefolia* (Spanish sage) enhances memory in healthy young volunteers, *Pharmacol Biochem Behav* 75:669-674, 2003.
65. Lim GP, Chu T, Yang F, et al: The curry spice curcumin reduces oxidative damage and amyloid pathology in an Alzheimer transgenic mouse, *J Neurosci* 21:8370-8377, 2001.
66. Szatmari SZ, Whitehouse PJ: Vinpocetine for cognitive impairment and dementia (Cochrane Review). In: *The Cochrane Library,* Issue 1, Chichester, UK, 2004, John Wiley & Sons.

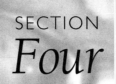

Medical Conditions

It has been become increasingly recognized that cardiovascular health is an important area of concern for women. Likewise, bone health and the prevention of osteoporosis are common concerns for women as they age. In the past it was assumed that effective hormonal treatments for the prevention of osteoporosis would also contribute to lowering the rate of incidence of cardiovascular disease. Unfortunately, the findings of recent large-scale studies have cast serious doubts on this approach and increased concerns about increased stroke and cancer risks.

Integrative approaches to the management of various medical conditions in women—among them disorders of the female reproductive and urinary tracts, including vaginal candidiasis, cervical dysplasia and cancer, urinary tract infection and incontinence, plus breast cancer—are emerging as viable alternatives for many women.

CHAPTER

14

Heart Disease

Cardiovascular disease, including coronary heart disease (CHD) and stroke, has become the leading cause of death among American women. Cardiovascular disease claims more women's lives than the next 16 causes of death combined, including all forms of cancer, chronic lung disease, pneumonia, diabetes, accidents, and acquired immunodeficiency syndrome. Although mortality trends for cardiovascular disease in men have decreased over the past 20 years, they have increased for women. Approximately half a million women sustain a myocardial infarction (MI) each year. More women (42%) than men (24%) die within 1 year of sustaining a recognized MI. Within 6 years, women (33%) are at greater risk than men (21%) of having a second MI.[1] Cardiovascular disease is of particular concern in minority communities, with death rates 69% higher among black women than among white women.

Although risk factors are the same for men and women (e.g., increased serum lipid concentrations, hypertension, obesity, sedentary lifestyle, smoking), some affect women differently than they do men. After age 45, cholesterol levels tend to plateau in men but increase steadily in women. By age 55, women often have higher cholesterol levels than men.[2] Although a high total cholesterol concentration does not appear to be as great a risk for women as it is for men, the combination of a low level of high-density lipoprotein (HDL) cholesterol and a high level of triglycerides (TGs) increases the risk of death in women from heart disease tenfold.[3] Research has shown that high systolic blood pressure and a high fasting blood glucose level are stronger risk factors for women than for men. Smoking increases risk in women two- to fivefold, significantly greater than the doubling in risk observed in men.[4]

Effective prevention strategies are critical because in women, the first cardiovascular event is often fatal. Health-care practitioners must emphasize individual risk-factor management *before* the onset of clinically apparent disease. Identification of risks and early intervention will produce other health benefits as well; risk factors for heart disease are also risk factors for other chronic diseases.

Prevention and Treatment Strategies

Other than a brief discussion of hormone replacement therapy (HRT), this section will not provide a detailed discussion of prescription-drug therapies for the treatment of cardiovascular disease. Undoubtedly, newer cholesterol-lowering medications have made a significant contribution in the prevention of CHD. In 1980, resins and niacin were the most commonly used lipid-lowering medications. By 1985, the use of fibrates had caused a decline in the use of niacin and resins. By 1989, 3-hydroxy-3-methylglutaryl-coenzyme A reductase inhibitor (HMG-CoA) statin drugs had replaced fibrates as the most frequently prescribed lipid-lowering medications.[5] By the mid- to late 1990s, several landmark trials had provided clear evidence that lipid-lowering therapy decreases cardiovascular events, including mortality. These studies included the Scandinavian Simvastatin Survival Study, the West of Scotland Coronary Prevention Study, and the Air Force/Texas Coronary Atherosclerosis Prevention Study.

By 2002, with the publication of the Heart Protection Study (HPS), the use of statin drugs for both the prevention and the treatment of CHD had become firmly established. The aim of the HPS, with more than 20,000 participants ranging in age from 40 to 80 years, was to determine whether statin therapy is of benefit to people who are at high risk for cardiovascular disease but have average to low levels of total cholesterol and low-density lipoprotein (LDL) cholesterol. High-risk patients (defined as those with previous CHD, diabetes, stroke, or peripheral vascular disease) were treated with simvastatin (40 mg/day), antioxidant vitamins (20 mg of β-carotene, 250 mg of vitamin C, and 600 mg of vitamin E daily), or placebo. The study showed that 40 mg/day of simvastatin reduced the risk of heart attack and stroke by one third. The HPS also provided the first definite evidence of benefit in older people (70 years or older, n = 5805) and women (n = 5082). Before the publication of the HPS, the beneficial effects of cholesterol reduction in women had been extrapolated almost entirely from research conducted in men. Because women tend to experience vascular disease at older ages than do men, this study is of special interest because it showed beneficial effects in both women and older populations. Among patients assigned to the antioxidant arm of the trial, the authors detected no change in the incidence of any of the end points and noted small but significant increases in blood levels of LDL cholesterol and TGs.[6]

Hormone Replacement Therapy and Cardiovascular Disease

For many years it was believed that HRT afforded postmenopausal women protection against cardiovascular disease. The main problem with this observation was that the majority of women prescribed HRT were healthy. Physicians generally considered women with certain risk factors, including hypertension, history of stroke, congestive heart failure, and smoking, to be poor candidates for HRT. This made observation data unclear; was the lower incidence of cardiovascular disease a result of HRT or because women taking HRT were generally healthy to begin with? A recently published metaanalysis of these observational trials, corrected for socioeconomic status, educational level, and coronary risk factors, failed to show any cardiac protection in women using HRT.[7]

Not only observational data led practitioners and researchers to believe in the beneficial effects of HRT on the heart. Biologically plausible mechanisms were also invoked. Estrogen has been shown to decrease the concentration of LDL cholesterol, increase the concentration of HDL cholesterol, diminish the inflammatory response to atherosclerosis, and exert a favorable effect on homocysteine levels. Yet estrogen has also been shown to increase TG levels and have an unfavorable effect on the level of C-reactive protein (CRP),[8] an independent risk factor for heart disease. Large clinical trials were needed to find the true benefit, if any, of HRT in cardiovascular disease.

Results from the Heart and Estrogen/Progestin Replacement Study (HERS), HERS Follow-Up (HERS II), and the Women's Health Initiative (WHI) have now challenged the belief that HRT is effective as a primary or secondary preventive strategy for healthy women and those with existing cardiovascular disease. The HERS study examined the effect of HRT (0.625 mg of conjugated estrogens plus 2.5 mg of medroxyprogesterone acetate per day) on coronary and noncoronary diseases in older postmenopausal women with preexisting CHD. In the initial HERS trial, 2763 postmenopausal women with established CHD were randomized to receive HRT or placebo. When the results were published in 1998, the risk for HRT appeared to exceed the benefit in women with established CHD; a higher rate of coronary death and nonfatal MI during the first year of the study was observed in women taking HRT.[9] The time trend was problematic; a 52% increase in coronary events was noted in the HRT group during the first year, but these adverse effects appeared to have disappeared by years 3 and 4, leading researchers to extend the follow-up period. Therefore more than 90% of the surviving HERS participants enrolled in HERS II for an additional 2.7 years' follow-up (mean). At the end of this follow-up period, researchers found no beneficial effect for HRT in women with established CHD. The authors concluded that HRT was not appropriate for use as a secondary prevention for coronary disease.

In July 2002, the arm of the WHI that had randomized women to receive either placebo or HRT (0.625 mg of conjugated estrogens plus 2.5 mg medroxyprogesterone acetate per day) was stopped prematurely because of an unacceptably increased risk of breast cancer.[10] The WHI is the largest primary prevention trial for HRT and cardiovascular disease undertaken to date. In addition to the increased risk of breast cancer, the study found a 29% increased risk of heart attack, a 41% increased risk of stroke, and double the risk of venous thromboembolism in women taking HRT. This study of healthy women showed no cardiovascular benefits of this combination hormone therapy and revealed that the coronary and stroke risks associated with its use make it inappropriate to initiate or continue HRT as a primary prevention for CHD.

Almost 11,000 women aged 50 to 79 years with a prior hysterectomy at baseline participated in the WHI estrogen-alone trial, which was designed to determine whether estrogen prevents heart disease in healthy older women. On March 1, 2004, the National Institutes of Health (NIH) informed study participants that they should stop study medications in the trial of conjugated equine estrogens (Premarin, estrogen-alone) versus placebo. Follow-up of participants will continue for several more years; follow-up studies will include ascertainment of outcomes and mammogram reports. When the study was stopped by the NIH, women, who now are an average age of almost 70 years and have had follow-up for approximately 7 years, were told that the current results show that estrogen alone does not appear to affect (either decrease or increase) coronary heart disease and appears to increase the risk of stroke.[10a]

The failure of HRT to protect women against the progression of existing coronary disease in HERS and HERS II, plus the failure of primary protection from cardiovascular disease in WHI, has, in part, led the U.S. Preventive Services Task Force to recommend that HRT not be routinely used for the prevention of chronic conditions in postmenopausal women.[11] As noted in other chapters of this book, it is important to remember that almost all of these studies were conducted with the use of a combination of conjugated estrogens and medroxyprogesterone acetate. This regimen has dominated in medical research, dramatically influencing the prescribing habits of physicians. It is unclear whether other estrogen/progesterone regimens would yield different results.

Lifestyle

Lifestyle interventions have been shown to substantially improve dyslipidemia, hypertension, and diabetes. Even women who require medications for these conditions benefit from nutritional counseling and exercise, and are often able to reduce the amount of medication needed, thereby reducing the incidence and severity of side effects and the cost of care.

Dietary intervention. A heart-healthy diet should be considered one of the primary therapeutic lifestyle interventions for anyone at risk of CHD. Researchers have demonstrated that diets high in fruit and vegetable intake reduce the risk of heart disease, stroke, and hypertension,[12,13] as well as many cancers.[14] Diet may reduce certain cardiovascular risks because of the wide variety of phytochemical compounds present in plants, a point that must be considered in the evaluation or recommendation of isolated vitamins and minerals and other supplements in the prevention or treatment of cardiovascular disease.

Dietary considerations for hypertension. The Dietary Approaches to Stop Hypertension (DASH) diet emphasizes fruits and vegetables (five to nine servings per day), low-fat dairy products (two to four servings per day), whole grains, poultry, fish, and nuts. Intake of saturated and trans fats, red meat, sweets, and sugar-containing beverages is limited. The DASH diet provides an abundance of naturally occurring potassium, magnesium, and calcium. A large study of the DASH diet revealed that it reduced systolic and diastolic blood pressure by 11.4 and 5.5 mm Hg, respectively, in patients with stage 1 hypertension. Black Americans experienced greater blood pressure reductions than did nonblack Americans.[15] This may be due to the fact that black Americans are more likely to be deficient in magnesium and potassium than whites; both of these nutrients are important in the maintenance of a healthy blood pressure, and this diet provides large amounts of both.

It is well known that some individuals are salt-sensitive and that the restriction of salt in the diet can help reduce blood pressure in some individuals. The DASH diet provides roughly 7.5 g/day of sodium, whereas the standard American diet averages 10 to 15 g. Although research on sodium restriction and hypertension has yielded conflicting results, depending on the population studied, most researchers agree that cutting back on salt is not likely to cause harm and may reduce blood pressure. Meta-analyses of randomized trials have shown that, on average, a reduction in sodium intake of 1.8 g/day is associated with systolic and diastolic blood pressure reductions of approximately 4 and 2 mm Hg, respectively, among individuals with hypertension.[16]

Research suggests that hypertensive individuals should limit their daily intake of sodium to 6 g/day. Considering that 1 tsp of salt contains 2.3 g of sodium, this is no easy goal. (The DASH diet is slightly more liberal.) The U.S. Surgeon General has recommended that a trial of sodium restriction be considered for anyone who (1) has a family history of hypertension, (2) is African-American, (3) is older than 45 years, (4) is overweight, or (5) has borderline hypertension.

Sodium restriction has been shown to prevent the development of hypertension in high-risk patients, and it may reduce the amount of medication required in older hypertensive patients. The Trials of Hypertension Prevention showed that sodium reduction, alone or in concert with weight loss, prevented hypertension by approximately 20%.[17] In the Trials of Nonpharmacologic Interventions in the Elderly, a reduction in salt intake, with or without weight loss, effectively reduced blood pressure and the need for antihypertensive medication in older patients.[18]

A 30-day randomized, controlled study of 412 adults with untreated systolic blood pressure of 120 to 160 mm Hg and diastolic blood pressure of 80 to 95 mm Hg showed that a combination of the DASH diet with reduced sodium intake was more effective than the DASH diet or sodium restriction alone.[19] The study also revealed that reduction of salt intake decreased blood pressure in men and women, blacks and whites, the young and old, and people with normal or high blood pressure.

Low- and high-fat diets. The battle between the proponents of high- and low-fat diets continues to rage across America. Most research has been focused on the beneficial effects of eating a diet low in saturated fat and, more recently, trans fatty acids. Saturated fat is the main fat found in animal products (e.g., beef, pork, dairy, poultry) and in coconut and palm oils. Contrary to popular belief, studies have shown that eating shellfish[20] and eggs[21] does not significantly affect the LDL cholesterol level. Although shellfish and eggs are high in cholesterol, they are low in saturated fat. Recently the public has added the words "trans fat" to its dietary vocabulary. Vegetable oils contain one or more double bonds between carbon atoms. When hydrogen is added to vegetable oils to cause the fat to become solid at room temperature (e.g., margarine), the hydrogens are added in the *trans* position (on the opposite sides of the longitudinal axis of the double bond). Trans fats increase levels of LDL cholesterol and TGs.[22] Many physicians recommend that cholesterol intake be limited to 300 mg/day and that consumption of saturated/trans fat be limited to 10% of total daily calorie intake.

Despite the data demonstrating that low-fat diets are beneficial to the cardiovascular system, low-carbohydrate, high-protein, high-fat diets have become increasingly popular in the pursuit of weight loss, cholesterol reduction, and treatment of metabolic syndrome. Despite this popularity and numerous positive anecdotal reports, only limited data have been published until recently. In one year-long multicenter controlled trial, 63 obese men and women were randomly assigned to consume a low-carbohydrate, high-protein, high-fat diet or a low-calorie, high-carbohydrate, low-fat diet. Subjects consuming the low-carbohydrate diet lost more weight than did subjects receiving the low-fat diet at 3 and 6 months, but the difference at 12 months was not significant.

After 3 months, no significant differences were found between the groups with regard to total or LDL cholesterol concentration. The increase in HDL cholesterol and decrease in TG concentrations were greater among subjects consuming the low-carbohydrate diet than among those receiving the conventional diet throughout most of the study. This may be of particular interest for women; low HDL and high TG levels are considered particularly serious risk factors. Both diets significantly decreased diastolic blood pressure and insulin response to oral glucose load. The authors concluded that the low-carbohydrate diet was associated with a greater improvement in some risk factors for CHD but noted that adherence was poor and attrition high in both groups.[23]

One concern about the long-term use of low-carbohydrate, high-fat diets is the lack of fiber and other key nutrients found in whole grains, fruits, and vegetables. Whole-grain products provide the body with complex carbohydrates, fiber, and other essential nutrients.

Populations that consume a diet high in grains and fiber have been shown to have a decreased risk of cardiovascular disease. It is clear that complex carbohydrates (e.g., bread, cereal, pasta) should be chosen over simple carbohydrates (e.g., soda, candy). Soluble fibers such as pectin, oat, and psyllium have been shown to reduce LDL and total cholesterol levels.

There is no question that more research must be conducted to determine which diet is best for individuals at risk for CHD. Indeed, some individuals may be more constitutionally predisposed to a high-protein, low-carbohydrate diet, whereas others do better with a low-fat, high–complex carbohydrate approach. But until longer and larger studies have been conducted to determine the long-term safety and efficacy of low-carbohydrate, high-protein, high-fat diets, it seems wise to keep total fat intake to 30% to 35% of the daily diet, with the bulk accounted for by monounsaturated fats (e.g., olive oil).

The Mediterranean diet and monounsaturated fats. Researchers have noted that people in countries bordering the Mediterranean Sea exhibit strikingly lower rates of heart disease, obesity, and cancer than their counterparts in the United States and other European countries. Original research on the Mediterranean diet stems from the study of villagers on the Greek island of Crete, whose diet emphasizes green vegetables, fruits, crusty breads, fish, and very little meat or cheese. Villagers typically drink wine with dinner. People living on Crete get more than 30% of their calories from fat, most of it from olive oil. Although this population has a relatively high-fat diet, the fat is mainly monounsaturated. Today the Mediterranean diet is actually a composite of the food habits of several countries and regions, including Spain, southern France, Italy, Greece, Crete, and parts of the Middle East. Unfortunately, many Americans believe they are consuming a Mediterranean diet when they eat huge portions of pasta with heavy cream sauce accompanied by a basket of white bread loaded with butter.

Studies have confirmed that diets low in saturated fat and rich in monounsaturated fats have a beneficial effect on endothelial function and lipid status. Monounsaturated fatty acids reduce the level of LDL cholesterol, but not HDL cholesterol, when they are used to replace saturated fat in the diet. A high intake of the polyunsaturated fatty acids found in other vegetable oils has been shown to reduce the HDL cholesterol level, about a 1% reduction for every 2% of total calories in which polyunsaturated fatty acids replace saturated or monounsaturated fatty acids.[24]

Soy protein and isoflavones. Soy provides a beneficial source of fiber and is naturally low in saturated fat and cholesterol. Epidemiologic data suggest an inverse relationship between the consumption of soy and risk of cardiovascular disease. Most clinical trials of soy have involved postmenopausal women. Research results vary, in part because different types of soy products have been used in these trials. Some trials of soy isoflavones have shown a decrease in the concentrations of total and LDL cholesterol plus an increase in the concentration of HDL cholesterol, whereas others have failed to show any beneficial effect on the lipid profile.[25]

The best documented evidence is the effect of soy protein on plasma lipids and lipoprotein concentrations, with reductions of approximately 10% in LDL cholesterol and small increases in HDL cholesterol concentrations. In addition to the beneficial effect on lipids, dietary soy protein appears to enhance flow-mediated arterial dilation in postmenopausal women.[26] A 1995 meta-analysis of 38 clinical trials involving soy showed that the consumption of soy protein in place of animal protein significantly decreases concentrations of total and LDL cholesterol and TGs, with no change in HDL cholesterol.[27] Although soy isoflavones contribute to the overall beneficial effects of soy, at this time it appears that it is primarily soy protein that plays the most significant role in lipid reduction.

The U.S. Food and Drug Administration found the evidence compelling enough to formally approve a health claim that allows the labels of foods containing at least 6.25 g of soy protein per serving (assuming four servings, or 25 g/day of soy protein) to state that the food reduces the risk of heart disease (Figure 14-1).

Fish and the omega-3 fatty acids. A growing body of evidence derived from epidemiologic data and clinical trials has consistently demonstrated that fish oil reduces TG concentrations, as well as the risk of a variety of cardiovascular events. The main beneficial components of fish oil are eicosapentaenoic acid (EPA) and docosahexaenoic acid (DHA).

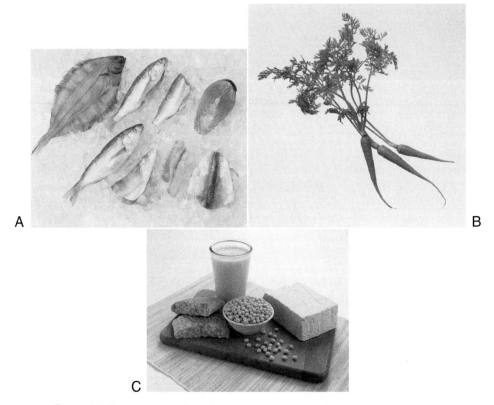

A

B

C

Figure 14-1 A variety of foods can be incorporated into a diet to help prevent heart disease. **A,** Oily fish, such as salmon, contain the omega-3 fatty acids that tend to lower the risk of heart disease. **B,** Carrots are key sources of carotenoids, which are useful for smokers who are prone to heart disease. **C,** Foods containing soy, such as soy milk and tofu, provide plant estrogens that reduce the risk of heart disease.

These fatty acids have a positive effect on vascular function, improving endothelial function through stimulation of nitric oxide, altering vascular tone by way of actions on selective ion channels, and maintaining vascular integrity.[28] Vascular integrity is maintained by making smooth muscle cells less responsive to proliferation.[29] EPA has several antithrombotic actions, including the inhibition of platelet-activating factor,[30] prostaglandin I_2, and thromboxane A_2, compounds involved in platelet aggregation and vasoconstriction.[31]

In concordance with the findings of basic science and animal research, clinical trials such as the Diet and Reinfarction Trial and the Indian Experiment of Infarct Survival have demonstrated reductions in cardiac death rates and the incidence of cardiac symptoms among patients taking fish oil.[32] The authors of a meta-analysis of 11 trials (comprising 15,806 patients) published between 1966 and 1999 concluded that omega-3 fatty acid–enriched diets reduce the risk of nonfatal MI, fatal MI, and sudden death among patients with CHD.[33] A recent Cochrane systematic review showed that fish oil supplementation reduced TG levels among patients with type 2 diabetes but also increased levels of LDL cholesterol, especially in individuals taking high doses. No beneficial or adverse effects on glycemic control were noted.[34] The American Heart Association now recommends the consumption of at least two servings of fish, especially salmon, per week.

The amount of omega-3 fatty acids needed to decrease serum TG levels, approximately 1 g/day, is easily obtained through the addition of fish to the diet. Administering as little as 0.21 g of EPA and 0.12 g of DHA per day in fish oil supplements has been shown to significantly decrease serum TG concentrations in subjects with hyperlipidemia.[35] Patients with primarily hypertriglyceridemia would appear to benefit from fish oil supplementation, however, those with increased LDL cholesterol and TG may be better off with combination therapy. The use of dietary interventions with lipid-lowering medications may be superior to treatment alone in patients with mixed forms of hyperlipidemia. A randomized, controlled 10-month crossover trial of 120 previously untreated hypercholesterolemic men ranging in age from 35 to 64 years showed that a modified Mediterranean-type diet rich in omega-3 fatty acids effectively potentiated the cholesterol-lowering effect of simvastatin, while countering the drug's insulin-increasing effect. Unlike simvastatin therapy alone, it did not decrease serum levels of β-carotene and coenzyme Q10 (CoQ10).[36]

Dyslipidemia often develops in patients who have undergone organ transplantation because of the long-term administration of corticosteroids and cyclosporine. Dietary interventions should be recommended and supported. However, if diet is not sufficient, combined treatment with low-dose pravastatin and fish oil has been shown to be more effective than pravastatin alone in improving the lipid profile after renal transplantation.[37]

A word of caution: Mercury levels in fish can range from 10 to 1000 ppb. Mercury, which finds its way into rivers, lakes, and oceans from coal-burning power plants and other industrial sources, is known to cause learning disabilities and developmental delays. Health care providers should recommend that patients eat fish high in omega-3 fatty acids that are least likely to contain methyl mercury—salmon, for instance. One 3-oz serving of salmon contains approximately 1.2 to 1.5 g of omega-3 fatty acids. Fish high in mercury, such as king mackerel and shark, should be avoided, especially by children and pregnant women. Mercury-free fish oil capsules are available for those who do not care for fish or are concerned about the presence of methyl mercury (and other pollutants). A recent study of 20 fish oil supplements taken from store shelves revealed that all were free of any detectable level of mercury (<1.5 ppb).[38] Fish oil supplements contain both DHA and EPA.

SOUND FISHY?

Inuit peoples consume more fat than just about any other people on the planet, yet they have a much lower incidence of heart disease. It seems that the secret lies in the amount of fish they consume. Omega-3 fatty acids are polyunsaturated fatty acids found in all seafood, including shellfish, oysters, and shrimp. The richest sources are salmon, tuna, mackerel, herring, sea bass, and trout. The American Heart Association now recommends that fish be eaten at least twice a week to prevent heart disease. Other research suggests that fish reduces the risk of stroke and improves mood. Although fish is a healthy, low-fat, protein-rich food, some types—most notably swordfish, shark, tilefish, king mackerel, and tuna steak—can be high in mercury. Consumption of these fish should be limited (and avoided altogether during pregnancy and early childhood).

Alcohol. Convincing evidence indicates that moderate consumption of alcohol (one or two drinks per day) reduces insulin resistance, decreases blood pressure, and increases the level of HDL cholesterol.[39] The authors of one metaanalysis found strong and consistent evidence linking moderate alcohol intake with increased HDL cholesterol and apolipoprotein A_1 levels and decreased concentration of fibrinogen. The authors calculated an overall predicted 24.7% reduction in risk of CHD associated with alcohol intake of 30 g/day in accordance with changes in these markers.[40] The findings of more recent research suggest that alcohol consumption is associated with a decreased probability of an increased level of CRP.[41]

Exactly what form of alcohol consumption offers the best protection against cardiovascular disease remains a matter of debate. Some researchers believe that any type of ethanol is beneficial,[42] whereas others contend that red wine specifically offers the most benefit.[43] The findings of one recent review of the clinical and experimental evidence suggest that red wine may offer greater cardiovascular protection than other types of alcoholic beverages.[44] This protection is thought to be conferred by the antioxidant, vasorelaxant, and antithrombotic properties of the polyphenolic compounds present in wine.[45]

We are well aware of the many problems associated with alcohol consumption—fetal alcohol syndrome, alcoholism, hypertension, and increased TG level, to name but a few. Research has shown that individuals who consume more than three drinks per day are more likely to experience harm than benefit.[46] The risk of breast cancer is increased among women who consume two or more servings of alcohol per day, causing some specialists to recommend that women limit themselves to an average of one daily serving of alcohol.[47] Individuals who enjoy having a glass of wine, a beer, or a mixed drink should be encouraged to consider it a part of a healthy lifestyle, but those who abstain from alcohol should not be encouraged to start drinking. It is important to note that many of the antioxidant compounds found in wine can also be found in purple grape juice.[48]

Smoking cessation. Undoubtedly, tobacco use is associated with an increased risk of cardiovascular disease, and there is no question that a reduction in smoking rates has been achieved in some countries through the implementation of strong legislative, fiscal, and educational programs. Yet, for social reasons, young women are beginning to smoke at an alarming rate in both developed and developing nations. This increase is associated in part with marketing in developing companies by tobacco companies, which use advertising that associates cigarette smoking with glamour, independence, power, and romance. The World Health Organization has estimated that the number of women smokers will triple over the next generation to more than 500 million and more than 200 million will die prematurely of tobacco-induced diseases.[49] A concerted effort to create a global strategy that educates and informs women about the health risks of smoking would help prevent an epidemic of heart disease and other tobacco-related diseases in the future.

Volumes of material address the complexity of smoking cessation, and I will not attempt to replicate them here. However, because this is a text on integrative approaches to health and well-being, it seems appropriate to comment on the use of two popular alternative treatments for this health problem. There are many reports of the successful use of acupuncture and acupressure to achieve smoking cessation. A Cochrane review published in 2002 identified 22 studies addressing this topic. The reviewers found that acupuncture was not superior to sham acupuncture in helping achieve smoking cessation at any time point. When acupuncture was compared with other antismoking interventions, no differences in outcome were found at any time point. The results with different acupuncture techniques failed to show that any particular method (e.g., auricular or nonauricular) was superior to control intervention.[50]

In spite of the clinical trials, many patients find acupuncture useful in their smoking cessation attempts. Given the safety of the intervention, there seems no reason to discourage a patient from using the method.

Hypnosis is another popular treatment used by patients and recommended by practitioners. Many anecdotal reports and uncontrolled studies claim effectiveness. A formal review of nine studies in which hypnotherapy was compared with 14 different control interventions revealed conflicting results for the effectiveness of hypnotherapy compared with no treatment or verbal advice. The reviewers concluded, "We have not shown that hypnotherapy has a greater effect on 6-month quit rates than other interventions or no treatment. The effects of hypnotherapy on smoking cessation claimed by uncontrolled studies were not confirmed by analysis of randomized controlled trials."[51]

Smoking cessation is a complex issue, and multiple approaches are often necessary. What works for one patient may not work for another. Practitioners should remain open to the many interventions that are safe and potentially effective for patients inclined to try them.

Weight loss

Exercise. Obesity is an urgent and growing health problem in the United States. The Office of the U.S. Surgeon General reports that the risks of overweight or obesity may soon cause as much disease and death as does cigarette smoking. The percent of women 55 to 75 years of age who are overweight, according to the National Institutes of Health criterion of a body mass index of 25 kg/m^2, is estimated to be between 53.9% and 55.8%.[52] Implementation of strategies to achieve optimal health, not necessarily a "normal" body weight, is probably the most effective approach for health care providers to take. It has been shown repeatedly that losing just 10 to 20 lb can significantly decrease cardiovascular risk in obese individuals (see Chapter 2).

Hypertension. Hypertension is two to three times more prevalent among overweight people than in lean individuals. Approximately 60% of people with hypertension are overweight. Clinical trials have demonstrated that a reduction in body weight also causes a reduction in blood pressure. A review of 11 weight-loss studies showed that the average reductions in systolic and diastolic blood pressure per kilogram of weight loss were 1.6 and 1.1 mm Hg, respectively.[53] In addition, a recent study demonstrated that weight loss not only reduces blood pressure but also decreases left ventricular wall thickness.

Blood pressure is reduced when excess body weight is lost, even if ideal body weight is not achieved. It is postulated that obese people have some degree of tissue resistance to insulin, resulting in hyperglycemia. As a result, more insulin is released into the bloodstream. Insulin directly stimulates the release of the adrenal catecholamine hormones, which increase vascular resistance and cause the kidneys to retain sodium. Sodium retention increases intravascular volume and ultimately results in higher blood pressure. High levels of insulin also thicken arterial smooth muscle, which leads to an increase in blood pressure. As excess weight is shed, much of the cellular resistance to insulin is lost, and catecholamine levels fall.

Lipids. Obesity is often associated with increased levels of TGs and low levels of HDL cholesterol.[24] It is thought that an increase in the TG level leads to increased catabolism of TG-rich HDL cholesterol, resulting in lower levels of HDL cholesterol.[54] Weight loss in most obese individuals increases the level of HDL cholesterol and decreases the TG level.[55] However, it is important to note that low-fat diets often reduce HDL cholesterol levels. For this reason, saturated fat should be replaced with monounsaturated fat in any weight loss program designed to increase HDL cholesterol levels.[56]

Heart health. In prospective studies, endothelial dysfunction has been associated with an increased incidence of cardiovascular events. The most effective nonpharmacologic approach for preventing endothelial dysfunction is aerobic physical activity, which can reduce oxidative stress associated with aging. Physical activity also improves endothelial dysfunction in patients with cardiovascular risk factors such as essential hypertension.[57]

Approximately 25% of women report engaging in no regular sustained physical activity, and this number is even higher among those 55 years and older. Unfortunately, health care providers often fail to adequately discuss and encourage patients to increase their daily activity. Data from the Nurses' Health Study indicate that simply walking 3 or more hours per week at a brisk pace can reduce the incidence of coronary events by 30% to 40%.[59] Exercise reduces concentrations of cholesterol and TGs, decreases blood pressure, and reduces the risk of stroke while helping maintain a healthy weight and fitness level. Regular exercise helps reduce abdominal fat, the type most associated with the development of diabetes and high blood pressure.

WALK IT OFF

More than 500,000 women die of heart disease each year in the United States, and the number of cases increases every year. What you may not know is that avoiding heart disease could be as easy as walking just 30 minutes a day. Studies have shown that walking briskly just 3 hours a week reduces a woman's risk of heart attack by roughly 40%. Exercise reduces cholesterol and TG levels, blood pressure, and the risk of stroke.

Dietary Supplements

Niacin. Niacin, or nicotinic acid, reduces serum concentrations of cholesterol and TGs. At the time of this writing it is currently the most effective drug for increasing the level of HDL cholesterol[59] and has been shown to reduce the incidence of coronary death and nonfatal MI.[60] Three grams per day of immediate-release niacin reduces LDL cholesterol level by an average of 20% to 25%, and doses of 1 g/day have been shown to increase the HDL cholesterol level by 15% to 20%. An extended-release prescription product, Niaspan (Kos Pharmaceuticals Inc., Miami, FL), decreased LDL cholesterol by 15% to 20% at its maximal dose of 2 g/day. Both the extended- and immediate-release products taken at doses as low as 1 g/day reduce TG concentrations by 20% to 35%.[61]

Niacin is sometimes combined with statin medication in patients with low HDL cholesterol. A 3-year double-blind, placebo-controlled study of 160 adults with atherosclerosis and low HDL cholesterol levels found that a combination of simvastatin and niacin improved HDL cholesterol levels, caused artery blockages to recede, and significantly decreased the incidence of heart complications compared with placebo.[62] Study patients received a combination of simvastatin and niacin alone, antioxidants alone (vitamins E, C, β-carotene, and selenium), simvastatin-niacin plus antioxidants, or placebo. Over the course of 3 years, the subjects who took simvastatin-niacin were 60% to 90% less likely than placebo patients to have a heart attack or stroke, require angioplasty, or die of causes related to heart disease. This study showed that the group receiving the combination plus antioxidants had less of an increase in HDL cholesterol, leading researchers to question the wisdom of combining antioxidants with statin therapy. The most that can be said from this part of the study is that this particular combination of antioxidants appeared to blunt some of the benefit of the simvastatin-niacin therapy. It should not be extrapolated to all patient populations and other statin treatments at this time.

The major limitation of the use of niacin as a lipid-lowering agent is its side effect profile, which includes vascular flushing with both immediate- and extended-release products. Taking a baby aspirin 30 minutes before taking niacin can minimize this effect. Alcohol and hot liquids tend to intensify the flushing, so avoiding these substances while taking the daily dose of niacin is advisable. Because the levels of liver function indicators may transiently increase, niacin should not be taken by anyone with liver disease. Sustained-release niacin has also been associated with severe liver toxicity when given in doses of more than 2 g/day. Niacin can worsen glycemic control in patients with diabetes and aggravate gouty arthritis.

Magnesium. Essential, or idiopathic, hypertension is a complex multifactorial disorder. The fundamental abnormality is increased peripheral resistance due primarily to changes in vascular structure and function. A considerable number of experimental, epidemiologic, and clinical studies point to the important role of magnesium in maintaining healthy vascular tone and function. Small changes in magnesium levels may have significant effects on cardiac excitability and vascular tone, contractility, and reactivity[63]; thus magnesium is often recommended as a nutritional component in the prevention and management of hypertension.

Magnesium deficiency, as well as abnormal magnesium metabolism, appears to play an important role in different types of cardiovascular diseases, including ischemic heart disease, congestive heart failure, sudden cardiac death, atherosclerosis, and several cardiac arrhythmias.[64] Low levels of dietary and serum magnesium have been associated with an increased prevalence of hypertension, insulin resistance, and diabetes. Studies suggest that magnesium deficiency among African-Americans is much more common than in other populations. This observation is important, given that this group has higher rates of diabetes, hypertension, and cardiovascular and renal disease.[65] Clinical trials of magnesium, as well as potassium, supplementation should be undertaken in this population to evaluate the effectiveness of these nutrients as a primary prevention and treatment strategy.

A metaanalysis of 20 trials comprising 1220 participants detected a dose-dependent reduction in blood pressure resulting from magnesium supplementation; however, the reduction was small. The pooled net estimates of blood pressure change were −0.6 (−2.2 to 1.0) mm Hg for systolic and −0.8 (−1.9 to 0.4) mm Hg for diastolic blood pressure. Magnesium has an apparent dose-dependent effect, with reductions of 4.3 mm Hg systolic (95% confidence interval [CI] 6.3-2.2; $P < 0.001$) and of 2.3 mm Hg diastolic (95% CI 4.9-0.0; $P = 0.09$) for each 10 mmol/day increase in magnesium intake.[66]

A common, inexpensive, and effective treatment for hypertension is the use of thiazide diuretics. However, these agents also increase the urinary excretion of magnesium and thus may exacerbate hypertension and increase the risk of arrhythmia. Patients taking thiazide diuretics should be encouraged to consume a diet rich in magnesium to offset any drug-associated loss or to take a dietary supplement that provides 200 to 500 mg/day magnesium. Good dietary sources for magnesium include green leafy vegetables, legumes, whole grains, broccoli, tofu, nuts, and seeds.

Potassium. Research on potassium supplementation clearly indicates that it is beneficial to the cardiovascular system, reducing blood pressure and preventing stroke.[67] A metaanalysis of 33 randomized, controlled trials comprising 2609 participants in which potassium supplementation was the only difference between the intervention and control groups showed potassium supplementation to be associated with a significant reduction in mean (95% CI) systolic and diastolic blood pressure of −3.11 mm Hg (−1.91 to −4.31 mm Hg) and −1.97 mm Hg (−0.52 to −3.42 mm Hg), respectively. Treatment effects appeared to be enhanced in studies in which participants were concurrently exposed to a high intake of sodium. The reviewers concluded, "Increased potassium intake should be considered as a recommendation for prevention and treatment of hypertension, especially in those who are unable to reduce their intake of sodium."[19]

Because of this evidence, the FDA in October 2000 authorized a new health claim, "Diets containing foods that are good sources of potassium and low in sodium may reduce the risk of high blood pressure and stroke." A recommended daily intake of 1600 to 3500 mg of potassium has been established, although athletes involved in prolonged, vigorous exercise and people taking diuretic therapy may require as much as 6000 mg/day.

Many fruits and vegetables, bananas in particular, are excellent sources of potassium, and a diet rich in these foods can provide a significant amount of potassium each day. An average-sized banana (120 g) contains 475 mg of potassium, providing almost 24% of the current recommended daily intake.

Coenzyme Q10. CoQ10, a highly lipophilic compound present in the inner mitochondrial membrane, is essential to the production of cellular energy in the form of adenosine triphosphate (ATP). CoQ10 is thought to prevent cellular damage during myocardial ischemia and reperfusion and has been used orally to treat various cardiovascular disorders, including angina pectoris, hypertension, arrhythmia, and congestive heart failure. A decreased plasma CoQ10/LDL cholesterol ratio may be associated with an increased risk of atherosclerosis.[68] CoQ10 deficiency can occur due to a failure of biosynthesis caused by gene mutation, inhibition of biosynthesis by HMG-CoA reductase inhibitors (statins), and, for unknown reasons in aging and cancer.[69]

Practitioners of natural and integrative medicine often recommend CoQ10 to patients with cardiovascular disease, as well as to those taking statin medications. A growing body of evidence suggests that under certain circumstances, the use of this dietary supplement can have a beneficial effect on the heart. In a year-long randomized, double-blind, controlled trial, orally administered CoQ10 (120 mg/day) reduced the incidence of total cardiac events (24.6% vs. 45.0%; $P < 0.02$), including nonfatal MI (13.7% vs. 25.3%; $P < 0.05$) and cardiac deaths in the intervention group compared with the control group (n = 73 in CoQ10 group, n = 71 in control group taking B vitamins).[70] A recent review of orally administered CoQ10 concluded that it "appears to be safe and well tolerated in the adult population. Issues concerning optimum target dosages, potential interactions, monitoring parameters, and the role of CoQ10 as a mono-therapeutic agent need to be investigated further. Favorable effects of CoQ10 on ejection fraction, exercise tolerance, cardiac output, and stroke volume are demonstrated in the literature; thus, the use of CoQ10 as adjuvant therapy in patients with CHF [congestive heart failure] may be supported."[71]

Interaction between warfarin and CoQ10 has been reported; however, a randomized, placebo-controlled study of 24 patients taking warfarin failed to find any alteration in International Normalized Ratio levels with daily doses of 100 mg CoQ10.[72] Doses used in clinical trials for cardiovascular disorders range from 30 to 300 mg/day; studies are needed to determine the optimal dose. At this time, most practitioners recommend 100 to 180 mg/day for patients with cardiovascular disease. As a side note, research on CoQ10 is being conducted in the area of Parkinson's disease and other neurologic disorders. Parkinson's disease is a degenerative disorder for which no treatment has been shown to slow the progression. A randomized, placebo-controlled study showed that CoQ10 slowed the progressive deterioration of function in patients with Parkinson's disease.[73] The best effect was seen in the group taking 1200 mg/day of the supplement, which was safe and well tolerated in the study.

L-Carnitine. L-Carnitine, an amino acid derivative, is essential for the intermediary metabolism of fatty acids. Carnitine is the shuttle that moves activated long-chain fatty acids across the inner mitochondrial membrane of a cell. These long-chain fatty acids do not readily traverse this membrane and therefore require this special transporter. A deficiency of carnitine can result in decreased movement of fatty acids into the mitochondria, with a subsequent reduction in energy production. Primary carnitine deficiency, although relatively rare, is caused by a defect in the plasma membrane carnitine transporter. Secondary carnitine deficiency is more common; it is associated with several inborn errors of metabolism and also caused by acquired medical or iatrogenic conditions (e.g., in patients taking valproate or zidovudine). In cirrhosis and chronic renal failure, carnitine biosynthesis is impaired or carnitine is lost during hemodialysis. Other chronic conditions such as diabetes mellitus, heart failure, and Alzheimer's disease can also cause carnitine deficiency.[74]

Long-chain fatty acids are an extremely important source of fuel for cardiac tissue. In some cardiac diseases such as ischemic cardiomyopathy, heart failure, hypertrophy, and dilated cardiomyopathy, ATP generation is diminished by impairment of fatty acid delivery to the mitochondria,[75] suggesting a role for carnitine supplementation. Preliminary research indicates that carnitine supplementation helps relieve skeletal muscle fatigue in patients with congestive heart failure.[76] Two reviews of the literature have found that carnitine appears to have beneficial effects on congestive heart failure[77] and angina.[78]

Carnitine may also be of benefit for patients with peripheral vascular disease, improving maximal walking distance. Supplementation with L-carnitine appears to be relatively safe at the doses typically used, generally 900 to 1500 mg/day. Side effects can include nausea, vomiting, diarrhea and abdominal cramping.

Antioxidants. The topic of antioxidants and cardiovascular disease has been a matter of controversy and debate for more than 50 years, particularly in the case of vitamin E. The strong antioxidant activity of vitamin E has been demonstrated in cellular, molecular, and animal experiments.[79] Vitamin E appears to protect cholesterol from oxidative damage, and animal studies, for the most part, have shown that it slows the progression of atherosclerosis.

Support for the role of antioxidant vitamins in heart disease prevention is based primarily on two large cohort studies published in 1993. In the Nurses' Health Study, researchers noted that among more than 85,000 middle-aged women, the risk of coronary artery disease was reduced by 40% in those who took vitamin E supplements compared with those who did not.[80] In the Health Professionals Follow-Up Study, more than 39,000 men ranging in age from 40 to 75 years were evaluated and monitored for 4 years. Researchers found a significant association between a high intake of vitamin E from supplements and a decreased risk of heart disease.[81]

Although these studies did not show cause and effect, it did appear that vitamin E intake and decreased risk of cardiovascular disease were correlated. However, recent prospective, controlled clinical trials of vitamin E, including the Cardiovascular Disease, Hypertension and Hyperlipidemia, Adult-Onset Diabetes, Obesity, and Stroke study; the Heart Outcomes Prevention Evaluation trial; the Secondary Prevention with Antioxidants of Cardiovascular Disease in End Stage Renal Disease trial; and the Heart Protection Study (HPS) present a confusing picture.[82] A meta-analysis of clinical trials showed that neither β-carotene nor vitamin E appeared to prevent all-cause or cardiovascular mortality in patients with known heart disease or those at risk for heart disease. Similarly, the use of these antioxidant vitamins did not affect the number of stroke events.[83]

A definitive decision has not yet been reached with regard to antioxidants. Several researchers have questioned the type of supplement, as well as the dose, used in many of the clinical trials. Most vitamin E studies used α-tocopherol supplementation. Some argue that a better test for vitamin E would be a supplement that contains a mixture of tocopherols (α-, β-, Δ-, γ-) and tocotrienols. Also, there must be some rationale for the dose used in the studies. Doses of 100 to 400 International Units/day are commonly used in studies, although most practitioners of natural medicine routinely prescribe 600 to 1000 International Units/day. Likewise, some researchers have called for a mixture of carotenoids, rather than isolated synthetic β-carotene.

Beyond Lipids

Physicians routinely check fasting lipid levels and treat the patient if levels are elevated because of the well-known increased risk of cardiovascular disease when cholesterol levels are high. If lipid levels are normal, no treatment is provided. However, this approach is problematic because many people with normal cholesterol levels experience cardiovascular events. Research has shown that inflammation is evident from the initiation through the progression of atherosclerosis, even if lipid levels are normal. Studies are now focused on assessing the potential for biochemical markers of inflammation to act as predictors of risk for coronary heart disease (CHD). Several large, prospective epidemiologic studies have consistently shown that CRP and interleukin-6 (IL-6) plasma levels are strong independent predictors of future cardiovascular events, both in patients with a history of CHD and in apparently healthy subjects.[84]

Of particular interest to women are the recent findings of 27,939 healthy women enrolled in the Women's Health Study, which showed that CRP is a stronger predictor of risk than is LDL cholesterol, predicts increased risk in subjects without overt hyperlipidemia, and adds prognostic information to risk scoring and LDL cholesterol categories.[85] Other data from this study show that a high sensitivity CRP level adds prognostic information to the diagnosis of metabolic syndrome. Taken together with data in men on the association of CRP with vascular risk, a strong argument can be made for screening in the primary prevention population.

A simple, reliable, standardized, inexpensive, high-sensitivity assay is available for measuring CRP. The patient does not have to fast, but he or she does have to be well. The test results will be inaccurate if the individual is sick; infection increases the concentration of CRP. Also, if the subject has an underlying inflammatory disorder, such as lupus or rheumatoid arthritis, the test cannot be used to assess cardiovascular risk. Most practitioners order the test twice, 2 weeks apart, and average the two scores.

Data from both men and women demonstrate that as weight progresses from normal to overweight to obese, CRP increases in a stepwise fashion. CRP levels are higher in obese subjects, probably because of increased insulin resistance. Interventions that alter insulin resistance, such as weight loss, exercise, and conjugated linoleic acid, also alter CRP.[86] A recent study found that obese women who ate a Mediterranean diet and increased their physical activity not only lost weight but also had a reduction in inflammatory markers such as CRP and IL-6.[87] Statins, but not aspirin, have been shown to reduce CRP levels.[88] A number of anti-inflammatory botanicals may influence CRP levels, but this area is unexplored at present.

Homocysteine. Homocysteine, an intermediate amino acid formed during the metabolism of methionine, has been shown to be an independent, modifiable risk factor for cardiovascular disease.[89] Plasma homocysteine is normally 12 μmol/L or less. An increased homocysteine level can play a role in the development of cardiovascular disease. A number of patients with established coronary artery disease have relatively normal lipid values and hyperhomocystinemia ($\geq$15 μmol/L). Researchers have noted that reductions in homocysteine levels after cardiac rehabilitation and exercise training led to a 20% to 30% reduction in overall coronary artery disease risk.[90] Furthermore, abnormal homocysteine concentrations are prevalent among patients with diabetes[91] and obesity,[92] both conditions associated with increased cardiovascular risk.

The three vitamins necessary for the metabolism of homocysteine are folic acid and vitamins B_6 and B_{12}. Increased homocysteine may be the result of a deficiency of folic acid, vitamin B_{12}, or, to a lesser extent, vitamin B_6.[93] Folic acid supplementation is a safe and effective method for reducing elevated homocysteine levels. Adequate intake of vitamins B_6 and B_{12} should be encouraged in the diet or in supplement form. Vitamin B_6 is found in meat, poultry, fish, legumes, peanuts, walnuts, oats, brown rice, and whole wheat. Vitamin B_{12} comes primarily from animal products. Non-animal sources of vitamin B_{12}, such as nutritional yeast, exist but vary widely in their B_{12} content. Vegans (vegetarians who do not consume diary products or eggs) should be encouraged to take a B_{12} supplement. Folic acid can be found in citrus fruits, tomatoes, green leafy vegetables, asparagus, broccoli, yeast, lentils, beans, eggs, beef, organ meats, whole grains, and enriched cereals.

At this time, it seems prudent to lower increased homocysteine levels as a secondary preventative measure in patients with coronary artery disease.

Botanicals. The role of plants in the treatment of cardiovascular disorders has been a long and impressive one. As with many other medical conditions, the first effective treatments for hypertension and congestive heart failure were derived from plants. Plant sterols have been shown to reduce cholesterol and are now added to numerous foods as part of a heart-healthy dietary approach. The monounsaturated fat in olive oil and multiple constituents within garlic have proved beneficial to the cardiovascular system when consumed as part of a healthy diet. Other botanicals—among them hawthorn, red yeast rice, and globe artichoke—are showing promise in a variety of cardiovascular conditions. The following brief overview lists only a few of the popular herbs being used by consumers and recommended by many practitioners of integrative medicine.

Garlic (Allium sativum). Garlic is perhaps the best known of the herbs for the cardiovascular system. Several meta-analyses have demonstrated a reduction in total cholesterol of 5% to 12% with garlic supplementation.[94] Although a short-term benefit of garlic in cholesterol reduction was noted in these reviews, long-term benefit has been questioned. Thirty-seven randomized trials, all but one in adults, consistently showed that compared with placebo, various garlic preparations caused small reductions in total cholesterol at 1 and 3 months (range of average pooled reductions 12.4 to 25.4 mg/dL). Eight placebo-controlled trials reported outcomes at 6 months; pooled analyses showed no significant reductions of total cholesterol with garlic compared with placebo. The reviewers stated that it was not clear whether statistically significant positive short-term effects, but negative longer term effects, were a result of systematic differences in studies with longer and shorter follow-up durations, fewer longer-term studies, or time-dependent effects of garlic.[95]

The benefits of long-term garlic consumption may not be directly related to lipid reduction. The antiatherogenic effects appear to be due to inhibition of platelet aggregation, inhibition of cholesterol biosynthesis, and enhanced fibrinolysis.[96] Garlic oil, aged garlic, fresh garlic, and garlic powder have been shown to inhibit platelet aggregation through their interference with the cyclooxygenase-mediated thromboxane-synthesis pathway.[97] Raw garlic inhibited cyclooxygenase activity noncompetitively and irreversibly.[98] After 26 weeks of garlic consumption, an 80% reduction in serum thromboxane was noted in healthy male volunteers eating 3 g of fresh garlic each day. Cooked garlic has less inhibitory effect on platelet aggregation than raw garlic.[99]

A 4-year study was conducted with 152 men and women with advanced plaque accumulation and one other cardiac risk factor (e.g., high cholesterol, hypertension). Patients were randomized to take 900 mg garlic (Kwai; Lichtwer Pharma AG, Berlin, Germany) or placebo for 48 months. High-resolution ultrasound was used to measure plaque in the carotid and femoral arteries at 0, 16, 36, and 48 months. At 48 months, a 2.6% reduction in plaque volume was noted in the garlic group, compared with a 15.6% increase in the placebo group ($P < 0.0001$).[100] These findings support the generally held belief that garlic has a preventive and mild therapeutic effect in atherosclerosis. Although these findings are encouraging, methodologic limitations prevent more concrete conclusions.

Garlic trials are often difficult to assess, given their short duration and the unpredictable release and inadequate definition of active constituents in the garlic preparations used. Most garlic supplements are standardized to "allicin potential" and are enteric-coated to prevent gastric acid inactivation of the allicin-producing enzyme, alliinase.[100a] An evaluation of garlic powder tablets used in clinical trials (1989 to 1997) found tremendous variation in the amount of allicin released using the validated U.S. Pharmacopoeia acid-disintegration test.

Older batches were more resistant to acid disintegration and released three times more allicin (44% vs. 15% of their potential; $P < 0.001$) than newer lots. Conflicting trial results may be the result of lower amounts of bioavailable allicin in some products.[101] A study found 23 of 24 brands available in the United States released just 15% of their allicin potential when subjected to the U.S. Pharmacopoeia testing method. Researchers in the field of garlic study have suggested that garlic powder supplements be standardized to dissolution allicin release and not allicin potential.[101] Clinical trials will be difficult to perform and difficult to interpret until the issue of dissolution and bioavailability of garlic products is adequately addressed.

Garlic is widely consumed around the globe as a spice, establishing its safety when used in rational amounts. Adverse effects of garlic reported in the literature include two cases of postoperative bleeding in patients taking garlic before surgery (during augmentation mammoplasty[102] and transurethral resection of the prostate gland).[103] Spontaneous spinal epidural hematoma has also been reported.[104] Three cases of hemorrhage with garlic have been reported; none of the patients was taking warfarin.[105] The American Herbal Products Association contraindicates the use of garlic in nursing mothers; however, serious adverse effects have not been reported in breastfed infants.[106] Interestingly, two studies found that infants nursed longer and ingested more breastmilk when their mothers consumed garlic capsules compared with infants being nursed by mothers taking placebo. No adverse effects were noted in the nurslings.[107]

Guggul (Commiphora mukul). The mukul myrrh tree grows in dry areas of India, Pakistan, and Afghanistan. For thousands of years, healers have used the resinous sap that exudes from the tree bark to control weight and treat other ailments. Since the 1960s, the bulk of research has focused on guggul's lipid-lowering activity.

Animal studies and small clinical trials demonstrate a reduction in total serum cholesterol, LDL cholesterol, very low-density lipoprotein (VLDL) cholesterol, and TGs and an increase in HDL cholesterol.[108] However, a recent rigorous randomized, placebo-controlled trial failed to find any significant lipid-lowering effect in 103 adults with hypercholesterolemia. The study provided standard dose guggulipid (1000 mg), high-dose guggulipid (2000 mg), or matching placebo three times daily for 8 weeks. The main outcome was a reduction in the LDL cholesterol level. Secondary outcome measures included levels of total cholesterol, HDL cholesterol, TGs, and directly measured VLDL cholesterol, as well as adverse events reports and laboratory safety measures including electrolyte levels and hepatic and renal function. Compared with participants randomized to placebo (n = 36), in whom levels of LDL cholesterol decreased by 5%, both standard dose (n = 33) and high-dose guggulipid (n = 34) increased levels of LDL cholesterol by 4% ($P = 0.01$ vs. placebo) and 5% ($P = 0.006$ vs. placebo), respectively, at 8 weeks, for a net positive change of 9% to 10%. No significant changes were detected in levels of total cholesterol, HDL cholesterol, TGs, or VLDL cholesterol in response to treatment with guggulipid on an intention to treat analysis. Although guggulipid was generally well tolerated, 6 participants treated with guggulipid experienced a hypersensitivity rash, compared with none in the placebo group.[109]

The use of guggul is contraindicated during pregnancy because of its purported uterine-stimulant properties.[110] Guggul has been reported to reduce the effectiveness of propranolol and diltiazem.[111] The crude herb is associated with many side effects, including abdominal pain, diarrhea, and rash. For this reason, guggul extracts standardized to 5%

guggulsterone content are generally preferred. The therapeutic dose is generally 500 mg taken thrice daily so as to provide a total of 75 of mg guggulsterone daily.

Globe artichoke (Cynara scolymus). The flower petals and fleshy flower bottoms of the globe artichoke have been eaten as a vegetable for many centuries. Artichoke leaf has been used as a treatment for dyspepsia and other gastrointestinal disorders since ancient times. Contemporary researchers have found that artichoke leaf extract may be beneficial for liver disorders, diabetes, and hyperlipidemia. In vitro research suggests that the leaf extract indirectly inhibits HMG-CoA reductase.[112] Artichoke extract also enhances biliary cholesterol excretion,[113] which may also contribute to its lipid-lowering effects.

A 1998 systematic review of artichoke leaf extract for cholesterol reduction identified only one high-quality, randomized, double-blind, placebo-controlled trial in 44 healthy volunteers. Artichoke extract was given at doses of 640 mg three times daily for 12 weeks. No differences were noted in total serum cholesterol levels compared with placebo; however, subgroup analysis did show a significant benefit for artichoke when baseline total cholesterol values were above 210 mg/dL.[114]

Since this review, a randomized, placebo-controlled, multicenter trial was undertaken in 143 patients with total cholesterol levels greater than 280 mg/dL. Patients were randomly assigned to receive either 1800 mg of artichoke dry extract per day (drug/extract ratio 25:1 to 35:1, aqueous extract, CY450) or placebo for 6 weeks. The decrease in total cholesterol and LDL cholesterol, respectively, in the treatment group was 18.5% and 22.9%, compared with 8.6% and 6.3% in the placebo group. The LDL/HDL ratio showed a decrease of 20.2% in the active group and 7.2% in the placebo group. No adverse events were noted.[115]

The adverse effects profile for artichoke is quite good. The only contraindication at this time is use in individuals with bile duct obstruction, because of the choleretic activity of the extract. Studies to date have been small or of short duration, making definitive conclusions about the use of artichoke leaf extract for lipid reduction impossible at this time.

Redyeast rice (Monascus purpureus). Red yeast rice is made by fermenting a type of yeast called *Monascus purpureus* over rice. It has a long history of use in traditional Chinese medicine and has been used to make rice wine and as a food preservative for maintaining the color and taste of fish and meat.[116]

Red yeast rice contains monacolin K, or what is more commonly referred to as mevinolin or lovastatin. Monacolin K inhibits HMG-CoA reductase; however, the small amount of monacolin K present in red yeast rice (roughly 0.2%) does not fully explain the beneficial lipid-lowering effect seen in limited clinical trials. Red yeast rice contains other potential lipid-lowering agents, among them 10 other monacolin analogues, omega-3 fatty acids, isoflavones, and plant sterols (β-sitosterol, campesterol, stigmasterol, and sapogenin).[117]

The most rigorous study to date was a randomized, double-blind, placebo-controlled study of 83 men and women that showed that individuals who took 2.4 g/day red yeast rice had significantly decreased cholesterol, from 250 to 208 mg/dL (17%) after 8 weeks of treatment compared to controls.[118] The LDL cholesterol level dropped from 173 to 134 mg/dL (22%) and TGs decreased from 133 to 118 mg/dL (12%), while HDL cholesterol remained the same. No significant differences between the two groups were noted with regard to total calories, total fat, saturated fat, monounsaturated fat, polyunsaturated fat, or fiber. No changes in liver function parameters or other serious adverse events were reported.

Two other small studies were presented at the 1999 American Heart Association meeting in Orlando, Florida. The first was a multicenter, open-label study in 187 subjects

(116 men, 71 women) with mild to moderate elevated total cholesterol and LDL cholesterol levels. This study showed that treatment with red yeast rice (2.4 g/day) reduced total cholesterol levels by more than 16%, LDL cholesterol levels by 21%, and triglyceride levels by 24%. HDL cholesterol levels also increased by 14%. Participants used the AHA Step 1 Diet throughout the study. After 4-weeks on this diet, red yeast rice was administered for 8 weeks. No change in the serum cholesterol level was noted after 1 month of dietary intervention. Eighteen percent of participants reported adverse effects with red yeast rice, which included headache, abdominal bloating, and gas.[119] The second, a study in older participants given red yeast rice, found significant reductions in total cholesterol and LDL cholesterol levels compared with those who received placebo over an 8-week period.[120]

The proprietary red yeast rice product used in the clinical trials, Cholestin (Pharmanex, Hong Kong), is no longer available as a dietary supplement in the United States. Merck, the pharmaceutical company that holds the patent for Mevacor (lovastatin), and Pharmanex engaged in a legal battle over allegations that red yeast rice was actually lovastatin being sold over the counter. Indeed, the dietary supplement does provide approximately 5 mg/day of this statin. After several years of legal actions in the courts, Pharmanex lost the fight and Cholestin was taken off the U.S. market. Since this time, Pharmanex has reformulated the Cholestin product with policosanol; it no longer contains red yeast rice. However, other red yeast rice products can still be found on the shelves of health food stores. The current cost for cholesterol-lowering drugs is roughly $120 to $300 per month, with an average monthly cost of $187.[121] The red yeast rice product used in the clinical trials costs approximately $25 to $35 per month.

Questions over safety have been raised given the fact that the dietary supplement contains small amounts of statins. However, adverse events have been limited to principally gastrointestinal upset. The dose used in clinical trials was 2.4 g/day taken in two divided doses.

Flavonoid-rich plants. Flavonoids (together with carotenoids) are partially responsible for the colors of flowers, fruit, and, sometimes, leaves. A wide variety of flavonoid classes are present in fruits, vegetables, and beverages such as tea and wine. Flavonoids exert antioxidant, antineoplastic, and antiinflammatory activity; extend the activity of vitamin C; and exert positive effects on the cardiovascular system.[122,123] Polyphenolic flavonoids are believed to reduce the risk of coronary artery disease through inhibition of platelet aggregation, reducing injury from ischemia and reperfusion, reducing plasma cholesterol levels and inhibiting LDL oxidation.[124,125] For instance, licorice extract (free of glycyrrhizin, the component associated with water retention and hypertension) and the isoflavane glabridin, a major polyphenolic compound found in licorice, were both shown to markedly inhibit LDL oxidation in 10 normolipidemic individuals in one study.[126]

Diets rich in plant polyphenols, such as red wine or tea, are thought to exert a beneficial effect on the cardiovascular system. Preliminary data exist to suggest that such plants may be considered part of a heart-healthy regimen. One of these flavonoid-rich herbs is hawthorn (*Crataegus oxyacantha, C. laevigata, C. monogyna*), a fruit-bearing shrub used in European and Asian medicine for the treatment of a variety of complaints including digestive disorders, dyspnea, urinary problems, and cardiovascular disease. People around the globe have consumed the fruit as a food and to produce wine and jams. Today a relatively large body of research is focused on the cardiovascular effects of hawthorn fruit, leaves, and flowers. Hawthorn is widely accepted in Europe as a treatment for mild cases of congestive heart failure and minor arrhythmias.

Hawthorn is rich in flavonoids, oligomeric procyanidins, and triterpenes, substances known to be beneficial to the cardiovascular system. In one metaanalysis, the evidence from randomized, double-blind, placebo-controlled trials using hawthorn extract mono-preparations for the treatment of congestive heart failure was assessed. In most studies, hawthorn was used as an adjunct to conventional treatment. Eight trials comprising 632 patients with chronic heart failure (New York Heart Association classes I-III) provided data that were suitable for metaanalysis. For the physiologic outcome of maximal work-load, treatment with hawthorn extract was more beneficial than placebo (weighted mean difference 7 Watt; 95% CI 3-11 Watt; $P < 0.01$; n = 310 patients). The pressure-heart rate product also showed a beneficial decrease (weighted mean difference –20; 95% CI –32 to –8; n = 264 patients) with hawthorn treatment. Symptoms such as shortness of breath and fatigue improved significantly with hawthorn treatment compared with placebo. Adverse events were infrequent, mild, and transient and included nausea, dizziness, and gastrointestinal complaints. The reviewers concluded that hawthorn extract offers significant benefit as an adjunct treatment for chronic heart failure.[127]

Herb-drug interaction between hawthorn and cardiac glycosides is almost universally listed in the herbal literature because it was thought that hawthorn potentiates the activity of cardiac glycosides. However, the European Scientific Cooperative on Phytotherapy[128] and the German Commission E[129] do not list hawthorn and cardiac glycosides as resulting in a possible herb-drug interaction. A randomized crossover trial involving 8 healthy volunteers evaluated digoxin 0.25 mg for 10 days and digoxin 0.25 mg with *Crataegus* special extract WS 1442 (hawthorn leaf with flower dry extract 5:1 [w/w], standardized to 18.75% oligomeric procyanidins; Schwabe Pharmaceuticals, Karlsruhe, Germany). Seventy-two–hour pharmacokinetic studies were also conducted. No statistically significant differences were noted in any measured pharmacokinetic parameters. After 3 weeks of concomitant therapy, hawthorn had not significantly altered the pharmacokinetic parameters for digoxin, suggesting that hawthorn and digoxin, at the dosages and in the dosage form studied, may be coadministered safely.[130]

The flowers, leaves, and fruit are considered to be the active parts of hawthorn. Most studies have involved two distinct preparations of hawthorn: Special extract WS 1442 contains 80 mg of hawthorn leaf with a 5:1 (wt/wt) dry flower extract standardized to 18.75% oligomeric procyanidins (15 mg) per capsule. Extract LI132 (Lichtwer Pharma GmbH, Berlin, Germany) contains 95 mg of hawthorn leaf, 55 mg of hawthorn fruit, and 45 mg of hawthorn flower, plus 30 mg of dry cold macerate 5:1 (wt/wt) of hawthorn leaf with flower per tablet. Crude preparations are likely to be quite effective; a considerable amount of the oligomeric procyanidins and flavonoids will be released into a properly prepared infusion or tincture.

Many questions remain regarding the use of this herb. How does hawthorn compare with standard therapies for congestive heart failure in terms of morbidity and mortality? Does the coadministration of hawthorn with digoxin or angiotensin-converting enzyme inhibitors enhance the effect of either drug therapy? Hawthorn is an intriguing herb with an excellent safety profile that merits additional research to determine its proper place in medicine.

Mind/body medicine. The overwhelming belief in the community at large is that certain types of people are at greater risk for heart disease than others. To more clearly evaluate the scientific data on the subject, an expert working group of the National Heart Foundation of Australia undertook an analysis of the currently available systematic reviews of major psychosocial risk factors to assess whether independent associations exist among any of the factors and the development and progression of CHD, or the occurrence of acute cardiac events. The expert group concluded (1) strong and consistent evidence supports an independent causal association among depression, social isolation, and lack of quality social support and the causes and prognosis of CHD; and (2) no strong or consistent evidence supports a causal association among chronic life stressors, work-related stressors (e.g., job control, demands, strain), type A behavior patterns, hostility, anxiety or panic disorders, and CHD.[131] Scientific agreement about the relationship between depression and CHD is considerable; however, debate continues regarding a potential connection between hostility/stress and heart disease with studies providing conflicting results.

Depression is associated with social changes, that may influence the development and course of cardiovascular disease—among them a diminishment in self-care motivation. Depression may also cause physiologic changes, such as nervous system activation, cardiac rhythm disturbances, systemic and localized inflammation, and hypercoagulability—all of which can negatively influence the cardiovascular system.[132] Patients with depression have been shown to have higher levels of IL-6,[133] a marker of inflammation and a strong independent predictor of cardiovascular disease. Men with the highest scores for both hostility and depression exhibited the highest levels of IL-6, suggesting an increased risk for cardiovascular disease.[134] Other researchers have found a relationship among hostility and time urgency/impatience and the development of hypertension, especially in young adults ages 18 to 30 years.[135]

Many of the lifestyle suggestions presented in this chapter are relevant here. Exercise, avoidance of tobacco, moderate consumption of alcohol, and a heart-healthy diet are essential in the prevention of cardiovascular disease. The data suggest that appropriate treatment of depression can help mitigate some of the risk for CHD. Helping patients deal with feelings of hostility may have a beneficial effect on blood pressure, as well as likely improving the overall quality of their lives and social interactions.

References

1. American Heart Association: *1999 Heart and stroke statistical update,* Dallas, TX, 1998, American Heart association: www.americanheart.org. Accessed September 2003.
2. Connelly P, MacLean D, Horlick L, et al: Plasma lipids and lipoproteins and the prevalenc of risk for coronary heart disease in Canadian adults, *Can Med Assoc J* 146:1977-1987, 1992.
3. *Women, heart disease and stroke in Canada: issues and options. Report no. CAT 50029722.* Ottawa, Ontario, Canada, 1997, Heart and Stroke Foundation of Canada.
4. Jonsdottir LS, Sigfusson N, Gudnason V, et al: Do lipids, blood pressure, diabetes, and smoking confer equal risk of myocardial infarction in women as in men? The Reykjavik Study, *J Cardiovasc Risk* 9:67-76, 2002.
5. Wang TJ, Stafford RS, Ausiello JC, et al: Randomized clinical trials and recent patterns in the use of statins, *Am Heart J* 141:957-963, 2001.
6. Heart Protection Study Collaborative Group: MRC/BHF Heart Protection Study of antioxidant vitamin supplementation in 20,536 high-risk individuals: a randomized placebo-controlled trial, *Lancet* 360:23-33, 2002.
7. Humphrey LL, Chan BK, Sox HC: Postmenopausal hormone replacement therapy and the primary prevention of cardiovascular disease, *Ann Intern Med* 20:273-284, 2002.
8. Kuller LH and the Women's Health Initiative: Hormone replacement therapy and risk of cardiovascular disease: implications of the results of the Women's Health Initiative, *Arterioscler Thromb Vasc Biol* 23:11-16, 2003.
9. Hulley S, Grady D, Bush T, et al: Randomized trial of estrogen plus progestin for secondary prevention of coronary heart disease in postmenopausal women. Heart and Estrogen/progestin Replacement Study (HERS) Research Group, *JAMA* 19:605-613, 1998.

10. Rossouw JE, Anderson GL, Prentice RL, et al: Risks and benefits of estrogen plus progestin in healthy postmenopausal women: principal results from the Women's Health Initiative randomized controlled trial, *JAMA* 288:321-333, 2002.
10a. Women's Health Initiative Participant Website: Information for physicians. Available at: http://www.whi.org/updates/advisory_ea_physicians.asp. Accessed March 18, 2004.
11. U.S. Preventive Services Task Force, Postmenopausal hormone replacement therapy for primary prevention of chronic conditions: recommendations and rationale, *Ann Intern Med* 137:834-839, 2002.
12. Key TJA, Thorogood M, Appleby PN, et al: Dietary habits and mortality in 11,000 vegetarians and health conscious people: results of a 17 year follow up, *BMJ* 313:775-779, 1996.
13. Ness AR, Powles JW: Fruit and vegetables and cardiovascular disease: a review, *Int J Epidemiol* 26:1-13, 1997.
14. Deleted in proof.
15. Svetkey LP, Simons-Morton D, Vollmer WM, et al, for the DASH Research Group: Effects of dietary patterns on blood pressure: subgroup analysis of the Dietary Approaches to Stop Hypertension (DASH) randomized clinical trial, *Arch Intern Med* 159:285-293, 1999.
16. Graudal NA, Galloe AM, Garred P: Effects of sodium restriction on blood pressure, renin, aldosterone, catecholamines, cholesterols, and triglyceride: a meta-analysis, *JAMA* 279:1383-1391, 1998.
17. Trials of Hypertension Prevention Collaborative Research Group: Effects of weight loss and sodium reduction intervention on blood pressure and hypertension incidence in overweight people with high-normal blood pressure: the Trials of Hypertension Prevention, Phase II, *Arch Intern Med* 157:657-667, 1997.
18. Whelton PK, He J, Cutler JA, et al: Effects of oral potassium on blood pressure: meta-analysis of randomized controlled clinical trials, *JAMA* 277:1624-1632, 1997.
19. Vollmer WM, Sacks FM, Ard J, et al: Effects of diet and sodium intake on blood pressure: subgroup analysis of the DASH-Sodium Trial, *Ann Intern Med* 135:1019-1028, 2001.
20. De Oliveira e Silva ER, Seidman CE, Tian JJ, et al: Effects of shrimp consumption on plasma lipoproteins, *Am J Clin Nutr* 64:712-717, 1996.
21. Vorster HH, Benade AJ, Barnard HC, et al: Egg intake does not change plasma lipoprotein and coagulation profiles, *Am J Clin Nutr* 55:400-410, 1992.
22. Lichtenstein AH, Ausman LM, Jalbert SM, et al: Effects of different forms of dietary hydrogenated fats on serum lipoprotein cholesterol levels, *N Engl J Med* 340:1933-1940, 1999.
23. Foster GD, Wyatt HR, Hill JO, et al: A randomized trial of a low-carbohydrate diet for obesity, *N Engl J Med* 348:2082-2090, 2003.
24. Grundy SM, Denke MA. Dietary influences on serum lipids and lipoproteins. *J Lipid Res* 31:1149-1172, 1990.
25. Demonty I, Lamarche B, Jones PJ: Role of isoflavones in the hypocholesterolemic effect of soy, *Nutr Rev* 61(6 pt 1):189-203, 2003.
26. Clarkson TB: Soy, soy phytoestrogens and cardiovascular disease, *J Nutr* 132:566S-569S, 2002.
27. Anderson JW, Johnstone BM, Cook-Newell ME: Meta-analysis of the effects of soy protein intake on serum lipids, *N Engl J Med* 333:276-282, 1995.
28. Abeywardena MY, Head RJ: Longchain n-3 polyunsaturated fatty acids and blood vessel function, *Cardiovasc Res* 52:361-371, 2001.
29. Pakala R, Pakala R, Benedict CR: Thromboxane A2 fails to induce proliferation of smooth muscle cells enriched with eicosapentaenoic acid and docosahexaenoic acid. *Prostaglandins Leukot Essent Fatty Acids* 60:275-281, 1999.
30. Panayiotou A, Samartzis D, Nomikos T, et al: Lipid fractions with aggregatory and antiaggregatory activity toward platelets in fresh and fried cod (*Gadus morhua*): correlation with platelet-activating factor and atherogenesis, *J Agric Food Chem* 48:6372-6379, 2000.
31. Nieuwenhuys CM, Feijge MA, Offermans RF, et al: Modulation of rat platelet activation by vessel wall-derived prostaglandin and platelet-derived thromboxane: effects of dietary fish oil on thromboxane-prostaglandin balance, *Atherosclerosis* 154:355-366, 2001.
32. Harris WS: Nonpharmacologic treatment of hypertriglyceridemia: focus on fish oils, *Clin Cardiol* 22(6 suppl):II40-II43, 1999.
33. Bucher HC, Hengstler P, Schindler C, et al: N-3 polyunsaturated fatty acids in coronary heart disease: a meta-analysis of randomized controlled trials, *Am J Med* 112:298-304, 2002.

34. Farmer A, Montori V, Dinneen S, et al: Fish oil in people with type 2 diabetes mellitus, *Cochrane Database Syst Rev* (3):CD003205, 2001.
35. Weber P, Raederstorff D: Triglyceride-lowering effect of omega-3 LC-polyunsaturated fatty acids: a review, *Nutr Metab Cardiovasc Dis* 10:28-37, 2001.
36. Jula A, Marniemi J, Huupponen R, et al: Effects of diet and simvastatin on serum lipids, insulin, and antioxidants in hypercholesterolemic men: a randomized controlled trial, *JAMA* 287:598-605, 2002.
37. Grekas D, Kassimatis E, Makedou A, et al: Combined treatment with low-dose pravastatin and fish oil in post-renal transplantation dislipidemia, *Nephron* 88:329-333, 2001.
38. Product Review: *Omega-3 fatty acids (EPA and DHA) from fish/marine oils* (posted 2001). Available at: www.consumerlabs.com. Accessed April 2004.
39. Eagles CJ, Martin U: Non-pharmacological modification of cardiac risk factors: Part 3. Smoking cessation and alcohol consumption, *J Clin Pharmacol Ther* 23:1-9, 1998.
40. Rimm EB, Williams P, Fosher K, et al: Moderate alcohol intake and lower risk of coronary heart disease: meta-analysis of effects on lipids and haemostatic factors, *BMJ* 319:1523-1528, 1999.
41. Stewart SH, Mainous AG, Gilbert G: Relation between alcohol consumption and C-reactive protein levels in the adult US population, *J Am Board Fam Pract* 15:437-442, 2002.
42. Gaziano JM, Hennekens CH, Godfried SL, et al: Type of alcoholic beverage and risk of myocardial infarction, *Am J Cardiol* 83:52-57, 1999.
43. Rifici VA, Stephan EM, Schneider SH, et al: Red wine inhibits the cell-mediated oxidation of LDL and HDL, *J Am Coll Nutr* 18:137-143, 1999.
44. Burns J, Crozier A, Lean ME: Alcohol consumption and mortality: is wine different from other alcoholic beverages? *Nutr Metab Cardiovasc Dis* 11:249-258, 2001.
45. Rotondo S, Di Castelnuovo A, de Gaetano G: The relationship between wine consumption and cardiovascular risk: from epidemiological evidence to biological plausibility, *Ital Heart J* 2:1-8, 2001.
46. Criqui MH: Do known cardiovascular risk factors mediate the effect of alcohol on cardiovascular disease? *Novartis Found Symp* 216:159-167, 1998; discussion, 167-172.
47. Mosca L, Grundy SM, Judelson D, et al: Guide to preventive cardiology for women: AHA/ACC Scientific Statement: Consensus Panel Statement, *Circulation* 99:2480-2484, 1999.
48. Stein JH, Keevil JG, Wiebe DA, et al: Purple grape juice improves endothelial function and reduces the susceptibility of LDL cholesterol to oxidation in patients with coronary artery disease, *Circulation* 100:1050-1055, 1999.
49. Wilson E: Young women and tobacco: hope for tomorrow, First International Conference on Women, Heart Disease and Stroke: Science and Policy in Action, May 7-10, 2000, Victoria, British Columbia, Canada. Available at: http://www.medscape.com/viewarticle/424901. Accessed April 2004.
50. White AR, Rampes H, Ernst E: Acupuncture for smoking cessation, *Cochrane Database Syst Rev* (2):CD000009, 2002.
51. Abbot NC, Stead LF, White AR, et al: Hypnotherapy for smoking cessation, *Cochrane Database Syst Rev* (2):CD001008, 2002.
52. Surveillance for five health risks among older adults: United States 1993-1997, *MMWR Morbid Mortal Wkly Rep* 48:89-130, 1999.
53. Stamler J: Epidemiologic findings on body mass and blood pressure in adults, *Ann Epidemiol* 1:347-362, 1991.
54. Rashid S, Uffelman KD, Lewis GF: The mechanism of HDL lowering in hypertriglyceridemic, insulin-resistant states, *J Diabetes Complications* 16:24-28, 2002.
55. Carmena R, Ascaso JF, Real JT: Impact of obesity in primary hyperlipidemias, *Nutr Metab Cardiovasc Dis* 11:354-359, 2001.
56. Gordon T, Ernst N, Fisher M, et al: Alcohol and high-density lipoprotein cholesterol, *Circulation* 64(3 pt 2):III63-III67, 1981.
57. Taddei S, Ghiadoni L, Virdis A, et al: Mechanisms of endothelial dysfunction: clinical significance and preventive non-pharmacological therapeutic strategies. *Curr Pharm Des* 9:2385-2402, 2003.
58. Manson JE, Hu FB, Rich-Edwards JW, et al: A prospective study of walking compared with vigorous exercise in the prevention of coronary heart disease in women, *N Engl J Med* 341:650-658, 1999.
59. Piepho RW: The pharmacokinetics and pharmacodynamics of agents proven to raise high-density lipoprotein cholesterol, *Am J Cardiol* 86(12A):35L-40L, 2000.

60. Crouse JR III: New developments in the use of niacin for treatment of hyperlipidemia: new considerations in the use of an old drug, *Coron Artery Dis* 7:321-326, 1996.
61. Expert Panel on Detection, Evaluation, and Treatment of High Blood Cholesterol in Adults: 2001 Executive summary of the third report of the National Cholesterol Education Program (NCEP) Expert Panel on Detection, Evaluation, and Treatment of High Blood Cholesterol in Adults (Adult Treatment Panel III), *JAMA* 285:2486, May 16, 2001. Available in its entirety at: hin.nhlbi.nih.gov/projects/slpprojectlayout4.asp?p=20. Accessed April 2004.
62. Brown BG, Zhao XQ, Chait A, et al: Simvastatin and niacin, antioxidant vitamins, or the combination for the prevention of coronary disease, *N Engl J Med* 345:1583-92, 2001.
63. Touyz RM: Role of magnesium in the pathogenesis of hypertension, *Mol Aspects Med* 24:107-136, 2003.
64. Chakraborti S, Chakraborti T, Mandal M, et al: Protective role of magnesium in cardiovascular diseases: a review, *Mol Cell Biochem* 238:163-179, 2002.
65. Fox CH, Mahoney MC, Ramsoomair D, et al: Magnesium deficiency in African-Americans: does it contribute to increased cardiovascular risk factors? *J Natl Med Assoc* 95:257-262, 2003.
66. Jee SH, Miller ER III, Guallar E, et al: The effect of magnesium supplementation on blood pressure: a meta-analysis of randomized clinical trials, *Am J Hypertens* 15:691-696, 2002.
67. Ascherio A, Rimm EB, Hernan MA, et al: Relation of consumption of vitamin E, vitamin C, and carotenoids to risk for stroke among men in the United States, *Ann Intern Med* 130:963-970, 1999.
68. Lu WL, Zhang Q, Lee HS, et al: Total coenzyme Q10 concentrations in Asian men following multiple oral 50-mg doses administered as coenzyme Q10 sustained release tablets or regular tablets, *Biol Pharm Bull* 26:52-55, 2003.
69. Crane FL: Biochemical functions of coenzyme Q10, *J Am Coll Nutr* 20:591-598, 2001.
70. Singh RB, Neki NS, Kartikey K, et al: Effect of coenzyme Q10 on risk of atherosclerosis in patients with recent myocardial infarction, *Mol Cell Biochem* 246:75-82, 2003.
71. Tran MT, Mitchell TM, Kennedy DT, et al: Role of coenzyme Q10 in chronic heart failure, angina, and hypertension, *Pharmacotherapy* 21:797-806, 2001.
72. Engelsen J, Nielsen JD, Hansen KF: Effect of coenzyme Q10 and Ginkgo biloba on warfarin dosage in patients on long-term warfarin treatment. A randomized, double-blind, placebo-controlled cross-over trial, *Ugeskr Laeger* 165:1868-1871, 2003.
73. Shults CW, Oakes D, Kieburtz K, et al: Effects of coenzyme Q10 in early Parkinson disease: evidence of slowing of the functional decline, *Arch Neurol* 59:1541-1545, 2002.
74. Evangeliou A, Vlassopoulos D: Carnitine metabolism and deficit: when is supplementation necessary? *Curr Pharm Biotechnol* 4:211-299, 2003.
75. Carvajal K, Moreno-Sanchez R: Heart metabolic disturbances in cardiovascular diseases, *Arch Med Res* 34:89-99, 2003.
76. Vescovo G, Ravara B, Gobbo V, et al: L-carnitine: a potential treatment for blocking apoptosis and preventing skeletal muscle myopathy in heart failure, *Am J Physiol Cell Physiol* 283:C802-C810, 2002.
77. Fugh-Berman A: Herbs and dietary supplements in the prevention and treatment of cardiovascular disease, *Prev Cardiol* 3(Winter):24-32, 2000.
78. Witte KK, Clark AL, Cleland JG: Chronic heart failure and micronutrients, *J Am Coll Cardiol* 37:1765-1774, 2001.
79. Dutta A, Dutta SK: Vitamin E and its role in the prevention of atherosclerosis and carcinogenesis: a review, *J Am Coll Nutr* 22:258-268, 2003.
80. Stampfer MJ, Hennekens CH, Manson JE, et al: Vitamin E consumption and the risk of coronary disease in women, *N Engl J Med* 328:1444-1449, 1993.
81. Rimm EB, Stampfer MJ, Ascherio A, et al: Vitamin E consumption and the risk of coronary heart disease in men, *N Engl J Med* 328:1450-1456, 1993.
82. Meagher EA: Treatment of atherosclerosis in the new millennium: is there a role for vitamin E? *Prev Cardiol* 6(Spring):85-90, 2003.
83. Roychoudhury P, Schwartz K: Antioxidant vitamins do not prevent cardiovascular disease, *J Fam Pract* 52:751-752, 2003.
84. Rattazzi M, Puato M, Faggin E, et al: C-reactive protein and interleukin-6 in vascular disease: culprits or passive bystanders? *J Hypertens* 21:1787-1803, 2001.

85. Ridker PM: High-sensitivity C-reactive protein and cardiovascular risk: rationale for screening and primary prevention, *Am J Cardiol* 92:17K-22K, 2003.
86. Clifton PM: Diet and C-reactive protein, *Curr Atheroscler Rep* 5:431-436, 2003.
87. Esposito K, Pontillo A, Di Palo C, et al: Effect of weight loss and lifestyle changes on vascular inflammatory markers in obese women: a randomized trial, *JAMA* 289:1799-1804, 2003.
88. Takeda T, Hoshida S, Nishino M, et al: Relationship between effects of statins, aspirin and angiotensin II modulators on high-sensitive C-reactive protein levels, *Atherosclerosis* 169:155-158, 2003.
89. Graham IM, Daly LE, Refsum HM, et al: Plasma homocysteine as a risk factor for vascular disease: the European concerted action project, *JAMA* 277:1775-1781, 1997.
90. Ali A, Mehra MR: Modulatory impact of cardiac rehabilitation on hyperhomocysteinemia in patients with coronary artery disease and "normal" lipid levels, *Am J Cardiol* 82:1543-1545, 1998.
91. Yeromenko Y, Lavie L: Homocysteine and cardiovascular risk in patients with diabetes mellitus, *Nutr Metab Cardiovasc Dis* 11:108-116, 2001.
92. Alexander JK: Obesity and coronary heart disease, *Am J Med Sci* 321:215-224, 2001.
93. Fallest-Strobl PC, Koch DD, Stein JH, et al: Homocysteine: a new risk factor for atherosclerosis, *Am Fam Phys* 56:1607-1612, 1997.
94. Ackermann RT, Mulrow CD, Ramirez G, et al: Garlic shows promise for improving some cardiovascular risk factors, *Arch Intern Med* 161:813-824, 2001.
95. Agency for Healthcare Research and Quality: *Garlic: effects on cardiovascular risks and disease, protective effects against cancer, and clinical adverse effects. Evidence Report/Technology Assessment no. 20.* Available at: www.ahrq.gov (posted October 2000). Accessed April 2004.
96. Legnani C, Frascaro M, Guazzaloca G, et al: Effects of a dried garlic preparation on fibrinolysis and platelet aggregation in healthy subjects, *Arzneimittelforschung* 43:119-122, 1993.
97. Lawson LD, Ransom DK, Hughes BG: Inhibition of whole blood platelet-aggregation by compounds in garlic clove extracts and commercial garlic products, *Thromb Res* 65:141-156, 1992.
98. Ali M, Thomson M: Consumption of a garlic clove a day could be beneficial in preventing thrombosis, *Prostaglandins Leukot Essent Fatty Acids* 53:211-212, 1995.
99. Ali M, Bordia T, Mustafa T: Effect of raw versus boiled aqueous extract of garlic and onion on platelet aggregation, *Prostaglandins Leukot Essent Fatty Acids* 60:43-47, 1999.
100. Koscielny J, Klussendorf D, Latza R, et al: The antiatherosclerotic effect of *Allium sativum*, *Atherosclerosis* 144:237-249, 1999.
100a. Low Dog T: Botanical medicine and cardiovascular disease. In Stein RA, Oz MC, editors: *Contemporary and alternative cardiovascular medicine*; Totowa, NJ, 2004, Humana Press.
101. Lawson LD, Wang ZJ, Papadimitriou D: Allicin release under simulated gastrointestinal conditions from garlic powder tablets employed in clinical trials on serum cholesterol, *Planta Med* 67:13-18, 2001.
102. Burnham BE: Garlic as a possible risk for postoperative bleeding, *Plast Reconstr Surg* 95:213, 1995.
103. German K, Kumar U, Blackford HN: Garlic and the risk of TURP bleeding, *Br J Urol* 76:518, 1995.
104. Rose KD, Croissant PD, Parliament CF, et al: Spontaneous spinal epidural hematoma with associated platelet dysfunction from excessive garlic consumption: a case report, *Neurosurgery* 26:880-882, 1990.
105. Vaes LP, Chyka PA: Interactions of warfarin with garlic, ginger, ginkgo, or ginseng: nature of the evidence, *Ann Pharmacother* 34:1478-1482, 2000.
106. Hale T: *Medications and mothers' milk,* Amarillo, Texas, 1999, Pharmasoft Medical Publishing, p 79.
107. Mennella JA, Beauchamp GK: The effects of repeated exposure to garlic-flavored milk on the nursling's behavior, *Pediatr Res* 34:805-808, 1993.
108. Nityanand S, Srivastava JS, Asthana OP: Clinical trials with gugulipid—a new hypolipidemic agent, *J Assoc Phys India* 37:323-338, 1989.
109. Szapary PO, Wolfe ML, Bloedon LT, et al: Guggulipid for the treatment of hypercholesterolemia: a randomized controlled trial, *JAMA* 290:765-772, 2003.
110. McGuffin M, Hobbs C, Upton R, et al: *American Herbal Products Association's Botanical Safety Handbook,* Boca Raton, Florida, 1997, CRC Press.

111. Dalvi SS, Nayak VK, Pohujani SM, et al: Effect of gugulipid on bioavailability of diltiazem and propanolol, *J Assoc Phys Ind* 42:454-455, 1994.
112. Gebhardt R: Multiple inhibitory effects of garlic extracts on cholesterol biosynthesis in hepatocytes, *Lipids* 28:613-619, 1993.
113. Kirchhoff R, Beckers CH, Kirchhoff GM, et al: Increase in choleresis by means of artichoke extract: results of a randomized placebo-controlled double-blind study, *Phytomedicine* 1:107-115, 1994.
114. Pittler MH, Ernst E: Artichoke leaf extract for serum cholesterol reduction, *Perfusion* 11:338-340, 1998.
115. Englisch W, Beckers C, Unkauf M, et al: Efficacy of artichoke dry extract in patients with hyperlipoproteinemia, *Arzneimittelforschung* 50:260-265, 2000.
116. Stuart MD: *Chinese Materia Medica—vegetable kingdom,* Taipei, Republic of China, 1979, Southern Materials Center.
117. McCarthy M: FDA bans red yeast rice product, *Lancet* 351:1637, 1998.
118. Heber D, Yip I, Ashley JM, et al: Cholesterol-lowering effects of a proprietary Chinese red-yeast-rice dietary supplement, *Am J Clin Nutr* 69:231-236, 1999.
119. Bonovich, K, Colfer H, Davidson M, et al: A multi-center, self-controlled study of cholestin in subjects with elevated cholesterol. American Heart Association, 39th Annual Conference on Cardiovascular Disease Epidemiology and Prevention, Orlando, Fla, March 1999.
120. Qin S, Zhang W, Qi P, et al: Elderly patients with primary hyperlipidemia benefited from treatment with a *Monacus purpureus* rice preparation: a placebo-controlled, double-blind clinical trial. American Heart Association, 39th Annual Conference on Cardiovascular Disease Epidemiology and Prevention, Orlando, Fla, March 1999.
121. Perreault S, Hamilton VH, Lavoie F, et al: Treating hyperlipidemia for the primary prevention of coronary disease: are higher doses of lovostatin cost-effective? *Arch Intern Med* 158:375-381, 1998.
122. Cook NC, Samman S: Flavonoids—chemistry, metabolism, cardioprotective effects, and dietary sources. *J Nutr Biochem* 7:66-76, 1996.
123. Manach C, Regerat F, Texier O, et al: Bioavailability, metabolism and physiological impact of 4-oxo-flavonoids, *Nutr Res* 16:517-544, 1996.
124. Aviram M, Fuhrman B: Polyphenolic flavonoids inhibit macrophage-mediated oxidation of LDL and attenuate atherogenesis, *Atherosclerosis* 137:S45-S50, 1998.
125. Xia J, Allenbrand B, Sun GY: Dietary supplementation of grape polyphenols and chronic ethanol administration on LDL oxidation and platelet function in rats, *Life Sci* 63:383-390, 1998.
126. Fuhrman B, Buch S, Vaya J, et al: Licorice extract and its major polyphenol glabridin protect low-density lipoprotein against lipid peroxidation: in vitro and ex vivo studies in humans and in atherosclerotic apolipoprotein E–deficient mice, *Am J Clin Nutr* 66:267-275, 1977.
127. Pittler MH, Schmidt K, Ernst E: Hawthorn extract for treating chronic heart failure: meta-analysis of randomized trials, *Am J Med* 114:665-674, 2003.
128. *Monographs on the medicinal uses of plant drugs,* Exeter, UK, 1997, European Scientific Cooperative on Phytotherapy.
129. Blumenthal M, Busse W, Goldberg A, et al, editors: *The complete German Commission E monographs: therapeutic guide to herbal medicines.* Boston, 1998, Integrative Medicine Communications.
130. Tankanow R, Tamer HR, Streetman DS, et al: Interaction study between digoxin and a preparation of hawthorn *(Crataegus oxyacantha),* *J Clin Pharmacol* 43:637-642, 2003.
131. Bunker SJ, Colquhoun DM, Esler MD, et al: "Stress" and coronary heart disease: psychosocial risk factors, *Med J Aust* 178:272-276, 2003.
132. Joynt KE, Whellan DJ, O'Connor CM: Depression and cardiovascular disease: mechanisms of interaction, *Biol Psychiatr* 54:248-261, 2003.
133. Glaser R, Robles TF, Sheridan J, et al: Mild depressive symptoms are associated with amplified and prolonged inflammatory responses after influenza virus vaccination in older adults, *Arch Gen Psychiatr* 60:1009-1014, 2003.
134. Suarez EC: Joint effect of hostility and severity of depressive symptoms on plasma interleukin-6 concentration, *Psychosom Med* 65:523-527, 2003.
135. Yan LL, Liu K, Matthews KA, et al: Psychosocial factors and risk of hypertension: the Coronary Artery Risk Development in Young Adults (CARDIA) study, *JAMA* 290:2138-2148, 2003.

CHAPTER

15

Breast Cancer

Breast cancer ranks as the leading cause of new cancers in women, accounting for approximately 31% of all cancers in women, compared with about 13% associated with lung and bronchus cancers.[1] In 2001, more than 192,000 new cases of breast cancer were diagnosed in American women. In terms of cancer mortality, breast cancer is the No. 2 cause of cancer deaths among women, comprising about 15% of all cancer deaths, second only to lung and bronchus cancers. Despite the overall decline in breast cancer mortality over the past decade, it is estimated that more than 40,000 deaths were attributed to the disease in 2003.

BREAST CANCER RISK

Women often hear that they have a 1 in 8 chance of developing breast cancer. This statement is based on statistics from the National Cancer Institute. If current rates stay constant, a female baby born today has a 1 in 8 chance of having breast cancer during her lifetime.[2] These statistics are broken down by age incidence in Table 15-1.

These probabilities are based on population averages. An individual woman's risk of breast cancer may be higher or lower depending on a variety of factors, including family history, genetic factors, reproductive history (age at menarche, age at first pregnancy, number of pregnancies, breastfeeding), the presence of certain types and features of benign breast disease, and other factors that are not yet fully understood. Non-Hispanic white, Hawaiian, and black women have the highest level of breast cancer risk. Some of the lowest levels of risk are found among Korean and Vietnamese women.[3]

The incidence of breast cancer has been increasing steadily since 1940, with global breast cancer rates increasing at a rate of approximately 2% per year. Several theories (explained below) have been proposed to explain this trend. Table 15-2 shows statistics for the various risk factors.

Genetic Predisposition

The risk for women with a first-degree relative (mother, sister, daughter) who has had breast cancer is 1.4 to 2.8 times greater than that of women with no such family history.[4]

Table **15-1**

Chances of developing breast cancer by age group

AGE GROUP (YR)	INCIDENCE OF BREAST CANCER
30–40	1 in 252
40–50	1 in 68
50–60	1 in 35
60–70	1 in 27
Ever	1 in 8

Gene mutations such as *BRCA1, BRCA2,* and *p53* have been linked to increased breast cancer risk. However, only 10% to 15% of all breast cancer cases appear to be genetically linked.

Dietary Factors

In 1997, the American Institute for Cancer Research and the World Cancer Research Fund concluded that adult diets high in polyunsaturated or monounsaturated fat may have no relationship to breast cancer risk, independent of any contribution to total fat intake, but diets high in saturated fat may increase the risk of breast cancer.[5] In a 2003 report

Table **15-2**

Risk factors for breast cancer*

RISK FACTOR	RELATIVE RISK
Family history of breast cancer	
One relative	1.4 to 2.8
Two relatives	4.2 to 6.8
Nulliparity	1.5 to 1.9
First child born after age 30	1.9
First menstrual period before age 12	1.2 to 1.3
Last menstrual period after age 55	1.5 to 2.0
Atypical hyperplasia on previous biopsy	2.2 to 5.0
Obesity	1.2
Postmenopausal estrogen replacement therapy	1.2 to 2.1
Alcohol use	
One drink per day	1.4
Two drinks per day	1.7
Three drinks per day	2.0

*Many women in whom breast cancer develops do not have any risk factor, other than age.

published in the *Journal of the National Cancer Institute*, researchers found that intake of animal fat, mainly from red meat and high-fat dairy foods, during the premenopausal years is associated with an increased risk of breast cancer.[6] Postmenopausal obesity and excessive alcohol consumption also appear to increase a woman's risk of breast cancer. A more detailed discussion of diet is presented later in this chapter.

Environmental Factors

Some researchers believe that prolonged exposure to pesticides, chlorinated solvents, ionizing radiation, and polychlorinated biphenyls (PCBs) contributes to the increased incidence of breast cancer.[7] Although evidence implicates organochlorine pesticide residues, this area is difficult to accurately assess and systematically review.[8]

Early Detection

Mammography has dramatically increased the clinician's ability to detect breast cancer. Some researchers argue that the incidence of breast cancer has not increased as dramatically as the numbers suggest but that this "increase" is related to increased rates of early detection. These numbers may reflect, in part, increased access and use of mammograms and the education of women in the performance of breast self-examination. However, increased rates of detection on mammography cannot account for all the long-term increase reported in breast cancer rates.[9]

Lifestyle Factors

Many women have delayed childbearing to a later age or have chosen not to have children, resulting in increased lifetime exposure to unopposed estrogen stimulation. Early age at the time of first pregnancy appears to be strongly protective against breast cancer. Some evidence suggests that late pregnancy actually promotes development of the disease. Breastfeeding also offers a protective effect. The longer a woman breastfeeds and the more babies she nurses, the lower her risk of breast cancer.[10] The growing trend toward later childbearing and the use of infant formulas may contribute to the increased incidence of breast cancer among women in industrialized nations.

CONVENTIONAL THERAPY

Conventional therapy remains the cornerstone of breast cancer treatment. Surgery, radiation, chemotherapy, hormonal therapy, or combinations of these treatments are used, depending on the size and stage of the cancer and the menopausal status, age, and overall health of the woman. Although it is beyond the scope of this chapter to adequately discuss the options for treatment now being offered, it is important to stress the advances being made in the field. New breast-imaging technology is improving the rates of early diagnosis, newer medications are offering a broader array of therapies, and the field of genomics offers the promise of understanding cancer biology and creating better targets for effective, less toxic treatments.

INTEGRATIVE MEDICINE

Several published reports indicate that women often turn to complementary and alternative medicine (CAM) after receiving the diagnosis of breast cancer (see Chapter 1). A study of predominantly non-Hispanic white women with breast cancer revealed that 64% reported regular use of vitamins and minerals and that 33% regularly used antioxidants, herbs, and health foods. Forty-nine percent of all participants regularly used prayer and spiritual healing, followed by support groups (37%) and humor or laughter therapy (21%). Approximately 27% of all participants used massage at least once after the diagnosis.[11] Traditional and ethnic medicine therapies were rarely used.

A survey of the types and prevalence of alternative therapies used by Latino, Chinese, black, and white women with breast cancer revealed that 48% had used at least one type of alternative therapy and approximately 33% had used two or more types after receiving the diagnosis of breast cancer but only 50% discussed this with their physicians. The most popular interventions were dietary therapies (27%), spiritual healing (24%), specialized diets (20%), physical methods (massage and acupuncture) (14%), herbal remedies (13%), psychological methods (9%), and megavitamins (8%). Black women were most likely to use a spiritual approach (36%), and Chinese women were most likely to use herbal remedies (22%). Women who used CAM tended to be younger and better educated, to have more private insurance, and a later stage of cancer at the time of diagnosis. More than 90% said they found alternative therapies helpful and, with the exception of homeopathy, would recommend these therapies to their friends.[12]

As these surveys suggest, a significant number of women with breast cancer reach out for CAM therapies during the course of treatment, primarily as a supplement to standard medical methods and as a strategy for avoiding passivity and feelings of hopelessness.[13] The following is a description of some of the popular remedies currently being recommended for the treatment or prevention of breast cancer.

Diet and Nutrition

High intakes of carotenoids have been associated with a lower risk of breast cancer in several epidemiologic studies. Dietary intake of vitamins A, C, and E; specific carotenoids; and fruits and vegetables were assessed in 83,234 women participating in the Nurses' Health Study. Consumption of five or more servings of fruits and vegetables per day was associated with a modestly lower risk of premenopausal breast cancer in the cohort as a whole with stronger risk reduction among those with a family history of breast cancer and alcohol consumption.[14] A study of women in Shanghai failed to reveal a relationship between breast cancer and total vegetable intake, but it did show declining risk with greater consumption of dark yellow-orange or green vegetables and white turnips. An inverse relationship was found between total fruit intake and breast cancer risk.[15]

A Canadian cohort study of 56,837 women showed that women who consumed high amounts of fiber had a 30% reduction in breast cancer risk compared with those who consumed low amounts of dietary fiber.[16]

Research suggests that it is not so much the amount of fat in the adult diet but, rather, the *type* of fat. The preponderance of evidence indicates that a high consumption of animal fat in the premenopausal years increases the risk of breast cancer. Common sense dictates that women should focus on a diet rich in fruits, vegetables, whole grains, low-fat dairy products, fish, and poultry several times a week and limit consumption of red meat to several times per month. Emphasis should be placed on monounsaturated and polyunsaturated fats, with generous use of olive oil. Although many debate the role of xenoestrogens in the diet, it seems wise to limit exposure to them through the consumption of organically grown foods and the consumption of fewer foods stored in plastic.

Phytoestrogens. Phytoestrogens, natural plant substances, are broken down into four main classes: phenolic, steroidal, saponin, and terpenoid. Phenolic phytoestrogens, found in the majority of vegetables, fruits, and some grains, are the most heavily researched group. Phenolic phytoestrogens can be divided into seven subfamilies: isoflavones, coumestans, flavones, flavonols, flavonones, lignans, and chalcones. Phytoestrogens exert both estrogenic and antiestrogenic effects depending on their concentration in the diet, levels of endogenous estrogens, and individual characteristics of the consumer, such as gender and menopausal status. Because of this dual action the use of phytoestrogens in the prevention of breast cancer and the safety of these substances in women with breast cancer remain subjects of debate among both alternative medicine practitioners and conventional researchers.

Phytoestrogens in soybeans inhibit breast cancer cell proliferation in vitro and breast cancer development in animal models.[17] It is hypothesized that phytoestrogens reduce the risk of breast cancer because their estrogenic activity is relatively weak compared with endogenous estrogens.[18] By binding to estrogen receptors in the premenopausal woman, phytoestrogens "turn down" estrogen production through negative feedback at the level of the hypothalamus and pituitary gland. In other words, when endogenous estrogen levels are high, phytoestrogens may have an antiestrogenic activity by preventing estrogen from binding to the estrogen receptor through competitive inhibition.

Other researchers have postulated that the anticarcinogenic effect of isoflavones is due to modulation of estrogen metabolism away from the production of potentially carcinogenic metabolites: 16α-(OH) estrone, 4-(OH) estrone, and 4-(OH) estradiol.[19] Genistein, an isoflavone present in many plants including soy and red clover, has been shown to inhibit a liver enzyme in rats that catalyzes the conversion of catechol estrogens to their electrophilic quinines. These compounds may be responsible for the genotoxicity of 4-hydroxylated estrogens.[20]

Human studies yield conflicting results with regard to shifting estrogen metabolism. A randomized crossover study of 18 postmenopausal women showed that daily consumption of 65 to 132 mg/day of isoflavones decreased the ratio of genotoxic to total estrogens.[21] Premenopausal Japanese women consuming a soy milk–supplemented diet for 3 consecutive months demonstrated a decrease in serum estrone and estradiol levels compared with those in the control diet group, although the difference was not statistically significant.[22] Another study failed to show any significant change in the duration of menstrual cycles, serum concentrations of sex hormones, or urinary estrogen-metabolite ratio among premenopausal women who supplemented their diets for 2 months with approximately 40 mg total isoflavones.[23] This daily dose of isoflavones is lower than the positive trial and may not have been sufficient. If isoflavones do shift urinary estrogen/metabolite ratios, the optimal dose and age for dietary intake remain to be determined.

An estrogen-independent mechanism may also account for some of the purported cancer-preventive effects of phytoestrogens. Genistein has been shown to reduce tyrosine kinase and inhibit angiogenesis.[24] Rats exposed to a carcinogen had a 40% lower rate of cancer when they were simultaneously given genistein.[25] The findings of in vitro and animal studies suggest that the inhibitory action of genistein on breast cancer cells is complex and only partially mediated by the alteration of estrogen receptor–dependent pathways.

Although preliminary data are intriguing, a recent review of the literature failed to support the hypothesis that a soy-rich diet in adult women is protective against the development of breast cancer, although immigrant and epidemiologic studies do suggest that soy is somewhat protective if consumed in early childhood and adolescence.[26] As of early 2003, 13 studies had been conducted to assess the direct relationship between individual adult dietary intake of soy products and the risk of breast cancer. Four of the 13 studies were prospective, and all failed to demonstrate statistically significant reductions in breast cancer. Four studies involved assessment of urinary isoflavone excretion, although three were case-control studies in which excretion was measured after breast cancer occurrence, thus seriously limiting causal interpretation of the results. The only prospective study involving urinary measurements before the occurrence of breast cancer showed a nonsignificant breast cancer risk reduction associated with high urinary excretion of isoflavones.[27] Three studies measured enterolactone (lignan) levels; two case-control studies showed a preventive effect with regard to breast cancer, but the only prospective study did not.[27] In a prospective population-based cohort study in Japan, frequent consumption of miso soup and isoflavones was associated with a reduced risk of breast cancer. The associations did not change substantially after adjustment for potential confounders, including reproductive and family history, smoking, and other dietary factors.[28] Population studies of the relationships between phytoestrogens and cancer are difficult to interpret because of the number of confounding factors. A great deal of complexity and diversity exists among phytoestrogens, making these compounds a challenge for researchers, as in vitro and in vivo studies often yield conflicting results. Specific cellular responses depend on the type of phytoestrogen, the concentration of estrogen receptors, co-activators, co-repressors, and duration of exposure. As one author states, "Overall, it is naïve to assume that exposure to these compounds is always good; inappropriate or excessive exposure may be detrimental."[29]

In addition to prevention, many women want to know if phytoestrogens are safe if they have a history of breast cancer. One review found that adult consumption of soy does not appear to affect the risk of breast cancer; nor does soy consumption affect the survival of breast cancer patients.[30] Based on in vitro and animal studies, women who enjoy eating soy and other phytoestrogen-rich foods should not be discouraged from consuming them in moderation after being treated for breast cancer. After this review was published, however, one in vitro study[31] and one animal study[32] demonstrated that genistein inhibits the antiproliferative effect of tamoxifen and increased the expression of estrogen-responsive genes, raising questions about isoflavone use by women undergoing treatment with this antiestrogen drug.

In summary, it appears that phytoestrogen/soy consumption early in life has a protective effect against breast cancer but that consumption later in life may not. Plant-based diets, however, offer many health benefits and should be encouraged for women of all ages.

Women with a history of breast cancer should not be concerned about the consumption of soy- and phytoestrogen-rich foods but should probably defer taking supplements containing isolated isoflavones.

Indole-3-carbinol (I3C). A large body of evidence suggests that generous consumption of fruits and vegetables offers protection against numerous cancers. One group of vegetables, the cruciferous variety, may be particularly protective against breast cancer. I3C is found in high concentrations in *Brassica* vegetables such as broccoli, cauliflower, Brussels sprouts, kale, collards, bok choy, and cabbage. Research increasingly suggests that dietary I3C prevents the development of estrogen-enhanced cancers of the breast, endometrium, and cervix. I3C inhibits the growth of human cancer cells in vitro and possesses anti-carcinogenic activity in vivo.[33] Exposure of various human breast cancer cell lines to I3C induces apoptosis—programmed cell death—of malignant cells.[34] Whereas estrogen increases the growth and survival of tumors, I3C appears to cause growth arrest and increased apoptosis, possibly ameliorating the harmful effects of estrogen.[35]

Researchers are working to more fully explain the mechanism(s) by which I3C may protect against breast cancer. One area being explored is I3C's effect on estrogen metabolism. Estrogens are metabolized via two irreversible competing pathways: 2-hydroxylation and 16-α-hydroxylation. Researchers have demonstrated that 16-α-hydroxylated metabolites have a high affinity for the estrogen receptor and low affinity for sex hormone–binding globulin, and are correlated with an increased incidence of mammary tumors in mice.[36] The 2-hydroxyestrone (2-OHE) metabolite is considered less biologically active and may inhibit angiogenesis.[37] These metabolites have opposing effects on estrogen receptor–positive breast cancer cells, with 16-OHE stimulating proliferation and 2-OHE showing no effect on cell growth.[38]

Estrogen metabolism may be altered by vegetables of the *Brassica* genus as a result of the presence of specific phytochemicals, indole glucosinolates. When these vegetables are cut or chewed, these phytochemicals are degraded by the plant enzyme myrosinase to a variety of indole structures.[39] When broken down in the body, these indoles induce the expression of P-450 enzymes (CY1A1) in hepatic and extrahepatic tissue,[40] inducing greater 2-hydroxyestrone (2HE) production and decreasing the pool of E1 available for conversion to 16-HE. In three small human interventional studies, daily administration of I3C pills (400 mg/day) or broccoli (500 g/day) significantly increased the urinary estrogen 2:16 value.[41]

Interestingly, no hormonal modulatory effect was seen among women with a rare mutant form of the CYP1A1 enzyme who were given oral I3C. This genetic disorder increases breast cancer risk 10-fold. This finding implies that CYP1A1 enzyme manipulation may be an important mechanism of action for I3C.[42]

The data have been inconsistent, however, with regard to the relationship between estrogen metabolites and breast cancer in women. One of the primary limitations is that many studies rely on measurements of estrogen metabolites made after the onset of breast cancer, which may be altered by the disease itself or by treatment.[43] Only two studies collected samples prospectively from women before the onset of cancer. One revealed that breast cancer was 30% less likely to develop in postmenopausal women in the highest tertile of the ratio of urinary 2-OHE to 16-OHE over follow-up periods as long as 19 years.[44] However, the number of breast cancer cases was considered too small (60 premenopausal, 42 postmenopausal) for the findings to be considered significant. The other study showed that the effect of the 2-OHE/16-OHE ratio differed with menopausal status: A low ratio was associated with a high breast cancer risk in premenopausal women but with a moderately decreased risk in postmenopausal women.[45]

Cigarette smoking,[46] physical exercise,[47] a high-protein diet,[48] and consumption of cruciferous vegetables, soy,[20] and omega-3 fatty acids[49,50] increase the ratio of 2-OHE to 16-OHE, whereas a high–saturated fat/low–soluble fiber diet decreases it.[51] Traditional lifelong Asian diets may protect against the development of breast cancer because they are rich in soy products (20% to 60% of daily protein provided by soy) and low in saturated fat.[52] Potential confounders were generally not accounted for in these studies,[43] making definitive conclusions about the true relationship of factors such as the ratio of 2-OHE to 16-OHE and breast cancer risk impossible at this time.

I3C may induce programmed cell death of breast cancer cells via its interaction with Bax, a cytosolic protein involved in the regulation of apoptosis. Thus I3C may be of therapeutic benefit for women with breast cancer by assisting in the regulation of the cell cycle and altering the expression of genes involved in the apoptotic pathway.[53]

The safety of doses up to 400 mg/day is reassuring. In a 4-week dose-ranging study, the only adverse effect noted was a slight increase in the concentration of the liver function enzyme alanine aminotransferase (which remained in the normal range) in 2 of 57 subjects.[45] No subject discontinued participation. Adverse effects noted at higher dosages (800 to 1200 mg/day) included imbalance and tremor.[48]

Preliminary data suggest that I3C supplementation is a promising preventive strategy for breast cancers, making it a prime candidate for research in human clinical trials, specifically among individuals who may be at high risk for breast cancer or with a history of the disease. It also remains a wise practice for women to increase their consumption of vegetables, with a special emphasis on those from the *Brassica* genus.

Flax. Although lignans are present in many plant foods, flax is by far the most significant source. One small study showed that daily consumption of 10 g of ground flax significantly increased the urinary 2:16 OHE-1 ratio in premenopausal women.[50] The significance of this urinary-estrogen ratio, as mentioned in previous sections of this chapter, in the development of estrogen-driven cancers remains a matter of controversy.

Dietary supplements

CoQ10. CoQ10, an antioxidant, was first isolated in 1957 from the mitochondria of beef heart and given the name ubiquinone. CoQ10 is an electron and proton carrier that assists in the production of energy (ATP) in the inner mitochondrial membrane.[54] Karl Folkers first investigated CoQ10 as a treatment for cancer in the early 1970s. As an adjuvant cancer therapy, CoQ10 is thought to protect normal tissues from free-radical damage caused by conventional cancer treatment. CoQ10 has been shown to increase phagocytosis and serum immunoglobulin G levels[55] while increasing resistance to bacterial, viral, and protozoal infections.[56] Some studies demonstrate that patients with cancer have low levels of CoQ10.[57]

The medical literature contains more than 125 references to the relationship between CoQ10 and cancer, 25 involve human studies and case reports. Clinical trials addressing survival of women with breast cancer showed prolonged survival among groups receiving CoQ10; however, the studies suffered from numerous methodologic flaws (no information on disease stage, no reporting on conventional therapies used, etc.).[58]

Four studies of disease regression all showed a positive effect. In one clinical series of 32 women with breast cancer and lymph node involvement, all women were treated with conventional therapy and then a 6-month nutritional program including 90 mg of CoQ10, 32.5 International Units of β-carotene, 2500 International Units of vitamin E, 2850 mg of vitamin C, 387 μg of selenium, 3.5 g of omega-3 fatty acids, and 1.2 g of γ-linolenic acid per day. After 18 months no participants had died, lost weight, or needed analgesics, and all 32 reportedly had stable disease.[59] The study did have its problems: 18 months is not long enough to adequately assess survival in women who underwent conventional therapy, and weight loss and the need for analgesics would only be expected in metastatic disease. Therefore, even though the results look promising, this report cannot be used as proof of efficacy. The authors published an updated report 2 years after the first follow-up.[60] All the patients were alive, without evidence of metastases. Regression of cancer, including the disappearance of residual cancer after surgery in one patient taking 300 mg of CoQ10 per day, was reported in 6 patients. Other reports describe regression of liver metastases and disappearance of malignant pleural effusions.[61]

Survival and disease recurrence outcomes among 90 women with unilateral nonmetastatic breast cancer diagnosed between 1989 and 1998 who had been prescribed megadoses of β-carotene, vitamin C, niacin, selenium, CoQ10, and zinc in addition to standard conventional cancer therapies were compared with matched controls. Controls were matched (2:1) to the vitamin and mineral–treated patients for age at the time of diagnosis, presence of axillary lymph-node metastasis, tumor stage and grade, estrogen-receptor status, year of diagnosis, and prescription of systemic therapy. Median follow-up of surviving patients was 68 months. Breast cancer–specific survival and disease-free survival times were not improved for the vitamin and mineral–treated group over those of the controls.[62]

In conclusion, the available data on CoQ10 as an adjuvant treatment in breast cancer are limited by methodologic flaws and incomplete reporting. However, CoQ10 does not appear to be harmful when used as part of a therapeutic protocol. With larger doses (600 to 1200 mg/day) patients may experience headache, fatigue, and heartburn. Because of the theoretical concern about interaction with warfarin (Coumadin), clotting times should be monitored in patients taking anticoagulant therapy. The dose used in most studies ranged from 90 to 360 mg/day.

Melatonin. Melatonin is a hormone secreted by the pineal gland in a diurnal rhythm, with the highest concentrations produced at night. Tryptophan is converted to serotonin, and serotonin is converted to melatonin. Secretion is stimulated by darkness and inhibited by light. Melatonin is a potent antioxidant, more potent than both glutathione and vitamin E.[63] Because of its highly lipophilic nature, melatonin readily crosses intracellular membranes into the nucleus, where it protects DNA and RNA from damage. Melatonin supplements are readily available in the United States without a prescription and have been widely used to stabilize or readjust sleep patterns, especially jet lag.[64]

Some evidence suggests that the pineal gland plays a role in the development of cancer. Calcification of the pineal gland has been associated with an increased incidence of breast cancer.[65] Serum levels of melatonin normally increase from 20 pg/mL in the morning to 70 pg/mL during sleep. The authors of one study reported that women with estrogen-receptor–positive breast tumors had low melatonin levels in nocturnal plasma but found no such changes in women with estrogen receptor–negative breast cancer.[66] Low serum melatonin levels have been associated with increased levels of reproductive hormones, particularly estradiol, resulting in increased growth and proliferation of hormone-sensitive cells in the breast. Chemically induced mammary tumorigenesis in animals has shown that activation of the pineal gland, with or without administration of melatonin, lengthens the latency and reduces the incidence and growth of tumors, whereas removal of the pineal gland usually has the opposite effect.[67] Melatonin inhibits cell growth and proliferation of estrogen receptor–positive MCF-7 cells in vitro,[68] and may also increase the expression of the *p53* tumor suppressor gene.[69]

Two articles published in 2001 suggest that women who sleep poorly at night or work night shifts are at increased risk for breast cancer. In the first article, data from the Nurses' Health Study were used to evaluate the relationship between rotating night shifts and breast cancer risk. The prospective cohort consisted of 78,562 women monitored for 10 years. The number of years spent working rotating night shifts was associated with a trend toward increased breast cancer. Women who worked 30 or more years of rotating night shifts had a 36% greater risk of breast cancer than women who had never worked rotating night shifts (relative risk 1.36, 95% confidence interval 1.04-1.78).[70] The second study involved breast cancer patients and control subjects who were matched for age and identified with the use of random digital dialing. The investigators wanted to evaluate night exposure to light by examining nine variables related to sleep habits, bedroom lighting, and night shift work. The study showed that women with breast cancer reported more nights per week of nonpeak sleep (2.2 nights; defined as not sleeping between 1 and 2 AM, the period of night when melatonin levels are typically highest) compared with control patients (1.7 nights). Breast cancer patients reported spending more years at jobs requiring at least 1 graveyard shift per week (4.5 years) than did control subjects (3.1 years). When hours of graveyard shift work per week was treated as a categorical variable, a trend toward increased risk with more hours per week was detected: Women who worked at least 5.7 graveyard shift hours per week had a greater than twofold increase in risk of breast cancer (odds ratio 2.3, 95% confidence interval 1.0-3.5). The authors concluded that graveyard shift work and nonpeak sleep reflect exposure to light during the night and that such light exposure may be linked to breast cancer risk.[71]

These studies suggest that the increased risk of breast cancer is, in part, due to a reduction in melatonin, which is caused by nighttime light exposure. Although this idea fits with in vitro and in vivo data indicating a correlation between melatonin levels and breast cancer, these studies are limited by several potentially significant confounders: Is it possible that women who work nights have lifestyle behaviors (other than working at night) that are different from those who work during the day? Information about stress levels, diet, alcohol and tobacco use, menopause status, weight, and other factors would be important to identify and examine.

A phase II study of 14 women with metastatic breast cancer who did not respond to tamoxifen (n = 3) or whose disease progressed after being initially stable (n = 11) evaluated the biologic and clinical effects of concomitant melatonin therapy. Melatonin was given orally at a dosage of 20 mg/day in the evening, every day, 7 days before the reinitiation of tamoxifen. Partial response was achieved in 4 of 14 patients (28.5%; median duration 8 months). The treatment was well tolerated in all cases. Mean serum levels of insulin-like growth factor 1 (a growth factor in breast cancer cells) decreased significantly during treatment. This decline was significantly higher in responders than in patients with stable disease or progression.[72]

In conclusion, given the current state of the science, the anticancer effects of melatonin should be studied in greater depth to clarify and elucidate whether, and when, this supplement should be considered in women with breast cancer, either as an adjuvant treatment (for women taking tamoxifen and/or experiencing progression) or as a preventive agent for certain groups (e.g., women working at night or at high risk). The optimal dose is not known, but is generally higher than the 3 to 5 mg taken for jet lag.

Herbal Treatments

Paclitaxel and related compounds. The taxanes (e.g., paclitaxel and docetaxel) are among the most beneficial drugs currently available for the treatment of breast cancer. Paclitaxel (Taxol) is extracted from the bark of the Pacific yew tree, *Taxus brevifolia*. The Food and Drug Administration approved paclitaxel for the treatment of ovarian cancer on December 29, 1992, and the treatment of breast cancer on April 15, 1994. The rate-limiting step for this therapy soon became apparent: It takes three or four 100- to 200-year-old yew trees to treat one cancer patient. The question was soon asked: Would it be necessary to sacrifice the Pacific yew forest and ecosystem to treat women with cancer?

Docetaxel (Taxotere) is extracted from the needles of the European yew tree, *T. baccata*, making the sacrifice of trees unnecessary. Other ornamental *Taxus* species have been found to contain anticancer compounds in their needles, making their harvest of economic benefit to growers and nurseries. Organic chemists continue to make headway with synthetic analogues.

The development of these drugs raises two important points: First, important and potentially lifesaving medicines remain to be found in the plant kingdom. Second, plant conservation is extremely important to ensure healthy ecosystems for the generations that will follow us.

Green tea (Camellia sinensis). Tea is the second most commonly consumed beverage, after water, in the world. Each year about 2.5 million tons of tea are manufactured from the dried leaves and leaf buds of the shrub *C. sinensis*. Black tea is fermented and dried. Green tea is steamed, rolled, and dried. Green tea, which accounts for about 20% of world production, is consumed principally in China and Japan, where it has been used as a beverage and medicine for more than 5000 years.

Although the precise composition of green tea varies with its geographic origin, time of harvest, and manufacturing process, dried tea leaves contain roughly 35% polyphenols, principally flavonols (including catechins), flavonoids, and flavondiols. Data compiled over the last 10 years have provided compelling evidence that these polyphenolic compounds exert protection against cancer. The polyphenolic antioxidant epigallocatechin-3-gallate (EGCG) is thought to be the primary constituent responsible for tea's cancer-protective properties.[73] Tea polyphenols selectively induce phase I and phase II metabolic enzymes that increase the formation and excretion of detoxified metabolites of carcinogens[74] and inhibit the interaction between estrogen and estrogen receptors in estrogen-responsive tumors in vitro.[75] Both black and green tea extracts have been shown to strongly inhibit neoplastic transformation in mouse mammary organ cultures.[76] EGCG inhibits the growth of breast cancer cell lines (MCF-7 and MDA-MB-231) but not that of normal breast epithelial cells in vitro.[77]

Green-tea drinkers in Asia have a significantly reduced risk of breast cancer, even after adjustments for age; specific Asian ethnicity; birthplace; age at menarche, parity, menopausal status, use of menopausal hormones; body size; intake of total calories; smoking, intake of alcohol, coffee, and black tea; family history of breast cancer; physical activity; and intake of soy and dark green vegetables. Although both green-tea and soy intake exerted significant, independent protective effects on breast cancer risk, the benefit of green tea was noted mainly among subjects who were low soy consumers.[78] Green-tea consumption was correlated with decreased recurrence of stage I and II breast cancer ($P < 0.05$ for crude disease-free survival) among 472 Japanese patients with stage I, II, and III disease. In a 7-year follow-up of patients with stage I and II breast cancer, the relative risk of recurrence was 0.564 (95% confidence interval 0.350-0.911) after adjustment for other lifestyle factors. No improvement in prognosis was observed in stage III breast cancer.[79]

It is anticipated that the growing body of basic science will lead to clinical trials assessing the role of green tea in the prevention of cancer. Given the safety of green tea and preliminary evidence of its health-generating properties, it is appropriate to think of this beverage as part of a healthy cancer prevention diet. Tea is low in caffeine compared with coffee. A 170-mL (6-oz) cup of tea contains an average of 34 mg of caffeine, compared with 115 mg in a similarly sized cup of brewed coffee. Decaffeinated teas are available for the caffeine-sensitive individuals and provide comparable levels of antioxidants. Green-tea extracts are also available in capsule form. Red bush tea (*Aspalathus linearis*), from South Africa, is naturally devoid of caffeine and has an antioxidant profile similar to that of green tea. What quantity of tea offers protection is still debated; however, two or three cups a day, together with a nutritious diet, is probably a good idea.

MAKE MINE TEA, PLEASE

The drinking of tea is an ancient tradition dating back 5000 years in China and India. These cultures have revered tea as an aid to good health, a claim that researchers are beginning to explore with increased interest. Investigators are especially interested in the polyphenols, antioxidant compounds, found in tea. Antioxidants are compounds that neutralize free radical molecules. These free radical molecules, which occur naturally in the body, can damage DNA, potentially leading to such ailments as cancer and heart disease. Scientific studies suggest that tea plays a role in maintaining a healthy cardiovascular system and preventing certain cancers. Tea has been shown to reduce the damage resulting from sun exposure and may even decrease the risk of skin cancer when applied topically. And here's one more enticing tidbit, in case you're still not sold on tea: Researchers have found that green tea increases metabolism, especially when consumed before a meal. Maybe it's time to exchange that mug of coffee for a cup of tea!

Ginger (Zingiber officinale). Chemotherapy-induced nausea and vomiting significantly reduces the quality of life and increases fatigue and anxiety. It also drives up the cost of health care delivery. Many herbalists recommend ginger as a treatment for this condition.

Ginger capsules, ginger tea, and ginger ale are often recommended to reduce chemotherapy-induced nausea.[80] Numerous studies have demonstrated the antiemetic effects of dried ginger rhizome in the treatment of hyperemesis gravidarum,[81] motion sickness,[82] and postoperative nausea.[83] The mechanism of action and constituent(s) responsible for the antiemetic activity of ginger are not completely understood. Several components of ginger—6-gingerol, 6-shogaol, and galanolactone—have been shown to exert anti–5-hydroxytryptamine (5-HT [serotonin]) activity in isolated guinea pig ileum. Galanolactone is a competitive antagonist predominantly directed at ileal 5-HT3 receptors.[84] Ginger may increase gastrointestinal motility and reduce feedback from the gastrointestinal tract to the central chemoreceptors.[85]

A randomized, double-blind study of patients experiencing vomiting secondary to chemotherapy with cyclophosphamide found that complete control of nausea was achieved in 62% of patients taking ginger, in 58% of those taking metoclopramide, and in 86% of those taking ondansetron. Complete control of vomiting was achieved in 68% of patients taking ginger, in 64% of those taking metoclopramide, and in 86% of those taking ondansetron. No adverse effects were attributed to ginger.[86]

In a 1987 clinical trial, 41 patients with leukemia were randomly assigned to receive oral ginger or placebo as an adjuvant therapy after the administration of intravenous prochlorperazine (Compazine). A significant reduction in nausea was reported among patients who took ginger compared with those who received placebo. However, only the abstract was published,[87] and efficacy is difficult to assess given the fact that patients were all pretreated with a recognized antiemetic.

In light of the strong historical use of ginger as an antiemetic and the growing body of scientific data supporting its efficacy, a double-blind, placebo-controlled, three-armed randomized clinical trial is being undertaken through the National Institutes of Health to assess the efficacy and safety of two dosage levels (1000 or 2000 mg/day orally) of ginger extract (standardized for 5% gingerols) in patients undergoing chemotherapy (cisplastin or Adriamycin).[88] Such research is needed to more appropriately assess efficacy, optimal dosage, and dosage form.

Ginger is quite safe when used in rational amounts. Concern has been raised regarding the effect of ginger on platelet function. A double-blind, randomized study of eight healthy male volunteers found no change in platelet function after the ingestion of 2 g of dried ginger compared with that seen after placebo.[89] The inhibition of thromboxane synthetase appears to occur only with higher doses; however, this phenomenon could be problematic for patients who are thrombocytopenic.

The antiemetic dosage is generally 250 to 500 mg dried ginger rhizome in capsule form, four times daily. Some people prefer to eat candied ginger, available at Asian grocery stores and health food stores.

Essiac. Essiac, a botanical mixture, has been widely used as a cancer treatment in Canada and the United States for more than 70 years. René Caisse (Essiac is her name spelled backward), a nurse from Ontario, Canada, promoted the original formula for the treatment of cancer after a woman was supposedly cured of breast cancer after taking this remedy, purportedly given to her by an Ojibwa medicine man. The four herbs in the original Essiac mixture are burdock root (*Arctium lappa*), Indian rhubarb (*Rheum palmatum, R. officinale*), sheep sorrel (*Rumex acetosella*), and slippery elm bark (*Ulmus fulva, U. rubra*). Between 1959 and 1978, Caisse worked with an American physician, Charles Brusch, to modify the recipe and promote its medicinal use as a cancer therapy. Four herbs—watercress, blessed thistle, red clover, and kelp—were added to the original recipe; Caisse and Brusch believed these additions potentiated the action of the formula while improving its taste. Flor-Essence (Flora Manufacturing and Distributing Ltd., Burnaby, British Columbia, Canada), purported to be the original eight-herb recipe developed by Caisse and Brusch, is widely available in health food stores. The original four-herb formula is still sold under the name Essiac and is also widely available. Numerous derivative products in the marketplace contain variations of both formulas.

During the 1920s and 1930s, Caisse treated many people with the oral and injectable forms of Essiac. At a public hearing held in March 1939, 49 of Caisse's 387 patients were allowed to testify. The Royal Cancer Commission concluded that of the eight patients with a confirmed diagnosis, two of the four recoveries might have been due to Essiac. Early mouse studies showed "definite and significant changes" in animals treated with Essiac compared with controls. From 1973-1976, Sloan-Kettering conducted animal studies using Essiac prepared by Caisse, with disappointing results. Caisse purportedly refused to divulge the ingredients in the formula to the National Cancer Institute or the Memorial Sloan-Kettering Cancer Center.

In 1978, Resperin Corporation entered into an agreement with Caisse and Brusch to produce and supply Essiac for a clinical trial in terminal cancer patients. In 1982, the Health Protection Branch closed the trial, citing inadequate manufacturing controls of consistency in batches and poor study design. No toxicity was noted during the trial period, but the data were inadequate to draw any conclusions about survival.

The Canadian Bureau of Human Prescription Drugs conducted a retrospective review of Caisse's patients on the basis of summaries provided by physicians who treated these individuals. Information was provided for 86 patients, all of whom had previously undergone conventional treatment. Forty-seven patients demonstrated "no benefit," 17 died, one showed subjective improvement, five had a reduced need for pain medication, four remained stable, and four demonstrated an "objective response"; the remaining eight patient charts could not be evaluated clinically. A follow-up of the eight patients whose disease was stable or who demonstrated an objective response showed that two had died and three had disease progression; in three, disease remained stable.[90]

Both the four- and eight-herb versions are widely used by cancer patients, although no clinical trials have been published in the medical literature at the time of this writing. Annual sales exceed $8 million. A survey conducted by the University of Texas Center for Alternative Medicine Research showed that 75% of 5051 cancer patient participants used Flor-Essence. Most respondents were women, and 22% of patients had breast cancer.[91] Another survey showed that 50% of cancer patients using Flor-Essence expected the herbal tonic to cure their cancers and 60% believed that the preparation would prolong their lives.[92]

The following is a brief summary of the herbs used in the original formulation.

Burdock (Arctium lappa). Burdock has been consumed as a vegetable and used medicinally for centuries. It has been used in Asian medicine to treat colds, coughs, and skin infections; European and American herbalists recommended it for rheumatism, gout, digestive disorders, and skin complaints. Historically, burdock was considered a reliable "blood purifier" and has made its way into formulas for a variety of chronic conditions. Burdock had some reputation, dating back to Hildegard of Bingen, the twelfth-century abbess and herbalist for the treatment of tumorous growths. Burdock root is also a component of the Hoxsey therapy, another controversial cancer treatment.

Contemporary research has been somewhat limited. Burdock has been shown to be protective of the liver in animals exposed to high levels of ethanol,[93] acetaminophen, and carbon tetrachloride.[94] Antioxidant and antiinflammatory activity has been identified.[95] Bactericidal and fungicidal activities have been noted, possibly accounting for the herb's widespread use in the treatment of skin conditions. Two animal studies from the 1960s showed that burdock exerted some antitumor activity[96,97]; however, in the 1970s, the National Cancer Institute and Memorial Sloan-Kettering failed to identify any antitumor effects exerted by burdock root (see previous text).

Rhubarb (Rheum palmatum). Rhubarb root has a long history of medicinal use, especially as a stimulant laxative. Emodin, an anthraquinone derivative in rhubarb, exerts antiproliferative effects in numerous cancer cell lines. It suppresses topoisomerase II activity and the proliferation of various tumor cell lines.[98] In vitro data demonstrate inhibitory activity against several breast cancer cell lines[99] and increased apoptosis in a human lung squamous-cell carcinoma line[100] and human cervical cancer cells.[101] Emodin also possesses antiviral, antimicrobial, immunosuppressive, hepatoprotective, antiinflammatory, and antiulcerogenic activity. Although intriguing, research at this time is basically limited to in vitro and animal data; no clinical trials have been carried out to evaluate the efficacy of rhubarb root against any cancer.

Sorrel (Rumex acetosella). The dried aerial parts of sheep sorrel have historically been used as a diuretic, febrifuge, and for the treatment of skin cancer. The plant contains anthraquinones, including emodin (see earlier mention under "Rhubarb"). Data are limited, although the research on emodin would hold true for sheep sorrel as well as rhubarb. The herb contains oxalates, making it inappropriate for someone with a history of renal oxalate stones.

Slippery elm (Ulmus fulva). Slippery elm has been used historically, and remains popular today, as a means of soothing the throat and gastrointestinal tract. The inner bark has also been used topically to treat skin inflammation. Slippery elm is rich in mucilage, which accounts for its soothing effect on the mucosa. Like many other plants, slippery elm contains β-sitosterol. This plant sterol has been shown to induce apoptosis[102] and to reduce metastasis of breast cancer cells in vitro.[103] Despite the popularity of this plant, no human or animal studies have been conducted to evaluate slippery elm's efficacy for any historical use. On the basis of its constituents, slippery elm is considered quite safe.

Although research on these herbal constituents is interesting, no compelling clinical evidence demonstrates that combinations of these herbs shrink tumors, prolong survival, or improve quality of life. There is no evidence that these herbs should be used as a sole therapy for cancer treatment. Sheep sorrel contains oxalic acid, something to be considered in patients with kidney stones. Rhubarb, an anthraquinone-containing laxative, can cause diarrhea and abdominal cramping. Given the vast number of cancer patients who use Essiac-type products, clinical trials are needed to assess what benefit, if any, Essiac or Flor-Essence provides.

St. John's wort (**Hypericum perforatum**). Many herbalists recommend St. John's wort for women experiencing depression after receiving the diagnosis of breast cancer. The most recent Cochrane review concluded, "There is evidence that extracts of Hypericum are more effective than placebo for the short-term treatment of mild to moderately severe depressive disorders."[104]

The mechanism by which this herb improves mood is not completely understood, nor are the active constituents well identified. (See Chapter 11 for a more detailed discussion of St. John's wort.) Combined with psychotherapy, hypnotherapy, support groups, or any combination of these approaches, St. John's wort may help women cope with the devastating psychologic pressure of dealing with breast cancer and its treatment.

However, questions have been raised regarding the concomitant use of St. John's wort and chemotherapeutic agents. St. John's wort has been shown to interact with irinotecan,[105] a chemotherapy drug used in the treatment of metastatic colorectal cancer, small cell lung cancer, and several other solid tumors. St. John's wort is known to interact with numerous other medications as well.

If St. John's wort is used, it should be discontinued before, or taken after, the completion of any chemotherapy treatment. The typical dose is 900 to 1800 mg/day of a standardized extract or its equivalent.

Astragalus (**Astragalus membranaceus**). Astragalus root has been shown to stimulate the immune system in vivo[106] and inhibit chemotherapy-induced immunosuppression in animals.[7] It is one of the main herbs used in Chinese *fu-zheng* therapy to enhance the immune system during chemotherapy and radiation therapy. (Fu-zheng is a form of traditional Chinese herbalism that literally means "to restore normalcy and balance to the body.") Astragalus is often prescribed in traditional Chinese medicine to those with low vitality, fatigue, weakness, and lack of appetite.[80] Research is lmited primarily to in vitro and animal models, and no rigorous randomized trials are available with which to evaluate the value of astragalus during chemotherapy. However, the herb is quite safe and is consumed regularly as part of the Asian diet: Astragalus root is often cooked in soup. The typical dose is 1000 to 2000 mg/day.

Massage Therapy

Lymphedema, an accumulation of protein-rich fluid, occurs in the arms of women treated for breast cancer when lymphatic drainage is interrupted because of axillary lymph node dissection, axillary radiation, or both. Women with lymphedema complain of heaviness, tightness, or swelling in the affected arm. After tumor involvement, infection, and axillary vein thrombosis have been ruled out, treatment should be directed at improving symptoms and easing discomfort.

Complex decongestive physiotherapy (CDP) is considered by many to be the standard of care. CDP combines compression bandages, manual lymphatic drainage (MLD, a specialized massage technique), exercise, and skin care with extensive patient education.[107] Compression wraps fit over the affected arm and help maintain or reduce the level of swelling. Studies have provided conflicting data regarding the use of MLD. One study showed beneficial effects in reduction of limb volume and dermal thickness with the use of MLD in breast cancer–related lymphedema,[108] whereas another that compared compression bandages, exercise, and skin care with and without MLD revealed no difference between the two groups.[109] MLD does not involve massage of the deep tissue; instead, gentle pressure is used to move fluid away from the affected area. Many licensed massaged therapists are trained in MLD and can teach women how to perform simple manual drainage at home. If a woman chooses to use this therapy, she should inquire about the massage therapist's training and experience.

Women with lymphedema should be instructed in proper skin care and advised to avoid (when possible) and treat promptly (when unavoidable) any cut, scrape, insect bite, skin irritation, or sunburn of the affected arm. Laboratory personnel and health-care providers should avoid medical procedures such as vaccination, blood draws, blood-pressure monitoring, and acupuncture in the arm with lymphedema. Symptoms can be exacerbated by the use of saunas, steam baths, or hot tubs; hot weather; and air travel. Women with lymphedema should be encouraged to maintain a healthy weight and get regular gentle exercise. Yoga or *tai chi* may help improve lymph flow. Swimming is a good choice of exercise because water provides even pressure all over the body.

Massage for well-being.   Many women with breast cancer find massage therapy to be relaxing, tension-relieving, and comforting. Quality of life therapies can be difficult to quantify but should never be overlooked or underestimated for those who are ill. Practitioners who can guide women to qualified massage therapists will most likely be deeply appreciated by their patients (Figure 15-1).

Mind/Body Approaches

Yoga, meditation, hypnosis, biofeedback, guided imagery, music therapy, breathing exercises, and prayer are increasingly being used by cancer centers to help individuals improve their quality of life. Biofeedback and hypnosis can help reduce nausea and pain. Prayer, meditation, and guided imagery may reduce stress and provide comfort. Several small studies have shown that mind/body interventions can reduce cancer-related pain,[110] and a nonrandomized crossover study revealed that guided imagery and biofeedback improved immune function (natural killer cell activity, numbers of peripheral blood lymphocytes).[111] Listening to music can have powerful therapeutic benefits. The right kind of music (whatever the patient enjoys) can ease anxiety, promote relaxation, and improve mood and appetite. Music is easily used in the hospital and home setting. Breast cancer support groups are beneficial for many women. A woman with breast cancer should be encouraged to reach out to friends and family—love is powerful medicine.

Acupuncture

Acupuncture is often used by cancer patients to obtain relief from the nausea and vomiting associated with chemotherapy.[112] The National Institutes of Health Consensus Development Conference on Acupuncture in 1997 stated that "there is clear evidence that needle acupuncture treatment is effective for postoperative and chemotherapy-induced nausea and vomiting, and for nausea of pregnancy and postoperative dental pain." The antiemetic effects of acupuncture may stem from an increase in hypophyseal secretion of β-endorphins and adrenocorticotrophic hormone, with subsequent inhibition of the

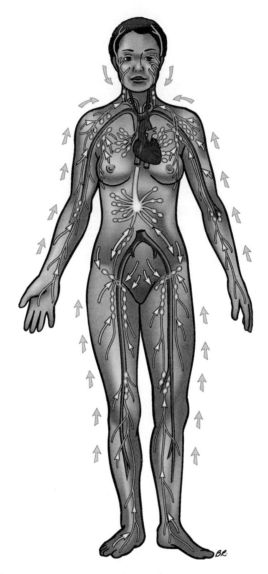

Figure **15-1** Direction of strokes for facilitating lymphatic flow. *(From Fritz S: Mosby's fundamentals of therapeutic massage, ed 3. St Louis, 2004, Mosby.)*

chemoreceptor trigger zone and vomiting center. Acupuncture also affects the upper gastrointestinal tract, decreasing acid secretion and repressing gastric arrhythmias.[113]

A three-arm, randomized, controlled trial of 104 women (mean age 46 years) with breast cancer compared the effectiveness of electroacupuncture with minimal needling and mock electrical stimulation or antiemetic medications alone in the control of emesis among patients undergoing a highly emetogenic chemotherapy regimen. Among women receiving high-dose chemotherapy, adjunct electroacupuncture was more effective in controlling emesis than was minimal needling or antiemetic pharmacotherapy alone, although the observed effect was of limited duration.[114]

Some oncology centers are making the services of licensed acupuncturists available on-site, and an increasing number of managed-care organizations and insurance companies are reimbursing for treatment.

BREAST CANCER/BREAST HEALTH RESOURCES

- Cancer Information Service of the National Cancer Institute
  800-4-CANCER (toll-free)
  http://cis.nci.nih.gov
- National Institutes of Health National Center for Complementary and Alternative Medicine (NCCAM) Clearinghouse
  888-644-6226 (toll-free); international 1-301-519-3153
  www.nccam.nih.gov
- National Breast Cancer Coalition
  202-296-7477
  www.stopbreastcancer.org
- SHARE (Self-help for women with breast cancer)
  English, 212-382-2111; Spanish, 212-719-4454
  www.sharecancersupport.org
- Y-ME National Breast Cancer Organization, Inc.
  800-221-2141 (toll-free)
  www.y-me.org
- Lesbian Community Cancer Project
  4753 North Broadway, Suite 602
  Chicago, IL 60640
  773-561-4662
  www.lccp.org
- Breast Cancer Action
  1280 Columbus Ave., Suite 204
  San Francisco, CA 94133
  415-243-9301
  www.bcaction.org
- National Women's Health Network
  202-628-7814, 202-347-1140
  www.nwhn.org

Adapted from Conry C: Evaluation of a breast complaint: Is it cancer? *Am Fam Phys* 49(2):445-450, 1994.

References

1. Greenlee RT, Hill-Harmon MB, Murray T, et al: Cancer statistics, 2001, *CA Cancer J Clin* 51: 15-36, 2001.
2. National Cancer Institute Surveillance, Epidemiology, and End Results Program: *Racial/ethnic patterns of cancer in the United States 1988-1992*. http://cis.nci.nih.gov/fact/pdfdraft/5_diag/fs5_6.pdf. Accessed April 2004.
3. National Cancer Institute Surveillance, Epidemiology, and End Results Program: *1997-1999*. http://cis.nci.nih.gov/fact/pdfdraft/5_diag/fs5_6.pdf. Accessed April 2004.
4. Harris JR, Lippman ME, Veronesi U, et al: Breast cancer I. *N Engl J Med* 327:319-328, 1992.
5. Richter WO: Fatty acids and breast cancer: is there a relationship? *Eur J Med Res* 8(8):373-380, 2003.
6. Cho E, Spiegelman D, Hunter DJ, et al: Premenopausal fat intake and risk of breast cancer, *J Natl Cancer Inst* 95:1079-1085, 2003.
7. Boik J: Cancer and natural medicine: a textbook of basic science and clinical research, Princeton, Minnesota, 1996, Oregon Medical Press.
8. Wolff SM, Toniolo PG, Lee EW, et al: Blood levels of organochlorine residues and risk of breast cancer, *J Natl Cancer Inst* 85:648-652, 1993.
9. Kopans DB, Marchant DJ, Osborne MP: Breast cancer: vigilance, not panic, *Patient Care* 15: 135-164, 1993.
10. United Kingdom National Case-Control Study Group: Breast feeding and the risk of breast cancer in young women, *BMJ* 307:17-20, 1993.
11. Lengacher CA, Bennett MP, Kip KE, et al: Frequency of use of complementary and alternative medicine in women with breast cancer, *Oncol Nurs Forum* 29:1445-1452, 2002.
12. Lee MM, Lin SS, Wrencsch MR, et al: Alternative therapies used by women with breast cancer in four ethnic populations, *J Natl Cancer Inst* 92:42-47, 2000.
13. Sollner W, Maislinger S, De Vries A, et al: Use of complementary and alternative medicine by cancer patients is not associated with perceived distress or poor compliance with standard treatment but with active coping behavior, *Cancer* 89:873-880, 2000.
14. Shumin Z, Hunter DJ, Forman MR, et al: Dietary carotenoids and vitamins A, C, and E and risk of breast cancer: *J Natl Cancer Inst* 91:547-556, 1999.
15. Malin AS, Qi D, Shu XO, et al: Intake of fruits, vegetables and selected micronutrients in relation to the risk of breast cancer, *Int J Cancer* 105:413-418, 2003.
16. Rohan TE, Howe GR, Friedenreich CM, et al: Dietary fiber, vitamins A, C, and E and the risk of breast cancer: a cohort study, *Cancer Causes Control* 4:29-37, 1993.
17. Barnes S, et al: Soybeans inhibit mammary tumors in models of breast cancer. In Pariza M, editor: *Mutagens and carcinogens in the diet*, New York, 1990, Wiley-Liss, pp 239-253.
18. Price KR, Fenwick GR: Naturally occurring oestrogens in foods: a review, *Food Addit Contam* 2:73-106, 1985.
19. Xu X, Duncan AM, Merz BE, et al: Effects of soy isoflavones on estrogen and phytoestrogen metabolism in premenopausal women, *Cancer Epidemiol Biomark Prev* 7:1101-1108, 1998.
20. Liehr JG, Ricci MJ: 4-Hydroxylation of estrogens as marker of human mammary tumors, *Proc Natl Acad Sci USA* 93:3294–3296, 1996.
21. Xu X, Duncan AM, Wangen KE, et al: Soy consumption alters endogenous estrogen metabolism in postmenopausal women, *Cancer Epidemiol Biomarkers Prev* 9:781-786, 2000.
22. Nagata C, Takatsuka N, Inaba S, et al: Effect of soymilk consumption on serum estrogen concentrations in premenopausal Japanese women, *J Natl Cancer Inst* 90:1830-1835, 1998.
23. Martini MC, Dancisak BB, Haggans CJ, et al: Effects of soy intake on sex hormone metabolism in premenopausal women, *Nutr Cancer* 34:133-139, 1999.
24. Knight D, Eden J: Phytoestrogens: a short review, *Maturitas* 22:167, 1995.
25. Lamartiniere C: *Genistein programs against mammary cancer*, presented at Dietary Phytoestrogens: Cancer Cause or Prevention? Herndon, Virginia, September 21-23, 1994, National Cancer Institute.
26. Adlercreutz H: Phytoestrogens and breast cancer, *J Steroid Biochem Mol Biol* 83(Dec):113-118, 2002.

27. Peeters PH, Keinan-Boker L, van der Schouw YT, et al: Phytoestrogens and breast cancer risk: review of the epidemiological evidence, *Breast Cancer Res Treat* 77:171-183, 2003.
28. Yamamoto S, Sobue T, Kobayashi M, et al: Soy, isoflavones, and breast cancer risk in Japan, *J Natl Cancer Inst* 95:906-913, 2003.
29. Davis SR, Dalais FS, Simpson ER, et al: Phytoestrogens in health and disease, *Recent Prog Horm Res* 54:185-210, 1999; discussion 210-211.
30. Messina MJ, Loprinzi CL: Soy for breast cancer survivors: a critical review of the literature, *J Nutr* 131(suppl 11):3095S-3108S, 2001.
31. Jones JL, Daley BJ, Enderson BL, et al: Genistein inhibits tamoxifen effects on cell proliferation and cell cycle arrest in T47D breast cancer cells, *Am Surg* 68:575-577; discussion 577-578, 2002.
32. Ju YH, Doerge DR, Allred KF, et al: Dietary genistein negates the inhibitory effect of tamoxifen on growth of estrogen-dependent human breast cancer (MCF-7) cells implanted in athymic mice, *Cancer Res* 62:2474-2477, 2002.
33. Brandi G, Paiardini M, Cervasi B, et al: A new indole-3-carbinol tetrameric derivative inhibits cyclin–dependent kinase 6 expression, and induces G1 cell cycle arrest in both estrogen-dependent and estrogen-independent breast cancer cell lines, *Cancer Res* 63:4028-4036, 2003.
34. Rahman KMW, Aranha O, Sarkar FH: Indole-3-carbinol (I3C) induces apoptosis in tumorigenic but not in nontumorigenic breast epithelial cells, *Nutr Cancer* 45:101-112, 2003.
35. Auborn KJ, Fan S, Rosen EM, et al: Indole-3-carbinol is a negative regulator of estrogen, *J Nutr* 133(suppl 7):2470S-2475S, 2003.
36. Fishman J, Martucci C: Biological properties of 16α-hydroxyestrone: implications in estrogen physiology and pathophysiology, *J Clin Endocrinol Metab* 51:611-615, 1980.
37. Fowke JH, Qi D, Bradlow HL, et al: Urinary estrogen metabolites and breast cancer: differential pattern of risk found with pre- versus post-treatment collection, *Steroids* 68:65-72, 2003.
38. Schneider J, Huh MM, Bradlow HL, et al: Antiestrogen action of 2-hydroxyestrone on MCF-7 human breast cancer cells, *J Biol Chem* 259:4840-4845, 1984.
39. McDanell R, McLean AEM: Chemical and biological properties of indole glucosinolates (gluco-brassicans): a review, *Food Chem Toxicol* 26:59-70, 1988.
40. Kall MA, Vang O, Clausen J: Effects of dietary broccoli on human *in vivo* drug metabolizing enzymes: evaluation of caffeine, estrone, and chlorzoxazone, *Carcinogenesis* 17:793-799, 1996.
41. Fowke JH, Longcope C, Hebert JR: Brassica vegetable consumption shifts estrogen metabolism in healthy postmenopausal women, *Cancer Epidemiol Biomarkers Prev* 9:773-779, 2000.
42. Taioli E, Bradlow HL, Sepkovic DW, et al: CYP1A1 genotype, estradiol metabolism and breast cancer in African-Americans, *Proc Annu Meet Am Assoc Cancer Res* 37:249, 1996.
43. Riza E, dos Santos Silva I, De Stavola B, et al: Urinary estrogen metabolites and mammographic parenchymal patterns in postmenopausal women, *Cancer Epidemiol Biomarkers Prev* 10:627-634, 2001.
44. Meilahn EN, De Stavola B, Allen DS, et al: Do urinary oestrogen metabolites predict breast cancer? Guernsey III cohort follow-up, *Br J Cancer* 78:1250-1255, 1998.
45. Muti P, Bradlow HL, Micheli A, et al: Estrogen metabolism and risk of breast cancer: a prospective study of the 2:6α ratio in pre- and postmenopausal women, *Epidemiology* 11:635-640, 2000.
46. Michnovicz JJ, Hershcopf RJ, Naganuma H, et al: Increased 2-hydroxylation of estradiol as a possible mechanism for the anti-estrogenic effect of cigarette smoking, *N Engl J Med* 315:1305-1309, 1986.
47. De Cree C, Van Kranenburg G, Geurten P, et al: 4-Hydroxycatecholestrogen metabolism responses to exercise and training: possible implications for menstrual cycle irregularities and breast cancer, *Fertil Steril* 67:505-516, 1997.
48. Anderson KE, Kappas A, Conney AH, et al: The influence of dietary protein and carbohydrate on the principal oxidative biotransformations of estradiol in normal subjects, *J Clin Endocrinol Metab* 59:103-107, 1984.
49. Osborne MP, Karmali RA, Hershcopf RJ, et al: ω3 fatty acids: modulation of estrogen metabolism and potential for breast cancer prevention, *Cancer Invest* 6:629-631, 1988.
50. Haggans CJ, Travelli EJ, Thomas W, et al: The effect of flaxseed and wheat bran consumption on urinary estrogen metabolites in premenopausal women, *Cancer Epidemiol Biomarkers Prev* 9:719-725, 2000.

51. Fowke JH, Longcope C, Hebert JR: Macronutrient intake and estrogen metabolism in healthy postmenopausal women, *Breast Cancer Res Treat* 65:1-10, 2001.
52. Barnes S: Evolution of the health benefits of soy isoflavones, *Proc Soc Exp Biol Med* 217:386-392, 1998.
53. Sarkar FH, Rahman KM, Li Y: Bax translocation to mitochondria is an important event in inducing apoptotic cell death by indole-3-carbinol (I3C) treatment of breast cancer cells, *J Nutr* 133(suppl 7):2434S-2439S, 2003.
54. Crane FL, Sun IL, Sun EE: The essential functions of coenzyme Q, *Clin Invest* 71(suppl):55-59, 1993.
55. Folkers K, Shizukuishi S, Takemura K, et al: Increase in levels of IgG in serum of patients treated with coenzyme Q10, *Res Comm Chem Pathol Pharmacol* 38:335-338, 1982.
56. Bliznakov EG: Coenzyme Q in experimental infections and neoplasia. In Folkers K, editor: *Biomedical and clinical aspects of coenzyme Q*, vol 3, New York, 1981, Elsevier, pp 325-334.
57. Folkers K, Osterborg A, Nylander M, et al: Activities of vitamin Q10 in animal models and a serious deficiency in patients with cancer, *Biochem Biophys Res Commun* 234:296-299, 1997.
58. Hoffer A: Orthomolecular treatment of cancer. In Quillin P, Williams RM, eds: *Adjuvant nutrition in cancer treatment*, Arlington Heights, IL, 1994, Cancer Treatment Research Foundation, pp 331-362.
59. Lockwood K, Moesgaard S, Hanioka T, et al: Apparent partial remission of breast cancer in high risk patients supplemented with nutritional anti-oxidants, essential fatty acids and coenzyme Q10, *Mol Asp Med* 15(suppl):231-240, 1994.
60. Lockwood K, Moesgaard S, Folkers K: Partial and complete regression of breast cancer in patients in relation to dosage of coenzyme Q10, *Biochem Biophys Res Commun* 199:1504-1508, 1994.
61. Lockwood K, Moesgaard S, Yamamoto T, et al: Progress on therapy of breast cancer with vitamin Q10 and the regression of metastases, *Biochem Biophys Res Commun* 212:172-177, 1995.
62. Lesperance ML, Olivotto IA, Forde N, et al: Mega-dose vitamins and minerals in the treatment of non-metastatic breast cancer: an historical cohort study, *Breast Cancer Res Treat* 76:137-143, 2002.
63. Reiter RJ, Melchiorri D, Sewerynek E, et al: A review of the evidence supporting melatonin's role as an antioxidant, *J Pineal Res* 18:1-11, 1995.
64. Lissoni P, Barni S, Tancini G, et al: A study of the mechanisms involved in the immunostimulatory action of the pineal hormone in cancer patients, *Oncology* 50:399-402, 1993.
65. Cohen M, Lippman M, Chabner B: Role of pineal gland in aetiology and treatment of breast cancer, *Lancet* 2:814-816, 1978.
66. Tamarkin L, Danforth D, Lichter A, et al: Decreased nocturnal plasma melatonin peak in patients with estrogen receptor-positive breast cancer, *Science* 216:1003-1005, 1982.
67. Sanchez-Barcelo EJ, Cos S, Fernandez R, et al: Melatonin and mammary cancer: a short review, *Endocrinol Relat Cancer* 10:153-159, 2003.
68. Czeczuga-Semeniuk E, Wolczynski S, Anchim T, et al: Effect of melatonin and all-trans retinoic acid on the proliferation and induction of the apoptotic pathway in the culture of human breast cancer cell line MCF-7, *Pol J Pathol* 53:59-65, 2002.
69. Mediavila MD, Cos S, Sanchez-Barcelo EJ: Melatonin increases P53 and P21 WAF1 expression in MCF-7 human breast cancer cells in-vitro, *Life Sci* 65:415-420, 1999.
70. Schernhammer ES, Laden F, Speizer FE, et al: Rotating night shifts and risk of breast cancer in women participating in the Nurses' Health Study, *J Natl Cancer Inst* 93:1563-1568, 2001.
71. Davis S, Mirick DK, Stevens RG: Night shift work, light at night, and risk of breast cancer, *J Natl Cancer Inst* 93:1557-1562, 2001.
72. Lissoni P, Barni S, Meregalli S, et al: Modulation of cancer endocrine therapy by melatonin: a phase II study of tamoxifen plus melatonin in metastatic breast cancer patients progressing under tamoxifen alone, *Br J Cancer* 71:854-856, 1995.
73. Mukhtar H, Ahmad N: Green tea in chemoprevention of cancer, *Toxicol Sci* 52(2 suppl):111-117, 1999.
74. Weisburger JH: Tea and health: the underlying mechanisms, *Proc Soc Exp Biol Med* 220:271-275, 1999.

75. Komori A, Yatsunami J, Okabe S, et al: Anticarcinogenic activity of green tea polyphenols, *Jpn J Clin Oncol* 23:186-190, 1993.

76. Steele VE, Kelloff GJ, Balentine D, et al: Comparative chemopreventive mechanisms of green tea, black tea and selected polyphenol extracts measured by in vitro bioassays, *Carcinogenesis* 21:63-67, 2000.

77. Vergote D, Cren-Olive C, Chopin V, et al: (–)–Epigallocatechin (EGC) of green tea induces apoptosis of human breast cancer cells but not of their normal counterparts, *Breast Cancer Res Treat* 76:195-201, 2002.

78. Wu AH, Yu MC, Tseng CC, et al: Green tea and risk of breast cancer in Asian Americans, *Int J Cancer* 106:574-579, 2003.

79. Nakachi K, Suemasu K, Suga K, et al: Influence of drinking green tea on breast cancer malignancy among Japanese patients, *Jpn J Cancer Res* 89:254-261, 1998.

80. Yance DR: *Herbal medicine, healing and cancer*, Chicago, Illinois, 1999, Keats Publishing, p 303.

81. Fissher-Rasmussen W, Kjaer SK, Dahl C, et al: Ginger treatment of hyperemesis gravidarum, *Eur J Obstet Gynecol Reprod Biol* 38:19-24, 1990.

82. Mowrey DB, Clayson DE: Motion sickness, ginger, and psychophysics, *Lancet* 1:655-657, 1982.

83. Phillips S, Ruggier R, Hutchinson SE: *Zingiber officinale* (ginger): an antiemetic for day case surgery, *Anesthesia* 48:715-717, 1993.

84. Huang QR, Iwamoto M, Aoki S, et al: Anti-5-hydroxytryptamine 3 effect of galanolactone, diterpenoid isolated from ginger, *Chem Pharm Bull (Tokyo)* 39:397-379, 1991.

85. Sharma SS, Gupta YK: Reversal of cisplatin-induced delay in gastric emptying in rats by ginger (*Zingiber officinale*), *J Ethnopharmacol* 62:49-55, 1998.

86. Sontakke S, Thawani V, Naik MS: Ginger as an antiemetic in nausea and vomiting induced by chemotherapy: a randomized, cross-over, double blind study, *Ind J Pharmacol* 35:32-36, 2003.

87. Pace JC: Oral ingestion of encapsulated ginger and reported self-care actions for the relief of chemotherapy-associated nausea and vomiting, *Dissertations Abstracts Int* 47:3297-3298, 1987.

88. *Trial of encapsulated ginger as a treatment for chemotherapy-induced nausea and vomiting*, available at www.clinicaltrials.gov. Accessed March 24, 2004.

89. Peirce A: *The American Pharmaceutical Association practical guide to natural medicine*, New York, New York, 1999, Stonesong Press, pp 288-292.

90. U.S. Congressional Office of Technology Assessment: *Essiac*, Washington, D.C., 1990, US Government Printing Office.

91. Richardson MA, T Sanders, C Tamayo et al. 2000. Flor-Essence™ herbal tonic use in North America: a profile of general consumers and cancer patients, *HerbalGram* 50:40-46, 2000.

92. Richardson MA: Research of complementary/alternative medicine therapies in oncology: promising but challenging, *J Clin Oncol* 17:38-43, 1999.

93. Lin SC, Lin CH, Lin CC, et al: Hepatoprotective effects of *Arctium lappa* Linne on liver injuries induced by chronic ethanol consumption and potentiated by carbon tetrachloride, *J Biomed Sci* 9:401-409, 2002.

94. Lin SC, Chung TC, Lin CC, et al: Hepatoprotective effects of *Arctium lappa* on carbon tetrachloride– and acetaminophen-induced liver damage, *Am J Chin Med* 28:163-173, 2000.

95. Lin CC, Lu JM, Yang JJ, et al: Anti-inflammatory and radical scavenge effects of *Arctium lappa, Am J Chin Med* 24:127-137, 1996.

96. Foldeak S, Dombradi G: Tumor-growth inhibiting substances of plant origin. I. Isolation of the active principle of *Arctium lappa*, *Acta Phys Chem* 10:91-93, 1964.

97. Dombradi C, Foldeak S: Screening report on the antitumor activity of purified *Arctium lappa* extracts, *Tumori* 52:173, 1966.

98. Jing X, Ueki N, Cheng J, et al: Induction of apoptosis in hepatocellular carcinoma cell lines by emodin, *Jpn J Cancer Res* 93:874-882, 2002.

99. Campbell MJ, Hamilton B, Shoemaker M, et al: Antiproliferative activity of Chinese medicinal herbs on breast cancer cells in vitro, *Anticancer Res* 22:3843-3852, 2002.

100. Lee HZ: Effects and mechanisms of emodin on cell death in human lung squamous cell carcinoma, *Br J Pharmacol* 134:11-20, 2001.

101. Srinivas G, Anto RJ, Srinivas P, et al: Emodin induces apoptosis of human cervical cancer cells through poly(ADP-ribose) polymerase cleavage and activation of caspase-9, *Eur J Pharmacol* 473:117-125, 2003.
102. Awad AB, Roy R, Fink CS: Beta-sitosterol, a plant sterol, induces apoptosis and activates key caspases in MDA-MB-231 human breast cancer cells, *Oncol Rep* 10:497-500, 2003.
103. Awad AB, Williams H, Fink CS: Phytosterols reduce in vitro metastatic ability of MDA-MB-231 human breast cancer cells, *Nutr Cancer* 40:157-164, 2001.
104. Linde K, Mulrow CD: St John's wort for depression, *Cochrane Database Syst Rev* (2):CD000448, 2000.
105. Mathijssen RH, Verweij J, de Bruijn P, et al: Effects of St. John's wort on irinotecan metabolism, *J Natl Cancer Inst* 94:1247-1249, 2002.
106. Zhao KS, Mancini C: Enhancement of the immune response in mice by *Astragalus membranaceus* extracts, *Immunopharmacology* 20:225-233, 1990.
107. Cheville AL, McGarvey CL, Petrek JA, et al: Lymphedema management, *Semin Radiat Oncol* 13:290-301, 2003.
108. Williams AF, Vadgama A, Franks PJ, et al: A randomized controlled crossover study of manual lymphatic drainage therapy in women with breast cancer–related lymphoedema, *Eur J Cancer Care (Engl)* 11:254-261, 2002.
109. Anderson L, Hojris I, Erlandsen M, et al: Treatment of breast cancer–related lymphedema with or without manual lymphatic drainage: a randomized study, *Acta Oncol* 39:399-405, 2000.
110. Spiegel D, Bloom JR: Group therapy and hypnosis reduce metastatic breast carcinoma pain, *Psychosomat Med* 45:333-339, 1983.
111. Gruber BL, Hersh SP, Hall NR, et al: Immunological responses of breast cancer patients to behavioral interventions, *Biofeedback Self Regul* 18:1-22, 1993.
112. Vickers AJ: Can acupuncture have specific effects on health? A systematic review of acupuncture anti-emesis trials, *J R Soc Med* 89:303-311, 1996.
113. Samuels N: Acupuncture for nausea: how does it work? *Harefuah* 142:297-300, 316, 2003.
114. Shen J, Wenger N, Glaspy J, et al: Electroacupuncture for control of myeloablative chemotherapy-induced emesis: a randomized controlled trial, *JAMA* 284:2755-2761, 2000.

16

Vaginal Health

During the reproductive years of a woman's life, yeast infections are a common cause of vaginitis. One study estimated that by age 25, more than half of all college women will have had at least one episode of vulvovaginal candidiasis (VVC).[1] Other researchers estimate that 75% of all women will experience at least one episode of VVC in their lifetimes and that 40% to 45% will have two or more episodes.[2] Generally, yeasts are present as commensal organisms that proliferate when changes in the vaginal environment become conducive to their growth. *Candida albicans* is the species most abundant in the vagina; however, *C. glabrata, C. tropicalis, C. krusei,* and *C. pseudotropicalis* are often present.[3] The blastospore and germinated hyphae are the two forms of *C. albicans* that infect the vagina. The blastospore attaches to the surface epithelial cells, whereas the hyphae invade the superficial layers of the vaginal epithelium, resulting in symptomatic vaginitis (Box 16-1).[4]

ORIGIN OF INFECTION

Many factors contribute to the proliferation of vaginal yeast. The use of broad-spectrum antibiotics reduces the number of beneficial lactobacilli in the vagina, yielding a favorable environment for the growth of *Candida* species.[4] Pregnancy, diabetes, and high-dose oral contraceptives can all increase the vaginal level of glycogen, which has been associated with an increased number of vaginal infections. High levels of estrogen directly stimulate the growth of yeast; a cytosolic receptor for estrogen has been found within *Candida* species.[5] Estrogen stimulates the germination of yeasts in vitro. Women may experience an increased incidence of vaginal yeast infections during the luteal phase of the menstrual cycle and pregnancy because of alterations in cell-mediated immunity. Individuals who are immunocompromised (as a result of medication or illness) are also at increased risk. Some researchers believe that sexual transmission plays a part in recurrent VVC (RVVC).[6] It is not known whether treating the sexual partners of women with RVVC would reduce the rate of recurrence.

Box **16-1**

Risk factors for vaginal candidiasis

Broad-spectrum antibiotics (penicillins, cephalosporins, tetracyclines)
Increased vaginal glycogen (pregnancy, high-dose oral contraceptives, diabetes mellitus)
Altered host immunity (acquired immunodeficiency syndrome, immunosuppressive drug therapy)
Local factors (increased vaginal warmth or moisture)
Increased urinary sugar (diabetes, excessive ingestion of dairy products and sucrose)

DIAGNOSIS

Women generally complain of vulvovaginal itching or burning and increased discharge. Examination usually shows vulvar erythema, and a white or yellow-white discharge may be noted. The diagnosis can be made through microscopic examination of the vaginal discharge after it has been suspended in 10% potassium hydroxide solution. This treatment facilitates the identification of yeast pseudohyphae by inducing lysis of cellular components of the discharge. The potassium hydroxide preparation is only about 60% sensitive in the detection of yeast forms, and the practitioner must be adequately skilled at microscopic technique. The absence of pseudohyphae therefore does not rule out yeast vaginitis. Some yeast strains do not produce hyphae or mycelia (e.g., *C. glabrata*). Culture of the discharge in Saboraud's medium will reveal many infections that might otherwise have been missed. Vaginal yeast cultures are not routinely performed because they are expensive and not always available, and many asymptomatic women have positive test results for *Candida*.

If a woman is having recurrent yeast infections (four or more infections in 1 year) a more complete evaluation is necessary to eliminate secondary causes (Box 16-2).

TREATMENT

Topical Antifungal Agents

Topical antifungal creams and suppositories that contain polyenes or imidazoles are the mainstay of treatment for VVC. The topical azole agents have been shown to be effective against *C. albicans* in vitro and are only minimally absorbed into the systemic circulation (Box 16-3).

Box **16-2**

When to obtain a vaginal culture

Recurrent VVC, before initiation of long-term therapy
Suspected acute VVC with negative microscopy findings
Failure of treatment to improve condition or eradicate yeast
Possible mixed infection with negative microscopy findings

Box 16-3

CDC 2002 guidelines for the treatment of sexually transmitted diseases: implications for women's health care[11]

INTRAVAGINAL AGENTS FOR UNCOMPLICATED VVC

Butoconazole 2% cream or 5 g intravaginally for 3 days* *or*
Butoconazole 2% cream 5 g (butaconazole [sustained-release]), single intravaginal application, *or*
Clotrimazole 1% cream 5 g intravaginally for 7-14 days[†] *or*
Clotrimazole 100-mg vaginal tablet for 7 days *or*
Clotrimazole 100-mg vaginal tablet, two tablets daily for 3 days *or*
Clotrimazole 500-mg vaginal tablet, one tablet in a single application *or*
Miconazole 2% cream, 5 g intravaginally for 7 days[†] *or*
Miconazole 100-mg vaginal suppository, one daily for 7 days[†] *or*
Miconazole 200-mg vaginal suppository, one daily for 3 days[†] *or*
Nystatin 100,000-U vaginal tablet, one daily for 14 days *or*
Tioconazole 6.5% ointment, 5 g intravaginally in a single application[†] *or*
Terconazole 0.4% cream, 5 g intravaginally for 7 days *or*
Terconazole 0.8% cream, 5 g intravaginally for 3 days *or*
Terconazole 80-mg vaginal suppository, one daily for 3 days

ORAL AGENT
Fluconazole 150-mg oral tablet, one tablet in single dose

[†]Over-the-counter preparations.

Studies note cure rates of 75% to 95% with clotrimazole (Mycelex), 63% to 91% with miconazole (Monistat), and 32% to 96% with nystatin.[7] Terconazole (Terazol) has cure rates similar to those of clotrimazole.[8]

Topical agents have been used extensively and are relatively benign. Side effects, which are site-specific, include itching, stinging, and irritation. Approximately 7% of women using topical antifungal creams report treatment-related vaginal discomfort.[9] Terconazole has been associated with rare side effects, such as fever and flulike symptoms, when used in high concentrations.[10] The risk of drug-drug interaction is low with topical creams, but these agents may reduce the effectiveness of barrier contraceptive methods. Only topical azole creams, not oral agents, are appropriate for use in pregnancy.

Recurrent infection. RVVC is typically defined as four or more episodes of VVC per year. It is estimated to occur in fewer than 5% of women. The pathogenesis of RVVC is poorly understood. Vaginal culture should be performed in patients with RVVC to confirm the clinical diagnosis and to identify unusual species, including non–*C. albicans* species, particularly *C. glabrata*. *C. glabrata* and other non–*C. albicans* species are found in 10% to 20% of patients with RVVC.[11]

Treatment with the standard antimycotic therapies is not as effective as for non–*C. albicans* species. Longer treatment with topical agents (7 to 14 days) or fluconazole given once and then repeated 3 days later may be sufficient for treatment; however, maintenance therapy may be necessary to prevent recurrence. Clotrimazole 500-mg vaginal suppositories may be used once per week as a first-line treatment. Fluconazole, 150 mg once per week, may be necessary. Although treatment with ketoconazole 100 mg/day is often recommended for as long as 6 months, caution must be exercised because this treatment causes hepatotoxicity in 1 patient per 10,000 to 15,000 people. Liver-function parameters must be regularly checked. Preliminary research suggests that boric acid is equivalent to the use of itraconazole for maintenance therapy in women with RVVC.[12]

Practitioners of integrative medicine often stress that women who experience RVVC need more than simple treatment with antifungal agents; the real focus should be on restoring a normal healthy vaginal flora that will prevent the proliferation of yeast.

Herbal, mineral, and probiotic treatment

Boric acid. The optimal treatment of non–*C. albicans* VVC remains unknown. Longer duration of therapy (7 to 14 days) with a topical azole drug is recommended as first-line therapy. If recurrence occurs, boric acid in a gelatin capsule may be administered vaginally once daily for 2 weeks as an effective treatment.[12a] Women can make their own boric acid capsules by purchasing boric acid powder (displayed in the eye care sections of most drugstores) and then packing it loosely into size 0 capsules (available at most pharmacies and health food stores). Many women with RVVC find that one capsule inserted vaginally at bedtime twice weekly is an effective maintenance therapy.

Garlic (Allium sativum). Fresh garlic vaginal suppositories are often recommended in lay self-care books for the treatment of VVC. Research demonstrates that garlic has antifungal activity. Aqueous bulb extracts of garlic had a minimal inhibitor concentration (MIC) value of 0.56 when tested against isolates of *C. albicans*.[13] Fresh garlic extracts are superior to garlic powder against *C. albicans*.[14] Aqueous garlic extract exerts its antifungal activity against *Candida* species by way of oxidation of the thiol groups present in essential proteins, causing inactivation of enzymes and subsequent microbial growth inhibition.[15]

Some practitioners advocate the insertion of a peeled garlic clove into the vagina for 8 to 12 hours (usually overnight) the treatment of VVC. No studies have been performed to evaluate the effectiveness of this therapy; however, given the in vitro data, there is no reason to believe that garlic would not have beneficial effect. One note of caution is necessary: Prolonged exposure of raw garlic to the vaginal mucosa may cause a burning sensation.

Goldenseal (Hydrastis canadensis). Many herbalists recommend a douche of goldenseal or Oregon grape root for the treatment of VVC. Goldenseal is one of the top 20–selling herbs in the United States, in spite of the fact that no clinical trials have been conducted to assess any use of this North American indigenous plant. Research has been directed mainly at the isolated constituent berberine, an alkaloid found in a number of plants, including goldenseal, barberry (*Berberis vulgaris*), Oregon grape (*Mahonia aquifolium*), and goldthread (*Coptis chinensis*), which has been shown to exert antimicrobial activity against several organisms. The protoberberines berberine and palmatine from *Coptis* species significantly inhibit the growth of a wide range of *Candida* species.[16] These protoberberines have been found to inhibit enzymes found only in fungi and that are involved in the synthesis of membrane sterols or cell wall chitin.[16] The MIC values of berberine hydrochloride are 1.0, 0.125, and 0.5 mg/mL against *C. albicans, C. tropicalis,* and *C. glabrata,* respectively. Berberine hydrochloride greatly inhibited the growth of *C. glabrata,* making research on berberine-containing herbs of specific interest for non–*C. albicans* infections and RVVC.[17]

Although vaginal suppositories would be the most direct treatment, herbalists generally recommend a douche consisting of 1 tsp of cut root simmered in 1 L of water for 10 minutes and then steeped for an additional 10 minutes. This mixture is strained and cooled. The patient is instructed to douche once a day for 3 to 5 days. The use of goldenseal is contraindicated during pregnancy by most authorities as it is thought to stimulate uterine contractions (similarly, douching is generally contraindicated during pregnancy).

Because goldenseal is an endangered species in several states, Oregon grape root, barberry, and goldthread are often substituted because they also contain berberine. Organically grown goldenseal is available and preferred over plants gathered in the wild (wildcrafted).

Pau d'arco (Tabebuia impetiginosa). Pau d'arco, also referred to as *lapacho,* is a large canopy tree native to the Amazon rainforest and other tropical parts of South and Latin America. Pau d'arco has a long and well-documented history of use by the indigenous peoples of the rainforest. It has been adopted by herbalists in Europe and the United States for the treatment of oral and vaginal yeast infections, as well as athlete's foot and ringworm. Pau d'arco contains several quinone compounds, including the naphthoquinone derivative lapachol (2%-7%). The quinoids are considered the most active parts of the herb. Research has shown that the constituent lapachol and other constituents such as the benzoic-acid derivatives exert antimicrobial activity against many organisms, including *Candida.*[18] No clinical trials have been conducted to establish therapeutic efficacy for any of the fungal conditions the herb is commonly used to treat.

Quality control has been a concern, with a variety of products being sold as pau d'arco. Often they are extremely poor-quality pau d'arco or are actually mahogany shavings, which are similar in odor and color to pau d'arco.[19] Reports of anti–vitamin K activity associated with prolonged bleeding have been noted with the isolated compound lapachol. Although this phenomenon has not been observed with crude herb preparations, most knowledgeable practitioners consider the simultaneous use of this herb and warfarin contraindicated. One ounce of herb is simmered in 1 pint of water for 15 minutes and then strained to yield a douche, which is used once daily for 3 to 5 days.

Tea tree (Melaleuca alternifolia). The tea tree is a small tree native to the northeast coast of New South Wales, Australia. The leaves are used to produce tea tree oil. The leaves themselves were used by indigenous Australians for the treatment of fever and wounds and as an infused beverage. The first written medical testimony on the tea tree, describing the use of tea tree oil in surgical wounds, was published in the *Medical Journal of Australia* in 1930. The oil was issued to soldiers during World War II as a disinfectant. Today, research has demonstrated that tea tree oil exerts considerable antifungal and antibacterial activity. Tea tree oil has been shown to be active against multiple *Candida* species, including fluconazole- and itraconazole-resistant strains, at MICs ranging from 0.25% to 0.50%.[20] Tea tree oil MICs against fluconazole-resistant isolates are comparable to those of fluconazole-susceptible isolates,[21] making the use of this agent intriguing not only as a primary treatment for candidiasis but also for resistant and non–*C. albicans* strains.

Although no trials are available for review, vaginal suppositories of tea tree oil are popular in the United Kingdom, and their use is becoming more widespread in the United States. One suppository is inserted vaginally before bed each night for 5 nights. Most suppositories contain 10% tea tree oil in a base of cocoa butter. Given the data so far, clinical trials of tea tree oil for the treatment of RVVC and antifungal-resistant strains of *Candida* are warranted.

Lactobacillus. *Lactobacillus* recolonization (through the use of yogurt or capsules) shows promise in the treatment of both yeast vaginitis and bacterial vaginosis, with little potential for harm. Because infection is associated with disruption of the vagina's normal commensal microflora, primarily a loss of lactobacilli, the exogenous application of lactobacilli appears to offer hope as an alternative to antimicrobial treatment.[22]

Although a great deal of basic science explains the "hows and whys" of using *L. acidophilus* for the prevention and treatment of vaginal candidiasis, clinical trials are few. Given the safety and relatively low cost of this type of therapy, more rigorous inquiry into its effectiveness is warranted.

A 12-month crossover trial of 33 women with RVVC showed a threefold decrease in the incidence of infections when patients consumed 8 oz of yogurt containing *L. acidophilus* each day. The mean number of infections per 6 months was 2.54 in the control arm and 0.38 in the yogurt arm ($P = 0.001$). Candidal colonization decreased from a mean of 3.23 per 6 months in the control arm to 0.84 in the yogurt arm ($P = 0.001$).[23] Weekly intravaginal application of *L. acidophilus* tablets has been found to be very similar in efficacy to clotramizole in a randomized, double-blind, placebo-controlled trial of human immunodeficiency virus–positive women monitored for a median of 21 months.[24]

Eating yogurt enriched with *L. acidophilus* seems a sensible approach to maintaining a healthy vaginal flora. Finding a quality *L. acidophilus* product may be more difficult. A recent analysis of 20 probiotic products whose labeling indicated that they contained *Lactobacillus* species revealed that 30% were contaminated with other organisms and that 20% contained no viable organisms. None of the products contained what their labels claimed.[25] Adherence to epithelial cells varies greatly among the *Lactobacillus* species and among different strains belonging to the same *Lactobacillus* species.[26] Additional work in basic science and appropriate formulation of products are necessary before this therapy can be fully integrated into a treatment regimen.

References

1. Geiger AM, Foxman B, Gillespie BW: The epidemiology of vulvovaginal candidiasis among university students, *Am J Publ Health* 85:1146-1148, 1995.
2. Klebanoff M, Carey JC, Hauth JC, et al: Failure of metronidazole to prevent preterm delivery among pregnant women with asymptomatic *Trichomonas vaginalis* infection, *N Engl J Med* 345:487-493, 2001.
3. King RD, Lee JC, Morris AL: Adherence of *Candida albicans* and other *Candida* species to mucosal epithelial cells, *Infect Immun* 27:667, 1980.
4. Sobel JD: Pathophysiology of vulvovaginal candidiasis, *J Reprod Med* 34(suppl):5722, 1989.
5. Rosenfeld WD, Clark J: Vulvovaginitis and cervicitis, *Pediatr Clin North Am* 36:489, 1989.
6. Spinillo A, Carratta L, Pizzoli G, et al: Recurrent vaginal candidiasis: results of a cohort study of sexual transmission and intestinal reservoir, *J Reprod Med* 37:343-347, 1992.
7. Eschenbach DA: Lower genital tract infections. In: Galask RP, Larsen B, editors: *Infectious diseases in the female patient*, New York, 1986, Springer-Verlag, p 163.
8. Thomason JL: Clinical evaluation of terconazole: United States experience, *J Reprod Med* 34(suppl):593, 1989.

9. Nixon SA: Vulvovaginitis: the role of patient compliance in treatment success, *Am J Obstet Gynecol* 165:1207-1209, 1999.
10. Tobin MJ: Vulvovaginal candidiasis: topical vs oral therapy, *Am Fam Phys* 51:1715-1720, 1995.
11. Sexually transmitted diseases treatment guidelines 2002, *MMWR Morbid Mortal Wkly Rep* 51:RR-6, May 10, 2002.
12. Guaschino S, De Seta F, Sartore A, et al: Efficacy of maintenance therapy with topical boric acid in comparison with oral itraconazole in the treatment of recurrent vulvovaginal candidiasis, *Am J Obstet Gynecol* 184:598-602, 2001.
12a. Sobel JD, Chaim W, Nagappan V, et al: Treatment of vaginitis caused by *Candida glabrata*: use of topical boric acid and flucytosine, *Am J Obstet Gynecol* 189:1297–1300, 2003.
13. Motsei ML, Lindsey KL, van Staden J, et al: Screening of traditionally used South African plants for antifungal activity against *Candida albicans*, *J Ethnopharmacol* 86:235-241, 2003.
14. Lemar KM, Turner MP, Lloyd D: Garlic (*Allium sativum*) as an anti-*Candida* agent: a comparison of the efficacy of fresh garlic and freeze-dried extracts, *J Appl Microbiol* 93:398-405, 2002.
15. Ghannoum MA: Studies on the anticandidal mode of action of *Allium sativum* (garlic), *J Gen Microbiol* 134(pt 11):2917-2924, 1988.
16. Park KS, Kang KC, Kim JH, et al: Differential inhibitory effects of protoberberines on sterol and chitin biosyntheses in *Candida albicans*, *J Antimicrob Chemother* 43:667-674, 1999.
17. Nakamoto K, Sadamori S, Hamada T: Effects of crude drugs and berberine hydrochloride on the activities of fungi, *J Prosthet Dent* 64:691-694, 1990.
18. Foster S, Tyler VE: *Tyler's honest herbal,* ed 4, Binghamton, NY, 1999, Haworth Herbal Press.
19. Ridley V: Pau d'arco (*Tabebuia spp*), *Br J Phytother* 5:118-123, 2001.
20. Mondello F, De Bernardis F, Girolamo A, et al: In vitro and in vivo activity of tea tree oil against azole-susceptible and -resistant human pathogenic yeasts, *J Antimicrob Chemother* 51:1223-1229, 2003.
21. Ergin A, Arikan S: Comparison of microdilution and disc diffusion methods in assessing the in vitro activity of fluconazole and *Melaleuca alternifolia* (tea tree) oil against vaginal *Candida* isolates, *J Chemother* 14:465-472, 2002.
22. Reid G: Probiotics for urogenital health, *Nutr Clin Care* 5:3-8, 2002.
23. Hilton E, Isenberg HD, Alperstein P, et al: Ingestion of yogurt containing *Lactobacillus acidophilus* as prophylaxis for candidal vaginitis, *Ann Intern Med* 116:353-357, 1992.
24. Williams AB, Yu C, Tashima K, et al: Evaluation of two self-care treatments for prevention of vaginal candidiasis in women with HIV, *J Assoc Nurses AIDS Care* 12:51-57, 2001.
25. Berman S, Spicer D: Safety and reliability of *Lactobacillus* dietary supplements in Seattle, Washington (abstract 37244), American Public Health Association 130th annual meeting, Philadelphia, PA, November 9-13, 2002.
26. Mastromarino P, Brigidi P, Macchia S, et al: Characterization and selection of vaginal *Lactobacillus* strains for the preparation of vaginal tablets, *J Appl Microbiol* 93:884-893, 2002.

CHAPTER

17

Cervical Dysplasia and Cancer

The incidence of cervical cancer has declined dramatically in the United States since 1950, primarily as a result of early detection through the use of the Papanicolaou, or Pap, smear. Mortality from cervical cancer has also been reduced by early treatment of precancerous lesions. Between 1973 and 1995, the Surveillance, Epidemiology, and End Results Program (sponsored by the National Cancer Institute) documented a 43% decrease in incidence and a 46% decrease in mortality from cervical cancer. Cervical cancer has declined from the leading cause of cancer mortality in women in the United States in the 1950s; it is now 13th on the list. The American Cancer Society estimates that about 12,200 cases of invasive cervical cancer will be diagnosed in 2003. Early diagnosis and treatment remain critical; the 5-year survival rate is roughly 92% for localized cancer. However, access to health care is not equal in the United States, leading to higher mortality rates among minority women and poor women.[1]

When the global situation is considered with regard to cervical cancer, it is apparent that early screening and treatment programs must be improved for the number of deaths from cervical cancer to be reduced. The development and implementation of an effective vaccine for the prevention of human papillomavirus (HPV) infection would also help reduce cervical cancer, especially in those areas where access to care is limited. Cervical cancer is still the second leading cause of cancer deaths among women worldwide and remains the leading cause of cancer death among women in Central America, Southwest Asia, and sub-Saharan Africa. See Box 17-1 for cervical cancer risk factors.

CAUSES OF CERVICAL CANCER
Human Papillomavirus

The HPVs comprise more than 100 different types of viruses; approximately 40 of these are transmitted sexually. In human beings, approximately 60 different types of papillomaviruses have been identified (Table 17-1).

For many years, researchers considered cervical cancer a sexually transmissible disease. It is extremely rare in nuns and is found most often in women with multiple male sexual partners. However, it was not until 1983 that the connection between HPV and cervical cancer was finally established, when HPV-16 was isolated from cervical cancer tissue. This

278

Box 17-1

Risk factors for cervical cancer in all populations

- Early age at time of first intercourse (<18 years)
- Multiple male sexual partners
- Mother took diethylstilbestrol (DES) during pregnancy
- History of sexually transmitted diseases, including HPV and human immunodeficiency virus
- Cigarette smoking (the incidence of cervical cancer is two to three times greater in smokers*
- Immunocompromise

*From Lyon J, Gardner J, West D, et al: Smoking and carcinoma *in situ* of the uterine cervix, *Am J Pub Health* 73:558-562, 1983.

same virus was found in tissue taken from cancers of the penis, vulva, and anal region. Fifty percent of these tumors contain HPV-16, 20% contain HPV-18, 10% contain HPV-33, and 10% contain various other HPV types. Clearly, 90% of all cervical cancers are linked to prior or current infection with HPV.[2] The National Institutes of Health Consensus Conference on Cancer of the Cervix and the World Health Organization have concluded that a cause-and-effect relationship exists between HPV and cervical cancer.

As viral DNA from HPV integrates into the host cell genome, the expression of viral E6 and E7 proteins can lead to the development of cervical cancer. The E6 and E7 proteins inactivate host proteins that normally control cell growth.[3] The latency period between the time of infection and cervical carcinogenesis is long (10 to 20 years),[4] leading researchers to theorize that other risk factors must be present for cancer to develop. As one author notes, HPV is a necessary but not sufficient cause for cervical cancer.[5] This situation opens the possibility that risk may be modified through various lifestyle and complementary modalities.

Chlamydia trachomatis

After HPV infection is taken into account, prior cervical infection with *C. trachomatis* is associated with an increased risk for the development of invasive cervical cancer. A large

Table 17-1

HPV	
VIRUS TYPE	ASSOCIATED LESION
HPV-1 and 4	Plantar warts
HPV-2, 7, 27, and 29	Common warts
HPV-3, 10, 26, and 28	Flat warts
HPV-5 and 8	Skin cancer (in those with epidermodysplasia verruciformis)
HPV-6 and 11	Genital warts
HPV-16, 18, 31, 33, 45, and others	Cervical cancers

study was undertaken to determine the role of *C. trachomatis* infection as a cause of invasive cervical cancer among women with HPV infection. A total of 499 women with invasive cervical cancer and 539 control patients from São Paulo, Brazil, and Manila, the Philippines, were included. *C. trachomatis* infection was found to double the risk of cervical cancer among HPV-positive women from both countries. It seems possible that cancer risk increases with higher *C. trachomatis* antibody titers.[6]

A longitudinal Swedish study showed a relative risk of 17.1 for cervical cancer associated with past *C. trachomatis* infection.[7] Other researchers have documented a causal relationship between HPV and *C. trachomatis* infections in the development of cervical neoplastic disease.[8] CT infection may act as a cofactor to HPV in the development of cervical cancer by modulating the host's immunity or by inciting chronic inflammation.[9] *C. trachomatis* infection increases the expression of HPV-16, suggesting that *C. trachomatis* has the ability to modify HPV activity.[10]

Oral Contraceptive Use

The long-term use of oral contraceptives has been linked to an increased risk of cervical cancer. A review published in the *Lancet* showed that, compared with those of women who had never used oral contraceptives, the relative risk of cervical cancer increased with longer duration of use. For durations of less than 5 years, 5 to 9 years, and 10 or more years, respectively, the relative risks were 1.1 (95% confidence interval 1.1-1.2), 1.6 (1.4-1.7), and 2.2 (1.9-2.4) for all women; and 0.9 (0.7-1.2), 1.3 (1.0-1.9), and 2.5 (1.6-3.9) for HPV-positive women. The results were broadly similar for invasive and in situ cervical cancers and in studies adjusted for HPV infection status, number of sexual partners, cervical screening, smoking, and use of barrier contraceptives.[11]

An important question is whether a link exists between the use of oral contraceptives and persistent HPV infection. Preliminary research has shown that high-risk–type HPV-16 stimulates the development of vaginal and cervical squamous cell carcinomas in transgenic mice exposed to slow-release pellets of 17β-estradiol. An oncoprotein of HPV-16 has been shown to bind to a tumor suppressor gene and stimulate its degradation. Steroid hormones are believed to increase the expression of HPV-16 oncogenes, which in turn bind to and degrade the tumor suppressor gene product, leading to carcinogenesis.[12]

Although these findings suggest a mechanism by which oral contraceptives may enhance the carcinogenic potential of HPV, a recent systematic review of 19 epidemiologic studies of the risks of genital HPV infection and oral contraceptive use failed to reveal any evidence of a strong positive or negative association between HPV infection and the use of oral contraceptives.[13] These data should be judged with some caution because of the heterogeneity of reports and confounders. Whether long duration of use increases the persistence of HPV infection remains uncertain.

The preceding information must be considered alongside the benefits of oral contraceptive use, which include an effective means of birth control and a reduction of ovarian cancer risk of up to 40% to 50%, especially when taken for at least 5 years. Unplanned pregnancies can be devastating, and ovarian cancer is the leading cause of death from all types of gynecologic cancer. Women should discuss the use of oral contraceptives with their health care provider, especially if they are at high risk (have a first-degree relative or genetic mutation) for ovarian cancer.

Vaccine for Human Papillomavirus

Intense research is currently under way to develop a reliable vaccine for the prevention of HPV and cervical cancer. A double-blind study randomly assigned 2392 women (ages 16 to 23 years) to receive three doses of placebo or HPV-16 virus-like–particle vaccine (40 µg per dose), given at day 0, month 2, and month 6. Genital samples to test for HPV-16 DNA were obtained at enrollment, 1 month after the third vaccination, and every 6 months thereafter. Women were referred for colposcopy according to a protocol. Biopsy tissue was evaluated for cervical intraepithelial neoplasia and analyzed for HPV-16 DNA with use of the polymerase chain reaction. The primary analysis was limited to women whose results were negative for HPV-16 DNA and HPV-16 antibodies at enrollment and HPV-16 DNA at month 7. Women were followed up for a median of 17.4 months after completing the vaccination regimen. The incidence of persistent HPV-16 infection was 3.8 per 100 woman-years at risk in the placebo group and 0 per 100 woman-years at risk in the vaccine group (100% efficacy; 95% confidence interval, 90-100; P <0.001). All nine cases of HPV-16–related cervical intraepithelial neoplasia occurred among the placebo recipients.[13a]

Several clinical trials investigating HPV vaccines are currently under way with the great hope that cervical cancer will soon go the way of smallpox and polio.

Genetic Factors

In light of the fact that cervical cancer never develops in a significant number of women with HPV infection, the role of genetics is being studied. Researchers have found an association between immune response genes and the risk of cervical cancer. Preliminary data suggest that the problem lies in a gene, or a cluster of genes, in the human leukocyte antigen region of chromosome 6, resulting in host immune responses to HPV infection that lead either to inherited susceptibility or resistance to the transforming properties of oncogenic papillomaviruses.[14]

SYMPTOMS OF CERVICAL CANCER

Early cervical cancer is usually asymptomatic. As the cancer advances, abnormal vaginal bleeding may occur, including spotting between menstrual periods, pink-tinged vaginal discharge, heavy menstrual periods, and bleeding after intercourse. Other symptoms include leg, back, or pelvic pain; swelling of the legs; and painful urination.

PREVENTION AND TREATMENT OF CERVICAL DYSPLASIA WITH NUTRITION AND DIETARY SUPPLEMENTS

This section focuses mainly on the evidence of safety and benefit for dietary supplements in the prevention and adjuvant treatment of cervical dysplasia. The appropriate guidelines for the current standard of care for the diagnosis, management, and treatment of abnormal Pap smear findings should be consulted.

Nutritional and Dietary Supplements

Nutritional deficiencies may be a cofactor in the development of cervical cancer. In general, research has demonstrated an inverse association between cervical cancer risk and dietary intake of dark green and yellow vegetables, vitamins C and E, and carotenoids. Researchers have examined the association of cervical cancer and diet for many years. Many of the early studies did not control for cigarette smoking, oral contraceptive use, or HPV infection. Oral contraceptives and cigarette smoking decrease serum levels of β-carotene, ascorbate, and folate, and these confounders must be adequately considered for a study to be valid. The following is a summary of the research available on nutrients that are thought valuable in the prevention of cervical cancer.

Carotenoids. A great deal of information is available on the inverse relationships between β-carotene and other carotenoids and the risk of invasive cervical cancer. Low serum levels of retinol (vitamin A) have been associated with increased risk, whereas high intake of carotenoids[15] and total vitamin A[16] has been associated with a lower risk of precancerous and cancerous cervical lesions.[17] Lycopene, a carotenoid found in tomatoes, pink grapefruit, watermelon, and other foods, may also offer protection against persistent HPV infection.[15] Higher levels of vegetable consumption have been associated with a 54% decrease risk of HPV persistence. A 56% reduction in the risk of persistent HPV was observed in women with the highest plasma lycopene concentration compared with women with the lowest plasma lycopene concentration.[18] Deficiency of β-carotene in cervical cells is believed to play a role in the development of cervical dysplasia,[19] and low plasma levels of β-carotene have been noted in women with cervical cancer.[20] A variety of mechanisms, including antioxidant protection, inhibition of viral gene expression, and modulation of immune response, have been proposed.[21]

In spite of the aforementioned research, clinical trials have not demonstrated a solid therapeutic role for β-carotene in the treatment of cervical dysplasia. A randomized, placebo-controlled, multicenter trial involving women with confirmed cervical intraepithelial neoplasia (CIN) was conducted in The Netherlands. Women received placebo (n = 141) or 10 mg/day β-carotene (n = 137) for 3 months. After 3 months, Pap smears, colposcopies, and, when necessary, biopsies were performed. Cervical cancer risk was comparable between the groups. Eighty-three percent of participants were available for evaluation at the end of the trial. Thirty-two percent of participants in both the control and treatment groups demonstrated regression to normal. No effect of β-carotene on the regression percentages was observed.[22] Potential confounders include lack of dietary control (the placebo group had a slightly higher intake of β-carotene in their daily diet than the supplemented group), the dose of β-carotene may have been too low, duration of therapy too short, and HPV status of women was not determined.

In a 1997 double-blind, placebo-controlled study, 98 women with moderate cervical dysplasia were randomly assigned to receive 30 mg/day of β-carotene or placebo for 9 months. Patients were evaluated at 3, 6, and 9 months by questionnaire, plasma levels of micronutrients, and findings of cervicovaginal lavage for the detection of HPV. Colposcopy with biopsy was performed at the conclusion of the trial in 69 women. Seventy percent of women in the placebo group were found during the baseline examination to have a lesion, compared with just 36% of the women in the treatment group. The treatment group demonstrated serum β-carotene levels several times greater than those in the placebo group; however, 25% of the control group took multivitamins containing β-carotene. More than 60% of the women in the placebo group who had initial lesions demonstrated regression to a lower grade lesion, and 47% demonstrated regression to normal. Only 23% of women in the treatment group demonstrated regression to normal. Independent risk factors for persistent CIN at 9 months included type-specific persistent HPV infection and continual HPV infection with high viral loads at baseline and 9 months. After controlling for these factors, the researchers found that the β-carotene and placebo groups did not differ in their risk for CIN after 9 months. CIN regression was not related to the serum β-carotene level.[23] Failure to control for dietary carotenoid intake and supplement use in this study is definitely a limitation.

A double-blind, placebo-controlled, randomized study involving dosages of 30 mg/day of β-carotene, 500 mg/day of vitamin C, or both, failed to show benefit over placebo in 141 women with CIN over a 2-year period.[24] A more recent double-blind, placebo-controlled trial of 103 women with relatively advanced cervical dysplasia (CIN stage 2 or 3) who were given either placebo or 30 mg/day β-carotene revealed no difference between the groups at the end of the 2-year trial.[25]

Although preliminary research suggested benefit, the data from these four randomized, placebo-controlled trials are not supportive of the theory that β-carotene increases the rate of regression in cervical dysplasia. However, methodological shortcomings of the clinical trials have been mentioned and must be considered when considering the totality of evidence to date. β-Carotene in supplement form has been found ineffective against the risk of other cancers. It may be that combinations of carotenoids and other antioxidants typically found in fruits and vegetables would be more effective. It may also be that the real strength of carotenoids is a lifelong exposure to prevent cervical abnormalities and not once the abnormalities are already present.

Folate and vitamin B$_{12}$. Folic acid is a cofactor in many biochemical processes. It is essential to the formation of thymidilate, which is the rate-limiting step in DNA synthesis. Low folic acid intake is thought to be associated with an increased risk of cervical cancer.[26] Some authors suggest that folic acid reduces the risk of cervical cancer by inhibiting the incorporation of HPV genes into chromosomal sites in affected cells.[27] Low red blood cell folate levels may be a risk factor for abnormal cytologic smears in cervical dysplasia and more severe lesions.[28]

One study randomly assigned 235 women with CIN I or CIN II to receive 10 mg/day of folate or placebo for 6 months. Clinical status, HPV-16 infection, and blood folate levels were assessed at 2-month intervals, and a punch biopsy was performed at the end of the study. Prevalence of HPV-16 infection at baseline was 16% among subjects in the upper range of red blood cell folate, compared with 37% in those in the low range. Serum folate levels in the treatment group increased significantly, and 85% of participants completed the trial. At the end of the trial, no significant differences were detected between the treatment and placebo groups with regard to dysplasia status, biopsy results, or prevalence of HPV-16 infection. Half of the women in each group had normal Pap smears, and two thirds had normal findings on cervical biopsy. The authors concluded that "folate deficiency may be involved as a co-carcinogen during the initiation of cervical dysplasia, but folic acid supplements do not alter the course of established disease."[29]

A 1995 double-blind, placebo-controlled study randomly assigned 331 women with biopsy-proven koilocytic atypia, mild CIN, or moderate CIN to receive oral folic acid (5 mg) or a similar-appearing placebo daily for 6 months. After a 1-month run-in period, cervical cytologic studies and colposcopy were repeated, and 45% of participants were found to be without detectable lesions; however, all of the participants continued the study. Pap smears, colposcopy, and assessment of serum vitamin levels (folate, retinol, alpha-tocopherol, β-carotene, and retinyl palmitate) were conducted at 3 and 6 months. No HPV analysis was performed. Median serum folate levels in the treatment arm at 3 and 6 months (29.0 and 20.0 μg/dL) were significantly higher than those in the placebo arm (7.8 and 7.1 μg/dL, respectively), and 79% of all participants finished the study. At the trial's conclusion, 7% of the treatment group and 6% of the placebo group demonstrated regression to a milder dysplasia or complete resolution.[30]

Although most research has been focused on folate, the relationship between folate and vitamin B_{12} in the synthesis, repair, and methylation of DNA suggests that it might be better to study folate along with vitamins B_6 and B_{12}. Homocysteine, which is produced during methionine metabolism, is often used as a marker of low folate and B_{12} levels. Vitamin B_{12} is a cofactor for methionine synthase, an enzyme that catalyzes the conversion of homocysteine to methionine and controls cellular folate uptake.[31]

Even in the face of clinical trials that fail to show that these vitamins are effective in the treatment of CIN, the basic science suggests that they may play a role in the prevention of cervical abnormalities, thus making recommendation of a multivitamin with folate and B vitamins for women of all ages a wise one.

Multivariate logistic regression analysis was used to determine the adjusted odds ratios for persistent HPV infection associated with individual nutrients among 201 women with persistent or intermittent HPV infection. Circulating levels of vitamin B_{12} were inversely associated with HPV persistence after adjustment for age, age at time of first intercourse, marital status, cigarette-smoking status, race, and body mass index. In addition, women with circulating levels in the highest tertile of vitamin B_{12} were less likely to have a persistent infection.[32] In a large, multiethnic community-based case-control study of invasive cervical cancer in five areas of the United States (183 cases, 540 controls), it was found that the risk of invasive cervical cancer was substantially and significantly greater in women in the upper three homocysteine quartiles.[33] Other researchers have shown that serum homocysteine is significantly predictive of the risk of invasive cervical cancer, reflecting folate, B_{12}, or B_6 inadequacy or genetic polymorphisms.[34]

Even in the face of clinical trials that fail to show that these vitamins are effective in the treatment of CIN, the basic science suggests that they may play a role in the prevention of cervical abnormalities, thus making recommendation of a multivitamin with folate and B vitamins for women of all ages a wise one.

Dihydroepiandrosterone (DHEA). Research on the therapeutic effects of DHEA has been conducted for more than 20 years. The role of this substance in dementia, memory, cancer, obesity, and aging continues to be investigated, with conflicting results. DHEA has been shown to exert chemopreventive and antiproliferative effects in human cancer lines[35]; however, little research has been focused on its role, if one exists, in cervical cancer. One pilot study addressed the potential role of DHEA in cervical dysplasia. In a pilot study 12 women with low-grade dysplasia confirmed by colposcopic examination were instructed to self-administer 150 mg/day of intravaginal micronized DHEA for up to 6 months.[36] Follow-up evaluations of the cervix were performed at 3 and 6 months along with serum levels of DHEA, DHEA-sulfate (DHEA-S), androstenedione, and testosterone. At the end of the study period, 10 of the 12 women (83%) had no evidence of dysplasia; the other 2 had normal colposcopic findings, but cytologic study revealed atypical cells of undetermined significance. The treatment was well tolerated. Androstenedione levels were increased at 3 months, whereas testosterone levels were unchanged over the course of treatment. No definitive conclusions can be made about the use of DHEA in cervical abnormalities given the current paucity of data.

Botanical Therapies

American mandrake **(Podophyllum peltatum).** Traditionally, American mandrake (Figure 17-1) was used as a bitter cathartic, emetic, and vermifuge by Native Americans. It was officially entered into the *United States Pharmacopoeia* in 1864. Podophyllin, a crude

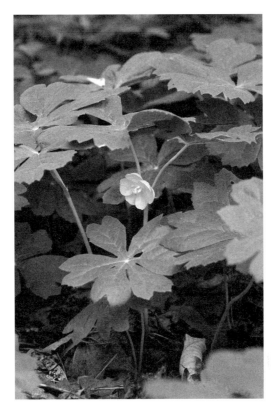

Figure 17-1 American mandrake *(Podophyllyum peltatum).* (*Courtesy Martin Wall Botanical Services.*)

resin obtained from the roots and rhizomes of wild mandrake, has been used for the treatment of genital warts since 1942 and is still commonly used for this purpose in conventional medicine.[37] Podophyllum resin is applied, usually in the practitioner's office, in a low concentration (0.5% podophyllotoxin) to small areas and washed off within 1 to 4 hours. Systemic toxicity is possible when the resin is applied to large areas or if it is left on the skin for longer than 6 hours. The use of the resin, or mandrake root, both internal and topical, is contraindicated during pregnancy because it is considered potentially embryotoxic and teratogenic.[38] This plant also provides the raw material for the production of anticancer drugs such as etoposide, teniposide, and etopophos.

Naturopathic and Herbalist Approaches

Many naturopathic physicians and herbalists recommend a variety of immune-enhancing, antiinflammatory, and antiviral botanicals for the treatment of mild to severe atypia. Depending on the source, one will find recommendations for myrrh, echinacea, usnea, lomatium, poke root, goldenseal, thuja, and yarrow (Box 17-2).

Naturopathic physicians often recommend treatment with a cervical escharotic, a caustic or corrosive substance that causes a thick, coagulated crust or slough (eschar) to form when it is applied, for patients with cervical dysplasia. This treatment typically contains

Box 17-2

Naturopathic Treatment Protocol for Mild Dysplasia (CIN1, Low-Grade Squamous Intraepithelial Lesion)

- Vitamin A vaginal suppositories nightly for 6 nights, *followed by*
- Herbal vaginal suppositories (myrrh, Echinacea, usnea, goldenseal, marshmallow, geranium, yarrow) nightly for 6 nights, *followed by*
- Repeat of the two treatments described above for an additional 12 days
- 6000 mg/day of vitamin C, 150,000 International Units/day of β-carotene, 10 mg of folic acid, multiple vitamin, lomatium isolate (5 drops twice daily), and tincture of red clover, dandelion root, licorice root, and goldenseal (2.5 mL twice daily for 3 months)

From Hudson T: *Women's encyclopedia of natural medicine,* Los Angeles, CA, 1999, McGraw-Hill.

zinc chloride and bloodroot (*Sanguinaria canadensis*), although other herbs may be added. The following naturopathic approach is commonly recommended for carcinoma in situ (CIN stage III):

- Escharotic treatment two times per week for 5 weeks, followed by
- Vitamin A vaginal suppositories nightly for 6 nights, followed by
- Herbal vaginal suppositories (myrrh, echinacea, usnea, goldenseal, marshmallow, geranium, yarrow) nightly for 6 nights
- Repetition of the two treatments with suppositories for an additional 12 days

Plus

- 10,000 mg/day of vitamin C, 200,000 International Units/day of β-carotene, and 10 mg/day of folic acid for 3 months, then 2.5 mg/day of folate and 400 μg/day of selenium
- Vegan diet for 3 months until follow-up[39]
- Multiple vitamin daily

The use of folate and β-carotene has been discussed elsewhere in this chapter. This protocol has not been subjected to any type of rigorous research to determine safety or efficacy. The choice of botanicals is interesting, though, and worthy of discussion.

Usnea (Usnea barbata, U. hirta). Usnea is a lichen, a thallophytic plant made up of an algae and a fungus growing in symbiotic association on a solid surface. Commonly referred to as "old man's beard," usnea hangs from the branches and trunks of trees like a gray-green beard. Many species of usnea are used medicinally, including *U. barbata*, *U. hirta*, and *U. florida*. Usnea has been used since ancient times in Egypt, Greece, and China, primarily as a treatment for wounds and as a remedy for indigestion.

The most extensively studied compound in this lichen is usnic acid. Usnic acid has documented antimicrobial activity against a number of human and plant pathogens, including multidrug-resistant strains of gram-positive bacteria such as *Streptococcus*, *Staphylococcus*, and *Mycobacterium*.[40] Usnic acid is being studied in the field of dentistry because research has shown it to be selective against *Streptococcus mutans* without inducing perturbing side effects on healthy oral flora.[40] Usnea appears to kill bacteria by disrupting metabolic function through uncoupling of oxidative phosphorylation at the inner mitochondrial membrane, effectively cutting off the organism's energy supply.[41] In addition, usnic acid exhibits antiviral, antiprotozoal, antiproliferative, antiinflammatory, and analgesic activity.[42] Preliminary research suggests that the antiviral activity of usnic acid results from inhibition of RNA transcription.[42]

Usnic acid may have a role in cancer therapy because of its antimitotic and antiproliferative action.[43] Usnic acid has also been shown to be a very effective UVB filter, making its incorporation in sunscreen products an interesting prospect.[44]

Herbalists often recommend usnea, generally in combination with other antimicrobials, for the treatment of pharyngitis and minor respiratory infections. Toxicity studies on hydroethanolic extracts of *U. barbata* and *U. hirta* have failed to show mortality with oral dosages of up to 32 g/kg body wt.[45] However, usnea has been shown to concentrate heavy metals from air pollution, making the sourcing of raw material very important.

At this time no data are available for review to help determine whether usnea would be effective in the treatment of HPV or whether it might increase the rate of regression in cervical dysplasia, although preliminary data suggesting antiviral and antiproliferative activity are intriguing.

Goldenseal (Hydrastis canadensis). Goldenseal, an indigenous North American herb, has emerged as one of the top 10 herbal supplements sold in the American marketplace.[46] Most research has been focused on the alkaloids (mainly berberine) present in the plant. Antimicrobial activity has been noted with the extract of goldenseal and the isolated alkaloids berberine, β-hydrastine, canadine, and canadaline.[47] In addition to demonstrating activity against *S. aureus, Escherichia coli*, and other microbes, crude methanol extracts of goldenseal root and rhizome have been shown to be active against multiple strains of *Helicobacter pylori*, which has been implicated in peptic ulcer disease.[48] Berberine possesses antiinflammatory and antipyretic activity.[49] The antiinflammatory activity appears to be due to inhibition of cyclooxygenase and possibly to inhibition of the enzyme that releases arachidonic acid from membrane phospholipids.[50] Preliminary data suggest that berberine inhibits certain tumor promoters[51] and inhibits angiogenesis,[52] making it a potentially beneficial substance in cancer therapy. However, medical science is a long way from fully understanding the mechanism by which berberine and goldenseal act, the most appropriate method of administration, the dosage, and what forms of cancer, if any, it might be effective against.

Given the popularity of this herb, surprisingly little research has been conducted on whole-plant extracts, and no clinical trials have been conducted to evaluate its efficacy for any clinical condition. Goldenseal has a long history of use for the treatment of gastrointestinal ailments, making its activity against *H. pylori* intriguing. Goldenseal was sometimes used in escharotic salves for skin cancers in the 19th century; however, only minimal evidence suggests an antineoplastic effect. No data indicate antiviral activity against HPV or any other virus.

Myrrh (Commiphora molmol, C. myrrha). Myrrh is an oleo gum resin obtained from the stems of various *Commiphora* species in northeastern Africa and Saudi Arabia,[53] where the herb is still commonly used by locals. *C. molmol* exerts antiinflammatory activity in both acute and chronic models of inflammation.[54] The oleo gum resin protects the gastrointestinal mucosa from damage induced by indomethacin and ethanol.[55] Analgesic activity has also been documented. Two compounds in the oleo gum resin, furanoeudesma-1,3-diene and curzarene, have morphinelike properties and interact with opioid receptors in the brain.[53] Local antiseptic activity is well documented,[56] providing scientific validity to its historical use in wound care by the physician Hippocrates more than 2000 years ago. In vitro research suggests cytotoxic and anticarcinogenic potential for *C. molmol*.[57] The German health authorities have approved the use of myrrh for inflammations of the oral and pharyngeal mucosa. Myrrh can be found in a number of toothpaste and mouthwash products in the United States.

The choice of myrrh in the naturopathic approach to cervical dysplasia is interesting. No data have been found to document antiviral activity, but, in light of the antiseptic, cytoprotective, and antiinflammatory effects of the herb, it may offer some therapeutic benefit. The use of myrrh at customary dosages (1 to 3 g/day) appears quite safe. Acute (24-hour) and chronic (90-day) oral toxicity studies on *C. molmol* oleo gum resin have been conducted in animals. Dosages in the acute study were 0.5, 1.0, and 3 g/kg; the long-term study dosage was 100 mg/kg per day. No significant difference was detected with regard to mortality in acute or chronic treatment compared with that in controls.[58]

Echinacea **(Echinacea purpurea, E. angustifolia, E. pallida).** Echinacea is one of the most popular herbs sold in the United States and Europe. It is used both as a single agent and in combination with other botanicals such as wild indigo (*Baptisia tinctoria*) or goldenseal. Research has been focused primarily on the use of various echinacea preparations for the treatment of upper respiratory infections, with most studies indicating some benefit when echinacea is taken early in the course of illness at a sufficient dosage.

Many studies have shown that echinacea extracts exert immunomodulatory activity. Activation of polymorphonuclear leukocytes and natural killer cells have been reasonably demonstrated.[59,60] Oral doses of *E. purpurea* (50 mg/kg) significantly increased circulating total white cell counts (mononuclear cells > granulocytes) and interleukin-2 levels over an 8-week period in animal studies.[61] Antiviral activity against herpes simplex-1 has been noted in vitro[62]; however, no statistically significant benefit was seen for *E. purpurea* extract among patients with recurring genital herpes.[63] In the 19th century, *E. angustifolia* was used both internally and externally for the treatment of skin lesions, cancerous growths, and foul mucous discharge.[64] Topically, *E. pallida and E. angustifolia* extracts inhibit inflammation in animal studies,[65] and promotion of wound healing has been noted with *E. angustifolia* in human subjects.[66] No published studies have addressed the use of echinacea in the treatment of cervical dysplasia, yet it is not surprising that it is included in the formula, given its historical use and contemporary reputation as an immune-enhancing agent.

Geranium **(Geranium maculatum, G. dissectum).** Geranium is commonly referred to as cranesbill or storksbill. The root has been used as an astringent for the treatment of diarrhea, wounds, and hemorrhoids for centuries. It remains popular as a douche for vaginal discharge, often in combination with other antimicrobial plants. Compounds from a related species, *G. caespitosum*, have been shown to potentiate the antibiotic activity of berberine, rhein, ciprofloxacin, and norfloxacin in vitro. Cellular concentrations of berberine were greatly increased in the presence of these compounds.[67] It may be that an active synergism occurs when goldenseal and geranium are applied topically together. Again, this is an interesting finding given the fact that geranium and cranesbill are often used in combination by herbalists and in this naturopathic protocol. The herb is quite safe when reasonably used.

Yarrow **(Achillea millefolium).** Known as soldier's woundwort, yarrow has been used since ancient times for the treatment of wounds and to staunch the flow of bleeding. Modern researchers have identified many compounds in the herb that exert antiseptic, analgesic, and hemostyptic activity, and the findings of animal studies verify the antiinflammatory activity of topical yarrow extract.[68] Other than a long and distinguished role in wound healing, no contemporary research indicates that yarrow would be of benefit in the treatment of cervical dysplasia. Indeed, given the longevity of use, it is odd that this herb has not been subjected to more clinical research.

Marshmallow **(Althaea officinalis).** Marshmallow was a favorite of Hippocrates. The herb was so valued that the root of its botanical name, *Althaea*, was taken from the Greek word *altho*, meaning "healing." Herbalists revere marshmallow for its soothing effect on irritated mucous membranes, a use that is approved by the German health authorities. The emollient effect is a result of the abundant polysaccharides, both in the leaf and the root, which also exert immune-enhancing and antibacterial activity. Research in human subjects for any clinical purpose, including the use of marshmallow as a topical agent in cervical dysplasia, is basically nonexistent.

Bloodroot **(Sanguinaria canadensis).** Bloodroot, known in early America as puccoon, was used as a red dye, insect repellent, vulnerary (wound-healing substance), expectorant, emmenagogue, antirheumatic, and powerful emetic. Physicians and herbalists carefully used it as an expectorant in the treatment of pneumonia, asthma, and emphysema. The dried rhizome of bloodroot was officially part of the *U.S. Pharmacopoeia* from 1820 through 1926 and was then featured in the National Formulary from 1926 through 1965 as an emetic and expectorant.

Bloodroot was used as a cancer treatment, primarily as an escharotic, during the 18th and 19th centuries. The popularity of this cancer remedy was mainly a result of the work of J. Weldon Fell, a New York physician who gained considerable notoriety in London using a paste made from the red sap of bloodroot, zinc chloride, flour, and water for the treatment of cancer. Patients at Middlesex Hospital were given two pills per day of a combination of bloodroot, hemlock, and arsenic iodide. Externally, a local treatment of the paste was applied. The hospital reported favorable effects; however, when reviewed today they are less than convincing.[69] After application of the paste, the tumor was said to become hard and could be removed in one piece with use of a process known as enucleation. Escharotic treatments became popular in Europe and the United States and remained so until the early 1900s.[70]

Researchers continue to explore potential antineoplastic compounds in bloodroot. Animal studies demonstrate a necrotizing effect on cancerous tissue when exposed to the alkaloids sanguinarine and chelerythrine present in bloodroot. The alkaloid sanguinarine exhibits a broad range of activity, including antimicrobial, antifungal, and antiinflammatory.[71] It interacts with nucleic acids and demonstrates cytotoxicity against various human tumor and normal cell lines. However, research suggests that sanguinarine exhibits no specificity for cancer cells, and its strong cytotoxicity is probably due to an early and severe glutathione-depleting effect, limiting the clinical usefulness of this isolated alkaloid in cancer treatment.[72]

Today, *Sanguinaria* is used mainly in mouthwashes and toothpastes to prevent tooth decay and gum disease. The alkaloids bind selectively to dental plaque, inhibiting 98% of the bacteria that contribute to plaque formation, bad breath, and gum disease at a concentration of 1 to 16 µg/mL.[71]

Bloodroot should not be used during pregnancy. It can cause severe vomiting with a dose as small as 1 g (5 mL of tincture). Total alkaloids in the root are 4% to 7%; of this 50% is sanguinarine. The lethal dose of orally administered sanguinarine chloride in rats has been documented as 1.66 g/kg.

Perspectives on Botanical Therapy

The protocol described above is being used by many naturopathic physicians for the treatment of cervical dysplasia and by some for the treatment of cervical cancer. At this time, only anecdotal information on efficacy is available. Escharotic agents were once a popular treatment for cancer, and evidence suggests antineoplastic activity with bloodroot. Some of the herbs possess antiinflammatory and antiviral activity, making direct application to the cervix an interesting idea. Given the cost and the amount of time involved, this is an area in which a high-quality study should be conducted. Cervical atypia and low-grade cervical dysplasia often spontaneously regress. Carcinoma in situ is not likely to regress spontaneously, and clinical trials should be conducted to definitively establish the value of this approach for women in this category.

References

1. Swan J, Breen N, Coates RJ, et al: Progress in cancer screening practices in the United States: results from the 2000 National Health Interview Survey, *Cancer* 97:1528-1540, 2003.
2. Syrjanen K: Spontaneous evolution of intraepithelial lesions according to the grade and type of the implicated human papillomavirus (HPV), *Eur J Obstet Gyn Reprod Biol* 65:45-53, 1996.
3. Munoz N, Bosch FX, de Sanjose S, et al: Epidemiologic classification of human papillomavirus types associated with cervical cancer, *N Engl J Med* 348:518-527, 2003.
4. Skyldberg B, Fujioka K, Hellstrom AC, et al: Human papillomavirus infection, centrosome aberration, and genetic stability in cervical lesions, *Mod Pathol* 14:279-284, 2001.
5. Heley S: Human papillomavirus: beware the infection you can't see, *Aust Fam Phys* 32:311-315, 2003.
6. Smith JS, Munoz N, Herrero R, et al: Evidence for *Chlamydia trachomatis* as a human papillomavirus cofactor in the etiology of invasive cervical cancer in Brazil and the Philippines, *J Infect Dis* 185:324-331, 2002.
7. Wallin KL, Wiklund F, Luostarinen T, et al: A population-based prospective study of *Chlamydia trachomatis* infection and cervical carcinoma, *Int J Cancer* 101:371-374, 2002.
8. Finan RR, Tamim H, Almawi WY: Identification of *Chlamydia trachomatis* DNA in human papillomavirus (HPV) positive women with normal and abnormal cytology, *Arch Gynecol Obstet* 266:168-171, 2002.
9. Tamim H, Finan RR, Sharida HE, et al: Cervicovaginal coinfections with human papillomavirus and *Chlamydia trachomatis, Diagn Microbiol Infect Dis* 43:277-281, 2002.
10. Fischer N: *Chlamydia trachomatis* infection in cervical intraepithelial neoplasia and invasive carcinoma, *Eur J Gynaecol Oncol* 23:247-250, 2002.
11. Smith JS, Green J, Berrington de Gonzalez A, et al: Cervical cancer and use of hormonal contraceptives: a systematic review, *Lancet* 361:1159-1167, 2003.
12. Moodley M, Moodley J, Chetty R, et al: The role of steroid contraceptive hormones in the pathogenesis of invasive cervical cancer: a review, *Int J Gynecol Cancer* 13:103-110, 2003.
13. Green J, Berrington De Gonzalez A, et al: Human papillomavirus infection and use of oral contraceptives, *Br J Cancer* 88:1713-1720, 2003.
13a. Koutsky LA, Ault KA, Wheeler SM, et al: A controlled trial of a human papillomavirus type 16 vaccine, *N Engl J Med* 347:1645-1651, 2002.
14. Gostout BS, Poland GA, Calhoun ES, et al: TAP1, TAP2, and HLA-DR2 alleles are predictors of cervical cancer risk, *Gynecol Oncol* 88:326-332, 2003.
15. Schiff MA, Patterson RE, Baumgartner RN, et al: Serum carotenoids and risk of cervical intraepithelial neoplasia in Southwestern American Indian women, *Cancer Epidemiol Biomarkers Prev* 10:1219-1222, 2001.
16. French AL, Kirstein LM, Massad LS, et al: Association of vitamin A deficiency with cervical squamous intraepithelial lesions in human immunodeficiency virus–infected women, *J Infect Dis* 182:1084-1089, 2000.
17. Shannon J, Thomas DB, Ray RM, et al: Dietary risk factors for invasive and in-situ cervical carcinomas in Bangkok, Thailand, *Cancer Causes Control* 13:691-699, 2002.
18. Sedjo RL, Doe DJ, Abrahamsen M, et al: Vitamin A, carotenoids and risk of persistent oncogenic human papillomavirus infection, *Cancer Epidemiol Biomarkers Prev* 11:876-884, 2002.
19. Palan P, Mikhail M, Basu J, et al: Beta carotene levels in exfoliated cervicovaginal epithelial cells in cervical intraepithelial neoplasia and cervical cancer, *Am J Obstet Gynecol* 167:1899-1903, 1992.
20. Palan P, Romney S, Mikhail M, et al: Decreased plasma beta-carotene levels in women with uterine cervical dysplasias and cancer, *J Nat Cancer Inst* 80(6):454-455, 1988.
21. Giuliano AR, Papenfuss M, Nour M, et al: Antioxidant nutrients: associations with persistent human papilloma virus infection, *Cancer Epidemiol Biomarkers Prev* 6:917-923, 1997.

22. deVet HC, Knipschild PG, Willebrand D, et al: The effect of beta-carotene and the regression and progression of cervical dysplasia: a clinical experiment, *J Clin Epidemiol* 44:273-283, 1991.
23. Romney SL, Ho GY, Palan PR, et al: Effects of beta-carotene and other factors on the outcome of cervical dysplasia and human papilloma virus infection, *Gynecol Oncol* 65:483-492, 1997.
24. Mackerras D, Irwig L, Simpson JM, et al: Randomized double-blind trial of beta-carotene and vitamin C in women with minor cervical abnormalities, *Br J Cancer* 79:1448-1453, 1999.
25. Keefe KA, Schell MJ, Brewer C, et al: A randomized, double blind, phase III trial using oral beta-carotene supplementation for women with high-grade cervical intraepithelial neoplasia, *Cancer Epidemiol Biomarkers Prev* 10:1029-1035, 2001.
26. Bernardi P, Pace V: Correlations between folic acid, human papilloma virus (HPV), and cervix neoplasms, *Minerva Ginecol* 46:249-255, 1994.
27. Butterworth CE Jr: Effect of folate on cervical cancer. Synergism among risk factors, *Ann N Y Acad Sci* 669:293-299, 1992.
28. Harper JM, Levine AJ, Rosenthal DL, et al: Erythrocyte folate levels, oral contraceptive use and abnormal cervical cytology, *Acta Cytol* 38:324-330, 1994.
29. Butterworth CE Jr, Hatch KD, Soong SJ, et al: Oral folic acid supplementation for cervical dysplasia: a clinical intervention trial, *Am J Obstet Gynecol* 166:803-809, 1992.
30. Childers JM, Chu J, Voigt LF, et al: Chemoprevention of cervical cancer with folic acid: a phase III Southwest Oncology Group Intergroup Study, *Cancer Epidemiol Biomarkers Prev* 4:155-159, 1995.
31. Alberg AJ, Selhub J, Shah KV, et al: The risk of cervical cancer in relation to serum concentrations of folate, vitamin B_{12}, and homocysteine, *Cancer Epidemiol Biomarkers Prev* 9:761-764, 2000.
32. Sedjo RL, Inserra P, Abrahamsen M, et al: Human papillomavirus persistence and nutrients involved in the methylation pathway among a cohort of young women, *Cancer Epidemiol Biomarkers Prev* 11:353-359, 2002.
33. Ziegler RG, Weinstein SJ, Fears TR: Nutritional and genetic inefficiencies in one-carbon metabolism and cervical cancer risk, *J Nutr* 132(suppl 8):2345S-2349S, 2002.
34. Weinstein SJ, Ziegler RG, Selhub J, et al: Elevated serum homocysteine levels and increased risk of invasive cervical cancer in US women, *Cancer Causes Control* 12:317-324, 2001.
35. Yoshida S, Honda A, Matsuzaki Y, et al: Anti-proliferative action of endogenous dehydroepiandrosterone metabolites on human cancer cell lines, *Steroids* 68:73-83, 2003.
36. Suh-Burgmann E, Sivret J, Duska LR, et al: Long-term administration of intravaginal dehydroepiandrosterone on regression of low-grade cervical dysplasia: a pilot study, *Gynecol Obstet Invest* 55:25-31, 2003.
37. Mayeaux EJ Jr, Harper MB, Barksdale W, et al: Noncervical human papillomavirus genital infections, *Am Fam Phys* 52:1137-1146, 1149-1150, 1995.
38. Karol MD, Conner CS, Watanabe AS, et al: Podophyllum: suspected teratogenicity from topical application, *Clin Toxicol* 16:283-286, 1980.
39. Hudson T: *Gynecology and naturopathic medicine: a treatment manual*, Beaverton, OR, 1992, TK Publications.
40. Cocchietto M, Skert N, Nimis PL, et al: A review on usnic acid, an interesting natural compound, *Naturwissenschaften* 89:137-146, 2002.
41. Abo-Khatwa AN, al-Robai AA, al-Jawhari DA: Lichen acids as uncouplers of oxidative phosphorylation of mouse-liver mitochondria, *Nat Toxins* 4:96-102, 1996.
42. Ingolfsdottir K: Usnic acid, *Phytochemistry* 61:729-736, 2002.
43. Campanella L, Delfini M, Ercole P, et al: Molecular characterization and action of usnic acid: a drug that inhibits proliferation of mouse polyomavirus in vitro and whose main target is RNA transcription, *Biochimie* 84:329-334, 2002.
44. Rancan F, Rosan S, Boehm K, et al: Protection against UVB irradiation by natural filters extracted from lichens, *J Photochem Photobiol B* 68:133-139, 2002.
45. Dobrescu D, Tanasescu M, Mezdrea A, et al: Contributions to the complex study of some lichens—*Usnea* genus. Pharmacological studies on *Usnea barbata* and *Usnea hirta* species, *Rom J Physiol* 30:101-107, 1993.
46. Li W, Fitzloff JF: A validated high performance liquid chromatographic method for the analysis of goldenseal, *J Pharm Pharmacol* 54:435-439, 2002.
47. Scazzocchio F, Cometa MF, Tomassini L, et al: Antibacterial activity of *Hydrastis canadensis* extract and its major isolated alkaloids, *Planta Med* 67:561-564, 2001.

48. Mahady GB, Pendland SL, Stoia A, et al: In vitro susceptibility of *Helicobacter pylori* to isoquinoline alkaloids from *Sanguinaria canadensis* and *Hydrastis canadensis, Phytother Res* 17:217-221, 2003.
49. Kupeli E, Kosar M, Yesilada E, et al: A comparative study on the anti-inflammatory, antinociceptive and antipyretic effects of isoquinoline alkaloids from the roots of Turkish *Berberis* species, *Life Sci* 72:645-657, 2002.
50. Huang CG, Chu ZL, Wei SJ, et al: Effect of berberine on arachidonic acid metabolism in rabbit platelets and endothelial cells, *Thromb Res* 106:223-227, 2002.
51. Nishino H, Kitagawa K, Fujiki H, et al: Berberine sulfate inhibits tumor-promoting activity of teleocidin in two-stage carcinogenesis on mouse skin, *Oncology* 43:131-134, 1986.
52. Wartenberg M, Budde P, De Marees M, et al: Inhibition of tumor-induced angiogenesis and matrix-metalloproteinase expression in confrontation cultures of embryoid bodies and tumor spheroids by plant ingredients used in traditional Chinese medicine, *Lab Invest* 83:87-98, 2003.
53. Evans WC: *Trease and Evans pharmacognosy,* 15th edition, London, UK, 2002, WB Saunders, pp 285-286.
54. Atta AH, Alkofahi A: Anti-nociceptive and anti-inflammatory effects of some Jordanian medicinal plant extracts, *J Ethnopharmacol* 60:117-124, 1998.
55. al-Harbi MM, Qureshi S, Raza M, et al: Gastric antiulcer and cytoprotective effect of *Commiphora molmol* in rats, *J Ethnopharmacol* 55:141-150, 1997.
56. El Ashry ES, Rashed N, Salama OM, et al: Components, therapeutic value and uses of myrrh, *Pharmazie* 58:163-168, 2003.
57. al-Harbi MM, Qureshi S, Raza M, et al: Anticarcinogenic effect of *Commiphora molmol* on solid tumors induced by Ehrlich carcinoma cells in mice, *Chemotherapy* 40:337-347, 1994.
58. Rao RM, Khan ZA, Shah AH: Toxicity studies in mice of *Commiphora molmol* oleo-gum-resin, *J Ethnopharmacol* 76:151-154, 2001.
59. Barrett B: Medicinal properties of Echinacea: a critical review, *Phytomedicine* 10:66-86, 2003.
60. Alban S, Classen B, Brunner G, et al: Differentiation between the complement modulating effects of an arabinogalactan-protein from *Echinacea purpurea* and heparin, *Planta Med* 68:1118-1124, 2002.
61. Cundell DR, Matrone MA, Ratajczak P, et al: The effect of aerial parts of Echinacea on the circulating white cell levels and selected immune functions of the aging male Sprague-Dawley rat, *Int Immunopharmacol* 3:1041-1048, 2002.
62. Binns SE, Hudson J, Merali S, et al: Antiviral activity of characterized extracts from echinacea spp. (Heliantheae: Asteraceae) against herpes simplex virus (HSV-I), *Planta Med* 68:780-783, 2002.
63. Vonau B, Chard S, Mandalia S, et al: Does the extract of the plant *Echinacea purpurea* influence the clinical course of recurrent genital herpes? *Int J STD AIDS* 12:154-158, 2001.
64. Felter HW, Lloyd JU: *King's American dispensatory,* Cincinnati, Ohio, 1898, Ohio Valley Co, pp 673-678.
65. Speroni E, Crespi-Perellino, Guerra M, et al: Skin effects of *Echinacea pallida* Nutt. root extract (oral presentation abstract), *Fitoterapia* 64(suppl 5):36, 1998.
66. Boon H, Smith M: *The botanical pharmacy: the pharmacology of 47 common herbs,* Kingston, Ontario, Canada, 1999, Quarry Health Books, pp 103-113.
67. Stermitz FR, Cashman KK, Halligan KM, et al: Polyacylated neohesperidosides from *Geranium caespitosum:* bacterial multidrug resistance pump inhibitors, *Bioorg Med Chem Lett* 13: 1915-1918, 2003.
68. Peirce A: *The American Pharmaceutical Association practical guide to natural medicines,* New York, New York, 1999, Stonesong Press, pp 679-682.
69. Report of the surgical staff of the Middlesex Hospital to the weekly board and governors, upon the treatment of cancerous diseases in the hospital on the plan introduced by Dr. Fell, *Boston Med Surg J* 482-485, 1857.
70. Naiman I: *Cancer salve and suppositories,* Cundiyo, New Mexico, 1994, Seventh Ray Press.
71. Bruneton J: *Pharmacognosy, phytochemistry, medicinal plants,* Paris, France, 1995, Lavoisier, pp 744-745.
72. Debiton E, Madelmont JC, Legault J, et al: Sanguinarine-induced apoptosis is associated with an early and severe cellular glutathione depletion, *Cancer Chemother Pharmacol* 51:474-482, 2003.

CHAPTER

18

Urinary Tract Infection

Urinary tract infections (UTIs) are one of the most common bacterial infections in human beings, accounting for more than 8 million patient visits per year.[1] Acute UTIs are primarily a disease of young, sexually active women. Approximately one in three women will experience at least one diagnosed UTI necessitating antibiotic treatment by the age of 24 years, and 40% to 50% of women will experience at least one UTI during their lifetimes.[2] The annual cost of health care services reaches $2 billion in the United States alone.[3]

UTIs have been traditionally classified according to the anatomic site of the infection. Examples of lower UTIs include cystitis, urethritis, and prostatitis; pyelonephritis and perinephric abscess are examples of upper UTIs. UTIs are also classified as complicated or noncomplicated. A noncomplicated UTI occurs in the absence of structural or neurologic abnormalities that would interfere with the normal flow of urine. A complicated infection may occur in either the upper or lower urinary tract but is accompanied by an underlying condition that increases the risk of a therapeutic failure. Examples include structural abnormalities of the urinary tract, physical obstruction or stricture, neurologic deficits that interfere with the normal flow of urine, and the presence of a urinary stone.

In women, most pathogenic bacteria travel an ascending route because of the short length of the female urethra and its proximity to the perianal area. On rare occasions, UTIs are caused by hematogenous spread of pathogens from a distant site of infection. The virulence of the microorganisms, the defense mechanisms of the individual, and the location of the infection all influence the course of the infection.

Bacterial adhesion allows many organisms the opportunity to gain a foothold in the urinary tract. Most gram-negative bacteria responsible for UTIs express molecules on their surfaces that allow them to attach themselves to the bladder mucosa. Type 1 fimbriae, produced by *Escherichia coli* and other cystitis-causing Enterobacteriaceae, are able to attach to mannose residues on cell membranes. It is these fimbriae that allow bacteria from the gut to attach to the perineum and vagina and thereby make their way to the urethra. Once the bacteria have attached themselves to the bladder mucosa, inflammation and clinical symptoms appear.

The urinary tract of an otherwise healthy individual is relatively resistant to bacterial infection. The urinary system has multiple redundant systems in place to help protect itself from microbial invasion. Normal bladder-emptying mechanisms impede bacterial multiplication. The low pH and high organic-acid concentration of urine make urine capable of inhibiting the growth and proliferation of numerous microorganisms.

The urinary frequency experienced during a UTI is, in part, a physiologic attempt by the body to flush out the microorganisms through increased diuresis. The epithelial cells of the bladder are coated with a type of mucus (uromucoid) that helps prevent the adherence of bacteria to the bladder wall. Tamm-Horsfall protein, produced in the kidney and secreted into the urine, binds specifically to type 1 fimbriated *E. coli*, the main cause of UTI of women.[4] Research has shown that the kidney produces defensins, antimicrobial peptides that play a pivotal role in nonspecific host defense.[5]

SYMPTOMS OF URINARY TRACT INFECTION

The chief presenting complaints for cystitis in healthy women are dysuria and urinary frequency and urgency without fever or constitutional symptoms. Approximately 20% of women report suprapubic pain. Flank pain, costovertebral-angle tenderness, fever, nausea, and vomiting are more often associated with pyelonephritis, although many patients with pyelonephritis also report lower UTI symptoms. Sometimes a vaginal infection can mimic the symptoms of UTI; however, a woman who complains of dysuria *without* vaginal discharge most likely has a UTI, not vaginitis.[6] When the primary complaint is discomfort during voiding, with virtually no symptoms of postvoid suprapubic pain or urinary frequency, the diagnosis of urethritis should be considered. Box 18-1 lists risk factors for UTI.

Box **18-1**

Risk factors for urinary tract infection
■ Sexual activity
■ Young age
■ Use of diaphragm or spermicide
■ Pregnancy
■ Incomplete emptying of the bladder caused by mechanical or neurogenic malfunction
■ Fecal incontinence
■ Neuromuscular disease
■ Catheterization
■ Medical instrumentation
■ Obstruction of urinary tract with resultant stasis
■ Fecal contamination caused by wiping of perineum from back to front
■ Renal abnormalities
■ Advanced age
■ Underlying disease, especially diabetes and immunocompromise

In women with urethritis, inflammation and infection are limited to the urethra and vagina. The origin of urethritis is usually a sexually transmitted pathogen such as *Chlamydia trachomatis, Ureaplasma urealyticum, Neisseria gonorrhoeae,* or *Trichomonas vaginalis.*[7]

DIAGNOSIS

The evaluation of urine for diagnostic purposes has been used since at least the time of Hippocrates. The color, amount of sediment, smell, and taste of urine assisted ancient healers in their understanding of illness. By the 1830s, microscopes were becoming available to the physician, and examination of the urine became more sophisticated. Today, dipsticks are used to test pH; the presence of ketones, protein, and glucose; specific gravity; and concentrations of bilirubin, urobilinogen, nitrite, leukocyte esterase (LE), and hemoglobin. Direct microscopic examination of fresh or Gram-stained urine and dipstick tests for LE and nitrites offer a quick and effective means of assessing acute, uncomplicated cystitis.

Pyuria without significant bacteriuria suggests urethritis. The LE test has a reported sensitivity of 75% to 96% and specificity of 94% to 98% in the detection of more than 10 leukocytes per high-power field.[8] The combination of positive nitrite and LE findings is highly suggestive of a UTI. If both of sets of results are negative, the negative predictive value is 98%, meaning that a UTI is extremely unlikely.[9] Urine cultures are often sent for further evaluation in young children, elders, pregnant women, symptomatic men, and anyone with suspected pyelonephritis before antimicrobial therapy is initiated.

A variety of organisms are capable of infecting the urinary tract. Gram-negative bacteria are the major offenders, with *E. coli* accounting for approximately 80% of infections in patients younger than 50 years.[10] Other gram-negative organisms include *Proteus, Klebsiella,* and *Enterobacter. Proteus* and *Klebsiella* are more common in those with urinary tract stones. *Serratia* and *Pseudomonas* are often associated with urinary obstruction and prolonged use of indwelling catheters. Infection can be due to gram-positive bacteria, especially *Staphylococcus saprophyticus,* which is frequently found in the urine of young women. If *Staphylococcus aureus* is found in a urine culture, one should maintain a high index of suspicion for kidney infection. Atypical organisms such as *U. urealyticum* and *Mycoplasma hominis* account for a small number of UTIs.

TREATMENT OF UNCOMPLICATED CYSTITIS

The treatment goals for uncomplicated cystitis are symptom relief, eradication of the offending organism, preventing damage to the kidney, and reducing the likelihood of recurrence. Antibiotics are the mainstay of conventional therapy. Mild illness in patients who are able to maintain oral hydration is generally managed on an outpatient basis with oral antibiotics and follow-up. Patients with more severe illness and those who cannot maintain oral hydration are typically hospitalized for administration of intravenous antibiotics and fluids, especially children younger than 1 year, the elderly, immunocompromised patients, men, and pregnant women.

The Infectious Diseases Society of America convened a committee to systematically review the data on antimicrobial therapy for UTIs and develop treatment guidelines for acute uncomplicated bacterial cystitis and acute pyelonephritis in women. The following is taken from the committee's recommendations regarding uncomplicated UTI[11]:

- Most antimicrobials given for 3 days are as effective as the same antimicrobial given for a longer duration. Trimethoprim-sulfamethoxazole, or trimethoprin alone, taken for 3 days is considered the current standard therapy.
- Fluoroquinolones are more expensive than trimethoprim-sulfamethoxazole and trimethoprim, and, in an attempt to postpone emergence of resistance to these drugs, they are not recommended as initial empiric therapy except in communities with high rates of resistance (i.e., 10%-20%) to trimethoprim-sulfamethoxazole or trimethoprim.

Antibiotic resistance is now a major factor in uncomplicated community-acquired UTIs. Resistance to trimethoprim-sulfamethoxazole approaches 18% to 22% in some regions of the United States, and nearly one in three bacterial strains causing cystitis or pyelonephritis is resistant to amoxicillin. Fortunately, for now, resistance to other agents, such as nitrofurantoin and the fluoroquinolones, has remained low, approximately 2%.[12] The fluoroquinolones, such as ciprofloxacin, ofloxacin, and levofloxacin, which exert broad-spectrum antibacterial activity against most gram-negative uropathogens, and the more recent members of this class, which are active against gram-positive uropathogens,[13] attain very high urinary concentrations, more than 100 times peak plasma levels, making them very effective in UTI treatment.

A 7- to 10-day regimen of oral fluoroquinolone is reasonable for outpatient management of mild to moderate pyelonephritis in the setting of a susceptible causative pathogen and rapid clinical response to therapy. Fluoroquinolones are the first-line treatment of acute uncomplicated cystitis in patients who cannot tolerate sulfonamides or trimethoprim, who live in geographic areas with an incidence of known resistance to trimethoprim-sulfamethoxazole of 10% to 20%, or who have risk factors for such resistance.[14] The use of fluoroquinolones is contraindicated in patients younger than 18 years because of the potential for joint toxicity, reported in experiments with young animals. Published pediatric series have shown that frequency of articular side effects varies with age: approximately 0.1% in adults and 2% to 3% in children.[15]

Nitrofurantoin has been used to treat uncomplicated cystitis for almost 50 years. Use of nitrofurantoin for the empiric treatment of mild cystitis is appropriate from a public health perspective as it does not share cross-resistance with the more commonly prescribed antimicrobials.[16] Nitrofurantoin is highly active against the most common uropathogens, *E. coli* and *S. saprophyticus*, and exerts some activity against several other uropathogens, including *Klebsiella* species. Nitrofurantoin is a urospecific drug that reaches high urine concentrations but does not have systemic antimicrobial activity.

TREATMENT CONSIDERATIONS FOR SPECIAL CIRCUMSTANCES
Pregnancy

Pregnancy causes a decrease in ureteral tone, peristalsis, and function of the vesicoureteral valves, all of which increase the risk for upper UTI. The immune system of a pregnant woman is modified to accommodate a semiallogeneic fetus, perhaps making gestational physiologic/immune adaptation an additional risk factor for UTI.[17] The incidence of asymptomatic bacteriuria (bacteria in the urine without clinical symptoms) is reported at 2% to 14% during pregnancy. Untreated asymptomatic bacteriuria can lead to fetal and maternal complications such as acute pyelonephritis, hypertension, anemia, preterm labor, low birthweight, and intrauterine growth retardation.[18] Approximately 20% to 30% of asymptomatic lower UTIs lead to pyelonephritis during pregnancy. Pregnant women with acute pyelonephritis may experience significant complications, including preterm labor, transient renal failure, acute respiratory distress syndrome, sepsis, shock, and hematologic abnormalities.[19] A 3- to 7-day course of antibiotic treatment for asymptomatic bacteriuria during pregnancy is clinically indicated to reduce the risk of pyelonephritis and preterm delivery. Routine screening for asymptomatic bacteriuria during pregnancy is cost-effective, particularly in high-prevalence populations.[20]

Children and Infants

Recurrent urinary tract infections (RUTIs) in children often cause greater morbidity and long-term consequences than they do in adults. UTIs in children can lead to pyelonephritis and, over time, renal scarring. Renal scarring can lead to impaired renal function, hypertension, and end-stage renal disease. A thorough medical evaluation is essential for any child with RUTIs.

Older Patients

UTIs are the second most common infection among noninstitutionalized older individuals (respiratory tract infections are most common). Factors that predispose a postmenopausal woman to UTI include urinary incontinence, cystocele, increased postvoiding residual urine, and a history of premenopausal UTI. Management of UTI in older individuals should generally involve urine culture followed by a longer course of treatment (7 to 14 days).

PREVENTION
Prevention of RUTIs

Since up to 30% of women will experience a recurrence within 3 to 4 months of an initial infection, prevention is an important goal. In the United States, more than 11 million women each year receive antimicrobials for the treatment of UTI, at a cost of more than $1.6 billion.[3] Both pharmacologic and nonpharmacologic approaches have been investigated. Although antimicrobials are effective in preventing recurrence of UTI, concerns have been raised about the risk of resistant bacteria. Practitioners often offer prophylactic antimicrobials to women who have more than three UTIs per year, to be used daily, at a low dose, or after sexual intercourse.

Nonpharmacologic Options

Dietary considerations. Dietary habits may be a risk factor for UTI recurrence in women, and dietary interventions may play a role in prevention. Frequent consumption of fresh juices, especially berry juices, and fermented milk products containing probiotic bacteria is associated with a decreased risk of UTI recurrence.[21] Clinical data, however, for these dietary interventions are mixed, although one could hardly argue against their use in the clinical setting given their safety and other health benefits.

Probiotics. *Lactobacillus* is part of a treatment category called *probiotic therapy* in which, microorganisms are administered to promote the health of the host. Advocates claim that selected strains of lactobacilli colonize the vagina and inhibit colonization by potential uropathogens. Three strains—*Lactobacillus rhamnosus* GR-1 and *L. fermentum* B-54 and RC-14—colonize the vagina and potentially act as a barrier to the ascension of uropathogens into the bladder.[23]

Although the basic science is sound, very little clinical research is available for review. Forty-seven women (18 to 50 years old) with RUTIs were randomly assigned to use a vaginal application of *Lactobacillus* or placebo twice weekly. No difference in infection rate was noted between the two groups.[24] A prospective, randomized study of 150 women compared cranberry-lingonberry juice with a *Lactobacillus* drink. The first group received 50 mL of cranberry-lingonberry juice concentrate (Maija, Marli, Finland) per day for 6 months, the second group received 100 mL of *Lactobacillus* GG drink (patented *L. rhamnosus* strain; Gefilus, Valio, Finland) 5 days a week for 1 year, and the third group served as an open control group. The cranberry-lingonberry juice contained 7.5 g of cranberry concentrate and 1.7 g of lingonberry concentrate in 50 mL of water with no added sugars, and the *Lactobacillus* drink contained 4×10^{10} colony-forming units of *Lactobacillus* GG per 100 mL. Women receiving the fruit juice had 20% fewer RUTIs than did the control and *Lactobacillus* groups. The *Lactobacillus* drink had no effect on UTI, and the researchers noted that it failed to colonize the periurethral area.[25]

The successful use of probiotics for treatment of any condition relies on a critical examination of the varying probiotic strains. Scientific evidence has shown that certain strains are more therapeutically effective than others. Adherence to epithelial cells varies greatly among the *Lactobacillus* species and among different strains belonging of the same species.[26] Not only must researchers verify the correct strains, but manufacturers must also be able to provide them to consumers in a stable formulation. A recent analysis of 20 probiotic products whose labels indicated that they contained *Lactobacillus* species showed that 30% of products were contaminated with other organisms and that 20% contained no viable organisms at all. None of the products contained what their labels claimed.[27]

Botanical therapies. Several botanicals are commonly used for the prevention or treatment of minor UTIs. The best known and researched of these botanicals is cranberry, although blueberry works in a similar fashion and may be more palatable from a patient's perspective. Other plant therapies include uva-ursi *buchu*, echinacea, and goldenseal. Herbal diuretics are often combined with urinary antiseptics to enhance their effects. Herbs purported to have diuretic activity include astragalus, rosemary, centaury, horsetail, dandelion, juniper nettle, boldo, celery root and seed, goldenrod, *ammi visnaga* fruit, and others. For the purposes of this chapter, only the botanicals most commonly used in the United States will be discussed in detail.

Cranberry (Vaccinium macrocarpon). The belief that drinking cranberry juice is beneficial in the prevention and treatment of UTIs is widespread. Indeed, many practitioners recommend it for the prevention of RUTIs. A growing body of basic science demonstrates that this fruit contains compounds that exert a beneficial effect on the urinary system. It was originally thought that acidification of the urine was the primary mechanism by which cranberry prevented infection, as bacteria favor an alkaline pH for growth.[28] This theory was questioned when a study of older patients failed to reveal any decrease in urinary pH with consumption of 1 L/day cranberry juice.[29] Yet another study of 12 healthy men (18 to 38 years old) showed that cranberry juice decreased urinary pH, and enhanced excretion of oxalic acid and uric acid when given 330 mL of the juice. Black currant juice increased urinary pH and the excretion of citric and oxalic acids. All changes were statistically significant.[30] Differing results might have occurred for a variety of reasons, including patient age, different concentration of cranberry solids in juice, and so on.

Regardless of whether cranberry alters urine pH, it is currently thought that cranberry exerts its antibacterial activity by preventing adhesion of bacteria to the bladder epithelium, preventing bacterial colonization of the urinary tract. Cranberry and blueberry, both of the *Vaccinium* genus, contain two groups of compounds that inhibit the adhesion activity of *E. coli*: Fructose inhibits type 1 fimbrial adhesion, and the proanthocyanidins inhibit P fimbrial adhesion of uropathogenic strains.[31]

Consumption of 15 ounces of cranberry juice cocktail resulted in interference with bacterial adhesion in a study of 22 participants. Urine samples were collected 1 to 3 hours after intake. Urine samples taken before ingestion of the juice served as a control. A series of six experiments were conducted. Urine from 15 of the 22 subjects showed significant inhibition of bacterial adherence ($P < 0.05$).[32]

An extensive review of the clinical trial literature by the Cochrane Collaboration was conducted to determine the evidence for the prevention of UTI. Five trials met the inclusion criteria (four crossover, one parallel). In four, the effectiveness of cranberry juice was compared with that of placebo juice or water, and in another, the effectiveness of cranberry capsules was compared with that of placebo capsules. Data from two of the five trials indicated that cranberries were effective in prevention of symptomatic or asymptomatic UTIs, but this result was not obtained in an intention-to-treat analysis.

Dropout rates were high, indicating that cranberry juice may not be an acceptable therapy when consumed over long periods of time. Overall, the quality of the five trials was poor; the sample sizes were small, making the reliability of the results somewhat questionable.[28] Of course, it remains difficult to assess how reliable a "placebo juice" is in a test of cranberry juice as the taste of cranberry juice is quite distinct and familiar.

Not included in this review is a recent trial conducted to assess the cost and efficacy of cranberry prophylaxis in adult women with RUTI. One hundred fifty sexually active women ages 21 through 72 years were randomized to spend 1 year in one of three: placebo juice and placebo tablets, placebo juice and cranberry tablets, or cranberry juice and placebo tablets. Tablets were taken twice daily and 250 mL of juice was taken three times daily. Outcome measures were (1) a decrease of greater than 50% in symptomatic UTIs per year (symptoms + $\geq$100,000 single organisms/mL) and (2) a decrease of greater than 50% in annual antibiotic consumption. Both cranberry juice and cranberry tablets decreased the number of patients experiencing at least one symptomatic UTI per year (20% and 18%, respectively) compared with placebo (32%; $P < 0.05$) in statistically signficant fashion. The mean annual costs of prophylaxis were $624 for cranberry tablets and $1400 for cranberry juice.[33]

Cochrane reviewers also addressed the effectiveness of cranberry in the treatment of UTI. A thorough search revealed no rigorous randomized trials that assessed the effectiveness of cranberry for the treatment of UTI.[28]

In the not-so-distant future, more definitive information about the efficacy of cranberry for prevention of RUTI should be available as more rigorous research is conducted in the United States. This information will include critical data on the most appropriate dose and acceptable dosage form. Research protocols with standardized products must be developed, and the issue of "placebo" controls in studies with cranberry juice must be addressed. The cranberry juices used in clinical trials have varied in their levels of cranberry solids, and European cranberry (*V. oxycoccos*) has occasionally been used instead of the more heavily researched American species (*V. macrocarpon*), although the generic term *cranberry* is simply used in most published results. How these species compare therapeutically has not been adequately investigated. Given the health benefits and safety of cranberries, it seems reasonable for otherwise healthy women to use cranberry products, if they choose, for the prevention of RUTI (Figure 18-1).

As with any therapy, patients should be instructed to contact a health care provider if symptoms consistent with infection develop so that appropriate treatment can be administered.

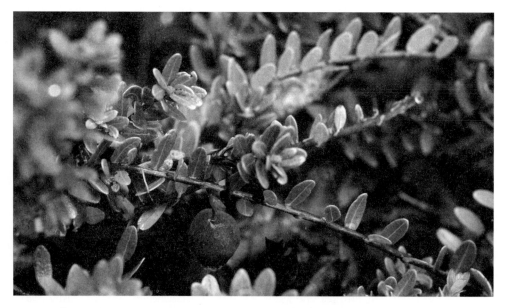

Figure 18-1 **Cranberry (***Vaccinium macrocarpon***).** (*Courtesy Martin Wall Botanical Services.*)

CRANBERRY

Newer research suggests that cranberry has health benefits beyond the urinary tract. Pilot studies found that cranberry helps prevent dental decay by interfering with bacterial adhesion. Similar to red wine and grape juice, cranberry may have a beneficial effect on the cardiovascular system. Additionally, preliminary data indicate that cranberry is effective against *Helicobacter pylori* (the organism associated with peptic ulcer disease), *Haemophilus influenzae* (an organism that is a common cause of ear and respiratory infections in children), and certain cancers.

Bearberry leaf (Arctostaphylos uva ursi). Bearberry leaves and preparations have long been used for the treatment of lower UTI and inflammation. The leaves contain 6% to 12% arbutin with small amounts of methylarbutin and free hydroquinone present.[34] The metabolites of arbutin are considered the primary constituents responsible for the herb's urinary antiseptic activity. Although it was originally thought that hydroquinone could only be liberated from arbutin in alkaline urine,[34] newer research challenges this hypothesis. It is now believed that deconjugation of hydroquinone is catalyzed by intracellular enzymes present in bacterial cytoplasm. Alkalinization of the urine does not appear to be a prerequisite for release of hydroquinone from arbutin.[35]

The urinary excretion of arbutin metabolites was examined in a randomized crossover study of 16 healthy volunteers after administration of a single oral dosage of bearberry-leaf dry extract, either as film-coated tablets or aqueous solution. With film-coated tablets, 64.8% of the arbutin dosage administered was excreted; with aqueous solution, 66.7% was excreted ($P = 0.61$). The maximal mean urinary concentration of hydroquinone equivalents was a little higher and peaked earlier in the aqueous solution group than in the group taking film-coated tablets, although this finding was not statistically significant. No significant differences between the two groups were found in the metabolite patterns detected (hydroquinone, hydroquinone-glucuronide, hydroquinone sulfate).[36] This researchs demonstrates that tea, tincture, and tablets are all appropriate dosage forms for bearberry.

Urine collected from healthy volunteers 3 hours after the ingestion of 1 g of arbutin was subjected to in vitro antibacterial testing. Antibacterial activity against *E. coli*, *Pseudomonas aeruginosa*, *Proteus mirabilis*, and *S. aureus* was noted[37]—important information given the causative organisms associated with UTI. So what about the use of bearberry for RUTI? Bearberry had a prophylactic effect on recurrent cystitis in a double-blind, prospective, randomized study of 57 women who had experienced at least three episodes of cystitis in the year preceding the study and at least one episode in the previous 6 months that had been successfully treated with antibiotics. Patients received either three tablets of UVA-E (containing a hydroethanolic extract of bearberry leaves with a standardized content of arbutin and methylarbutin and dandelion root and leaves) or placebo three times daily for 1 month. Patient follow-up was 12 months. At the end of the year, none of the patients in the bearberry group had experienced a recurrence of cystitis, compared with 23% of women in the placebo group ($P < 0.05$).[38]

Despite the virtual absence of controlled clinical trials, bearberry leaves are endorsed by the European Scientific Cooperative on Phytotherapy and the German Commission E for minor infection/inflammatory disorders of the lower urinary tract. The dosage recommended by these authorities is that which provides 400 to 800 mg/day arbutin, divided into two or three doses. This is equivalent to 1.5 to 2.5 g in infusion or cold aqueous extract or 2 to 4 mL of a tincture (1:5) taken three times daily.

The use of bearberry is contraindicated during pregnancy[39] because of the potential for hydroquinone toxicity in the fetus. In bone marrow, hydroquinone produces microtubulin dysfunction,[40] and exposure of human lymphocytes and cell lines to hydroquinone has been shown to cause various forms of genetic damage.[41] The use of bearberry is also contraindicated during lactation.[42] Gastrointestinal irritation, nausea, and vomiting may occur because of the plant's high tannin content.[43] Most authorities recommend limiting the use of bearberry to 2 weeks at a time, as long-term safety data are not available.

Buchu (Barosma betulina, Agathosma betulina). The leaves of *buchu*, a small South African shrub, have been traditionally used as a diuretic and are considered an effective urinary antiseptic by many herbalists. No clinical trials have been conducted to evaluate the efficacy of *buchu* in the prevention or treatment of UTI, and a recent study of the essential oil (10 μL, undiluted) demonstrated very low activity against *E. coli*, *Saccharomyces cerevisiae*, and *S. aureus*.[44]

The use of *buchu* is contraindicated during pregnancy,[45] as the essential oil contains traces of the hepatotoxin (R)-(+)-pulegone, a monoterpene oxidized by the cytochrome P450 system to reactive metabolites (i.e., menthofuran) that can cause acute liver injury.[46] Prolonged or high dosages of *buchu* should be avoided.

The use of *buchu* is also contraindicated in subjects with kidney inflammation[39] because of purportedly irritating nature of the volatile oils on the renal tubules. *Buchu* leaf can cause gastrointestinal irritation as a result of its essential-oil and tannin content.

Commercially available *buchu* leaf is often a combination of B. crenulata (L.) Hook, B. serratifolia Willd, and B. betulina. These species contain varying amounts of diosphenol, the constituent purportedly responsible for the diuretic activity of *buchu*,[47] and pulegone, which may be hepatotoxic in sufficient doses. Concentrations of pulegone vary widely among species, but it accounts for roughly 32% of the essential oil, which is present at concentrations of about 1.5% to 2.5% in the leaf.[45] *Buchu* is probably not harmful when used in small dosages for a short duration (7 days); however, the lack of data supporting its usefulness in the treatment of UTI makes it a poor therapeutic option.

Cornsilk (Zea mays). The use of corn and cornsilk for afflictions of the kidney and bladder can be traced back to the Incas. Parke-Davis introduced a cornsilk product in the 1880s for the treatment of urinary pain and spasm. Physicians of the time believed that cornsilk was useful in the treatment of minor urinary complaints, although many debated whether it was more of a urinary demulcent than diuretic. Although some older data supported a diuretic activity, more contemporary research failed to find any significant diuretic activity when the aqueous extract given in oral dosages of 5 g/kg to guinea pigs[48]; nor did it increase 12- to 24-hour urine output in dogs.[49] The *British Herbal Compendium* lists cornsilk as both a mild diuretic and a urinary demulcent. The German Commission E also recognizes the use of cornsilk as a mild diuretic. Cornsilk is quite safe and is often included in herbal formulas designed to ease the pain of cystitis. No contraindications are found in the literature.

Dandelion (Taraxacum officinale). The diuretic activity of dandelion has been recognized for many centuries, hence its old common names urinaria and piss-a-bed.[50] The root and leaf were used as bitter stomachics and cholagogue. The German Commission E, *British Herbal Compendium*, and French authorities all recognize dandelion as a diuretic. Diuretic activity, which has been documented in animals,[51] is believed to be due to the high potassium content of the herb.

Dandelion is extremely safe; its leaves have been used as salad greens for millennia. However, many authorities consider the use of dandelion contraindicated in the presence of obstruction of the bile duct, gallbladder empyema, and ileus because of the cholagogic and choleretic effects of the herb.[42]

Goldenseal (Hydrastis canadensis). Goldenseal is one of the top 20–selling herbs in the United States, in spite of the fact that no clinical trials of this indigenous plant have been conducted for any medical condition. Research has been directed primarily at the isolated constituent berberine, an alkaloid found in several plants, including goldenseal, barberry (*Berberis vulgaris*), Oregon grape (*Mahonia aquifolium*), and goldthread (*Coptis chinensis*). Antimicrobial activity has been suited for goldenseal extract and the isolated alkaloids berberine, β-hydrastine, canadine, and canadaline.[52] Activity against *S. aureus* and *E. coli* has been documented,[52] and crude methanol extracts of goldenseal root and rhizome have been shown to be very active against multiple strains of *H. pylori*.[53]

The major question about the use of goldenseal for UTI is the extent to which berberine and other alkaloids are absorbed across the intestine. Researchers have postulated that P-glycoprotein contributes to the poor intestinal absorption of berberine and that the use of P-glycoprotein inhibitors might increase its therapeutic utility.[54] A recent study found berberine and several of its metabolites in present urine samples obtained from five volunteers after they took berberine chloride 0.9 g/day orally for 3 days.[55] At this time, the question of absorption of the crude herb remains unanswered. Other constituents of the plant may enhance or inhibit its absorption.

The use of goldenseal is contraindicated during pregnancy by almost all authorities. The 50% lethal dose of berberine in human beings is 27.5 mg/kg.[56] Long-term animal studies noted depression of cardiac function, dilation of blood vessels, stimulation of uterine and intestinal smooth muscle, and respiratory depression with sustained intravenous dosages of 2 mg/kg berberine. Lower dosages caused stimulation of cardiac and respiratory function and depression of intestinal peristalsis.[57] Newall states that overdose of the isolated alkaloids berberine and hydrastine can result in upset stomach, nervousness, depression, convulsions, paralysis, and death from respiratory failure.[58] However, no deaths or severe adverse effects from oral use of goldenseal could be found in the medical literature. Goldenseal contains 2.5% to 6.0% alkaloids, and the recommended dosage is 1 g thrice daily, resulting in a daily dosage of 180 mg berberine or 0.3 mg/kg/day for a 70-kg individual. Although the question of efficacy beyond the gastrointestinal tract remains unanswered, goldenseal appears to be relatively safe when used in otherwise healthy individuals at the recommended dosage.

Summary

Given the vast number of women who experience UTIs and the growing incidence of microbial resistance, the need for appropriately studied alternative options is obvious. Probiotics, cranberry, and blueberry appear to be promising agents for the prevention of

RUTIs; however, the most appropriate dosage, form, and availability of consistent product remain to be determined. Botanicals such as bearberry certainly merit more research, in light of the preliminary data and these herbs' long history of use. The use of acupuncture for a variety of medical problems is growing in the United States and Europe, and rigorous clinical trials are necessary to determine whether it has a role in the prevention of RUTIs. Basic science research is needed to understand the mechanism(s) by which these approaches may work.

The findings of a small number of clinical trials suggest that acupuncture is beneficial in the prevention of RUTI in women,[22] although larger studies are required before formal recommendations can be made.

References

1. Ambulatory care visits to physician offices, hospital outpatient departments, and emergency departments: United States, 1997. Vital and Health Statistics series 13, no. 143. Atlanta, Georgia, November 1999, National Center for Health Statistics, Centers for Disease Control and Prevention, Department of Health and Human Services.
2. Foxman B: Epidemiology of urinary tract infections: incidence, morbidity, and economic costs, *Am J Med* 112:1S-10S, 2002.
3. Foxman B, Barlow R, D'Arcy H, et al: Urinary tract infection: self-reported incidence and associated costs, *Ann Epidemiol* 10:509-515, 2000.
4. Pak J, Pu Y, Zhang ZT, et al: Tamm-Horsfall protein binds to type 1 fimbriated *Escherichia coli* and prevents *E. coli* from binding to uroplakin Ia and Ib receptors. *J Biol Chem* 276:9924-9930, 2001.
5. Nitschke M, Wiehl S, Baer PC, et al: Bactericidal activity of renal tubular cells: the putative role of human beta-defensins, *Exp Nephrol* 10:332-337, 2002.
6. Cunha B: Urinary-tract infections: current issues in diagnosis and treatment, *Antibiotics for Clinicians* 2(suppl 2):3-4, 1998.
7. Kurowski K: The woman with dysuria, *Am Fam Phys* May 1, 1998. Available at: http://www.aafp.org/afp/980501ap/kurowski.html. Accessed April 2004.
8. Hooton TM, Stamm WE: Diagnosis and treatment of uncomplicated urinary tract infection, *Infect Dis Clin North Am* 11:551-581, 1997.
9. Kiel DP, Moskowitz MA: The urinalysis: a critical appraisal, *Med Clin North Am* 71:607-624, 1987.
10. Stamm WE, Hooton TM: Management of urinary tract infections in adults, *N Engl J Med* 329:1328-1334, 1993.
11. Warren JW, Abrutyn E, Hebel JR, et al: Guidelines for antimicrobial treatment of uncomplicated acute bacterial cystitis and acute pyelonephritis in women. *Clin Infect Dis* 29:745-758, 1999.
12. Gupta K: Addressing antibiotic resistance, *Dis Mon* 49:99-110, 2003.
13. Naber CK, Hammer M, Kinzig-Schippers M, et al: Urinary excretion and bactericidal activities of gemifloxacin and ofloxacin after a single oral dose in healthy volunteers, *Antimicrob Agents Chemother* 45:3524-3530, 2001.
14. Schaeffer AJ: The expanding role of fluoroquinolones, *Dis Mon* 49:129-147, 2003.
15. Gendrel D, Chalumeau M, Moulin F, et al: Fluoroquinolones in paediatrics: a risk for the patient or for the community? *Lancet Infect Dis* 3:537-546, 2003.
16. Hooton TM: The current management strategies for community-acquired urinary tract infection, *Infect Dis Clin North Am* 17:303-332, 2003.
17. Nowicki B: Urinary tract infection in pregnant women: old dogmas and current concepts regarding pathogenesis, *Curr Infect Dis Rep* 4:529-535, 2002.
18. Uncu Y, Uncu G, Esmer A, et al: Should asymptomatic bacteriuria be screened in pregnancy? *Clin Exp Obstet Gynecol* 29:281-285, 2002.
19. Gilstrap LC III, Ramin SM: Urinary tract infections during pregnancy, *Obstet Gynecol Clin North Am* 28:581-591, 2001.

20. Locksmith G, Duff P: Infection, antibiotics, and preterm delivery, *Semin Perinatol* 25:295-309, 2001.
21. Kontiokari T, Laitinen J, Jarvi L, et al: Dietary factors protecting women from urinary tract infection, *Am J Clin Nutr* 77:600-604, 2003.
22. Alraek T, Soedal LI, Fagerheim SU, et al: Acupuncture treatment in the prevention of uncomplicated recurrent lower urinary tract infections in adult women, *Am J Public Health* 92:1609-1611, 2002.
23. Reid G: Probiotic therapy and functional foods for prevention of urinary tract infections: state of the art and science, *Curr Infect Dis Rep* 2:518-522, 2000.
24. Baerheim A, Larsen E, Digranes A: Vaginal application of lactobacilli in the prophylaxis of recurrent lower urinary tract infection in women, *Scand J Prim Health Care* 12:239-243, 1994.
25. Kontiokari T, Sundqvist K, Nuutinen M, et al: Randomised trial of cranberry-lingonberry juice and *Lactobacillus GG* drink for the prevention of urinary tract infections in women, *BMJ* 322:1571, 2001.
26. Mastromarino P, Brigidi P, Macchia S, et al: Characterization and selection of vaginal *Lactobacillus* strains for the preparation of vaginal tablets, *J Appl Microbiol* 93:884-893, 2002.
27. Berman S, Spicer D: Safety and reliability of *Lactobacillus* dietary supplements in Seattle, Washington (abstract 37244), American Public Health Association 130th annual meeting. Philadelphia, PA, November 9–13, 2002.
28. Jepson RG, Mihaljevic L, Craig J: Cranberries for preventing urinary tract infections, *Cochrane Database Syst Rev* (3):CD001321, 2001.
29. Nahata MC, Cummins BA, McLeod DC, et al: Effect of urinary acidifiers on formaldehyde concentration and efficacy with methenamine therapy, *Eur J Clin Pharmacol* 22:281-284, 1982.
30. Kessler T, Jansen B, Hesse A: Effect of black currant, cranberry and plum juice consumption on risk factors associated with kidney stone formation, *Eur J Clin Nutr* 56:1020-1023, 2002.
31. Zafriri D, Ofek I, Adar R, et al: Inhibitory activity of cranberry juice on adherence of type 1 and type P fimbriated *Escherichia coli* to eucaryotic cells, *Antimicrob Agents Chemother* 33:92-98, 1989.
32. Sobota AE: Inhibition of bacterial adherence by cranberry juice: potential use for the treatment of urinary tract infection, *J Urol* 131:1013-1016, 1984.
33. Stothers L: A randomized trial to evaluate effectiveness and cost effectiveness of naturopathic cranberry products as prophylaxis against urinary tract infection in women, *Can J Urol* 9:1558-1562, 2002.
34. Bradley PR, editor: *British herbal compendium*, vol 1, Dorset, UK, 1992, British Herbal Medicine Association, pp 211-213.
35. Siegers C, Bodinet C, Ali SS, et al: Bacterial deconjugation of arbutin by Escherichia coli, *Phytomedicine* 10(suppl 4):58-60, 2003.
36. Schindler G, Patzak U, Brinkhaus B, et al: Urinary excretion and metabolism of arbutin after oral administration of *Arctostaphylos uvae ursi* extract as film-coated tablets and aqueous solution in healthy humans, *J Clin Pharmacol* 42:920-927, 2002.
37. *Monographs on the medicinal uses of plant drugs*, fascicule 5, Exeter, UK, 1997, European Scientific Cooperative on Phytotherapy.
38. Larsson B, Jonasson A, Pianu S: Prophylactic effect of UVA E in women with recurrent cystitis: a preliminary report, *Curr Ther Res Clin Exp* 53:441-443, 1993.
39. McGuffin M, Hobbs C, Upton R, et al: *The American Herbal Products Association's botanical safety handbook*, Boca Raton, FL, 1997, CRC Press.
40. Whysner J, Verna L, English JC, et al: Analysis of studies related to tumorigenicity induced by hydroquinone, *Regul Toxicol Pharmacol* 21:158-176, 1995.
41. Smith MT, Zhang L, Jeng M, et al: Hydroquinone, a benzene metabolite, increases the level of aneusomy of chromosomes 7 and 8 in human CD34–positive blood progenitor cells, *Carcinogenesis* 21:485-490, 2000.
42. Blumenthal M, Goldberg A, Brinckmann J, et al, editors: *Herbal medicine: expanded Commission E monographs*, Newton, Massachusetts, 2000, Integrative Medicine Communications, pp 389-393.

43. Paper DH, Koehler J, Franz G: Bioavailability of drug preparations containing a leaf extract of *Arctostaphylos uva ursi (Uvae ursi folium), Planta Med* 59(suppl 7):A589, 1993.
44. Lis-Balchin M, Hart S, Simpson E: Buchu (*Agathosma betulina* and *A. crenulata,* Rutaceae) essential oils: their pharmacological action on guinea-pig ileum and antimicrobial activity on microorganisms, *J Pharm Pharmacol* 53:579-582, 2001.
45. Bradley PR, editor: *British herbal compendium,* vol 1. Dorset, UK, 1992, British Herbal Medicine Association.
46. Khojasteh-Bakht SC, Chen W, Koenigs LL, et al: Metabolism of (R)-(+)-pulegone and (R)-(+)-menthofuran by human liver cytochrome P-450s: evidence for formation of a furan epoxide, *Drug Metab Dispos* 27: 574-580, 1999.
47. Evans WC: *Trease and Evans' pharmacognosy,* ed 14, London, UK, 1996, WB Saunders, p 272.
48. Al-Ali M, Wahbi S, Twaij H, et al: *Tribulus terrestris:* preliminary study of its diuretic and contractile effects and comparison with *Zea mays, J Ethnopharmacol* 85:257-260, 2003.
49. Doan DD, Nguyen NH, Doan HK, et al: Studies on the individual and combined diuretic effects of four Vietnamese traditional herbal remedies (*Zea mays, Imperata cylindrica, Plantago major and Orthosiphon stamineus*), *J Ethnopharmacol* 36:225-231, 1992.
50. Motherby G: *A new medical dictionary; or general repository of physic. Containing an explanation of the terms, and a description of the various particulars relating to anatomy, physiology, physic, surgery, materia medica, chemistry, etc.,* ed 2, London, UK, 1785, Johnson, under Dens Leonis.
51. Racz-Kotilla E: The action of *Taraxacum officinale* extracts on the body weight and diuresis of laboratory animals, *Planta Med* 26:212-217, 1974.
52. Scazzocchio F, Cometa MF, Tomassini L, et al: Antibacterial activity of *Hydrastis canadensis* extract and its major isolated alkaloids, *Planta Med* 67:561-564, 2001.
53. Mahady GB, Pendland SL, Stoia A, et al: In vitro susceptibility of *Helicobacter pylori* to isoquinoline alkaloids from *Sanguinaria canadensis* and *Hydrastis canadensis, Phytother Res* 17:217-221, 2003.
54. Pan GY, Wang GJ, Liu XD, et al: The involvement of P-glycoprotein in berberine absorption, *Pharmacol Toxicol* 91:193-197, 2002.
55. Pan JF, Yu C, Zhu DY, et al: Identification of three sulfate-conjugated metabolites of berberine chloride in healthy volunteers' urine after oral administration, *Acta Pharmacol Sin* 23:77-82, 2002.
56. McGuffin M, Hobbs C, Upton R: *American Herbal Products Association botanical safety handbook,* Boca Raton, Florida, 1997, CRC Press, pp 136-138.
57. Osol A, Farrar GE: *The dispensatory of the United States of America,* ed 25, Philadephia, 1955, Lippincott.
58. Newall CA, Anderson LH, Phillipson JD: *Herbal medicines: a guide for health-care professionals,* London, UK, 1996, Pharmaceutical Press, pp 151-152.

CHAPTER

19

Bone Health and Osteoporosis

Osteoporosis, literally "porous bones," is one of the most common disorders faced by older women in our society today. The National Institutes of Health Development Consensus Panel on Osteoporosis Prevention, Diagnosis, and Therapy states, "Osteoporosis is defined as a skeletal disorder characterized by compromised bone strength predisposing a person to an increased risk of fracture. Bone strength primarily reflects the integration of bone density and bone quality."[1] This panel was formed in response to the significant impact osteoporosis has the health of older Americans (Box 19-1).

Rapid growth in both bone size and strength occurs during childhood, but growth is not complete until an individual is approximately 30 years old. Bone mass attained early in life is perhaps the most important determinant of lifelong skeletal health. After the third decade, bone resorption accelerates, with a loss of 0.5% bone mass per year.[2] At this time, no accurate measure of overall bone strength exists.

Box 19-2 lists the risk factors for osteoporosis that have been identified.[3]

Low bone mass is associated with female sex, advanced age, estrogen deficiency, white race, low weight and body mass index, family history of osteoporosis, smoking, and history of fracture. Consumption of alcohol and caffeine-containing beverages has been inconsistently associated with decreased bone mass.

Box **19-1**

Osteoporosis statistics

- Ten million Americans currently have osteoporosis
- Eighteen million more have low bone mass, which increases the risk of osteoporosis
- One of two American women and one of eight American men will experience an osteoporosis-related fracture in their lifetimes
- Osteoporosis causes 1.5 million fractures each year: 700,000 vertebral, 300,000 of the hip, and 250,000 of the wrist, as well as more than 300,000 other fractures

Box **19-2**

Risk factors for osteoporosis

- History of osteoporosis-related fracture after age 50
- Current low bone mass
- History of osteoporosis-related fracture in a first-degree relative
- Female sex
- Slenderness or small frame
- Advanced age
- Family history of osteoporosis
- Estrogen deficiency as a result of menopause, especially that which begins early or is surgically induced
- Abnormal absence of menstrual periods (amenorrhea)
- Anorexia nervosa
- Low lifetime calcium intake
- Use of certain medications (e.g., corticosteroids, anticonvulsants)
- Low testosterone level (in men)
- Sedentary lifestyle
- Current cigarette smoking
- Excessive use of alcohol
- White or Asian race, although people of African and Hispanic descent are also at significant risk

DIAGNOSIS OF OSTEOPOROSIS

A bone mineral density (BMD) test is generally performed on anyone at high risk for osteoporosis. The dual-energy x-ray absorptiometry (DEXA) scan is regarded as a safe and accurate method for evaluating bone density. The National Osteoporosis Foundation recommends that the following women receive a DEXA:

- Postmenopausal women younger than 65 years with at least one risk factor: oral steroid use, thyroid problems, eating disorders, amenorrhea lasting 3 months or longer, family history of osteoporosis, smoking, alcoholism, very thin frame, low calcium intake
- Postmenopausal women who have sustained a bone fracture
- Any woman older than 65 years
- Premenopausal women with any of these risk factors should seek advice about obtaining a scan.

The World Health Organization has provided guidelines based on bone mass measurements. Osteopenia is defined as a BMD T-score (T-score is the number of standard deviations [SD] above or below the young adult mean) of 1.0 to 2.5 SD below the mean for healthy adults.[4] Osteoporosis is defined as a BMD T-score at least 2.5 SD below the mean. For every SD below normal, the risk of fracture doubles. As with most diagnostic tests, these numbers are part of a continuum, and a T-score of –2.2 SD below the mean should be appropriately addressed to reduce the risk of fracture even if, by strict definition, it does not meet the criteria for the diagnosis of osteoporosis.

TREATMENT
Hormone Replacement Therapy

Bone tissue is quite sensitive to estrogens. It is not entirely understood why women demonstrate accelerated bone loss with menopause; it has been shown that estrogen replacement therapy arrests bone loss.[5] Estrogen's beneficial effect on bone may be due to its ability to increase calcitonin levels, leading to decreased bone resorption. Estrogen receptors are also present on osteoblast bone-forming cells, resulting in a relative increase in collagen production.[6] Mean bone mass is increased by about 5% and bone remodeling is reduced to premenopausal levels with estrogen therapy. This effect persists for the duration of therapy.[7]

Observational and retrospective data suggest a 50% reduction in the incidence of vertebral, hip, and forearm fractures with estrogen replacement therapy.[8] Although researchers have believed for years that estrogen reduces the risk of fractures, it was not until the publication of the Women's Health Initiative (WHI) study that more reliable data were available to support this observation. In this study, the risk of hip and spinal fracture in women who received a combination of conjugated equine estrogen and progestin was reduced by 34%.[9] However, to prevent a fracture, a woman must be willing to accept a greater risk of other diseases, such as heart disease, stroke, and breast cancer, especially because the hormones must be taken for a long period. The unfavorable risk/benefit profile of hormone replacement therapy (HRT) strongly limits its use for prevention of osteoporosis, given that other medications have been shown to reduce the incidence of fractures.[10] The combination therapy used in the WHI was stopped before its completion because of the unacceptable numbers of adverse effects (breast cancer, stroke, blood clots).

The estrogen-only arm of the WHI was designed to determine whether estrogen prevents heart disease in healthy older women. Hip fractures were the major secondary outcome, and breast cancer the major possible risk. When the study was stopped by the NIH in early 2004 because of increased risk of stroke and no effect on heart disease, it also found a decreased risk of hip fracture and no increased breast cancer.[11] Increasing numbers of researchers are exploring the effectiveness of very low-dose estrogen for the reduction of the incidence of fractures in postmenopausal women. The findings of a 3-year randomized, placebo-controlled study of postmenopausal women taking low-dose 17β-estradiol appear promising. Healthy women (n = 167), older than 65 years at the time of enrollment, were randomized to receive either 0.25 mg/day of micronized 17β-estradiol (n = 83) or placebo (n = 84); all women who had not undergone hysterectomy received 100 mg/day of oral micronized progesterone for 2-week periods every 6 months. Mean bone mineral density (BMD) increased at all sites in participants taking low-dose estrogen, compared with placebo ($P < 0.001$). The researchers noted increases in BMD of 2.6% for the femoral neck, 3.6% for the total hip, 2.8% for the spine, and 1.2% for the entire skeleton. The levels of two markers of bone turnover, N-telopeptides of type 1 collagen and bone alkaline phosphatase, decreased significantly ($P < 0.001$) in participants taking low-dose estrogen, whereas concentrations of estradiol, estrone, and sex hormone–binding globulin increased. The adverse effects profiles of the two groups were similar: Specifically, no statistically significant difference was noted with regard to breast tenderness, changes in endometrial thickness or pathologic effects, or annual mammography results.[12] Although this study did not determine whether the incidence of fractures was reduced, the findings are encouraging. It is also interesting to note that oral micronized progesterone was used at 6-month intervals instead of being taken daily or on a monthly basis. If low-dose estrogen can offer protection for the bone, without increased risk of stroke or cancer, this should be more fully explored given the number of baby boomer women who will be confronted with osteoporosis in the near future.

Raloxifene

Raloxifene was the first selective estrogen receptor modulator on the American market. Raloxifene mimics the effects of estrogen on the skeleton and cardiovascular system while functioning as an estrogen antagonist in breast and endometrial tissue. It was approved for the prevention of postmenopausal osteoporosis in 1997 and for the treatment of postmenopausal osteoporosis in 1999. Randomized, placebo-controlled trials in postmenopausal women with osteoporosis have shown that raloxifene increases bone density over 12 to 36 months.

The authors of the Multiple Outcomes of Raloxifene Evaluation (MORE) trial studied the effects of placebo and raloxifene 60 or 120 mg/day in 7705 postmenopausal women with osteoporosis. All women received 500 mg of calcium and 400 to 600 International Units of cholecalciferol daily; follow-up was conducted from 1994 through 1998 at 180 clinical centers in the United States and Europe. Those taking 60 or 120 mg of raloxifene had fewer new fractures (6.6% and 5.4%, respectively) than those taking placebo (10.1%), but the actual incidence of fracture did not differ significantly between treatment groups.[13] No statistically significant difference was observed between the treatment and placebo groups for nonvertebral fractures.

In addition to its effect on bone, raloxifene substantially reduces the risk of estrogen receptor–positive breast cancer. In the MORE study, women taking either dose of raloxifene had 76% fewer breast cancers diagnosed than those women taking the placebo.

The most common adverse effects of raloxifene in clinical trials are hot flashes and leg cramps; the most serious adverse effect is venous thromboembolism. Women in the MORE trial who received raloxifene had three times the number of venous thromboembolism events than those in the placebo group, and the authors estimated that one case would occur for every 155 women treated with raloxifene for 3 years.[14] Women with a history of thromboembolism and those who are at increased risk should not be prescribed raloxifene.

Bisphosphonates

Several antiresorptive agents have been used successfully in the treatment of postmenopausal osteoporosis. Bisphosphonates inhibit bone resorption through their effect on osteoclasts.[15] Recent trials of these agents have revealed evidence of efficacy in the prevention of both vertebral and nonvertebral fractures.

Alendronate (Fosamax), an analogue of pyrophosphate, is adsorbed onto the hydroxyapatite of bone, resulting in the inhibition of bone resorption. It was the first bisphosphonate approved by the U.S. Food and Drug Administration (FDA) for the prevention and treatment of osteoporosis. The Fracture Intervention Trial, a randomized, placebo-controlled trial involving 6459 postmenopausal women with low femoral neck BMD, demonstrated an approximate 50% decrease in the risk of new vertebral, hip, and wrist fractures in women who reported at least one preexisting vertebral fracture at baseline.[16] In this study, women received supplemental calcium and vitamin D if their dietary intake was insufficient. The daily alendronate dose was 5 mg during the first 2 years and 10 mg during the third and fourth years of the study. In addition to fracture reduction, a small increase in BMD (4% to 8%) was noted.

Risedronate is the second bisphosphonate approved for use in osteoporosis. Data from the Vertebral Efficacy with Risedronate trial (2458 patients) showed a 41% reduction in the incidence of new vertebral fractures and a 39% reduction in the incidence of non-vertebral fractures with a dose of 5 mg/d.[17] In a study of 5445 women ages 70 to 79 years with documented low BMD, a significant reduction in the incidence of hip fracture was documented.[18]

Alendronate and risedronate are good alternatives for women with osteoporosis or those who are at high risk. Patients should be encouraged to take the medication with a full 8 oz of water, while sitting upright, first thing in the morning, 30 minutes before breakfast, to enhance absorption and reduce esophageal irritation, which is the drug's main side effect. The FDA has approved alendronate 5 mg/day and 35 mg once weekly for the prevention of osteoporosis; the treatment dosage is 10 mg/day or 70 mg once weekly. The FDA has also approved risedronate for the prevention and treatment of osteoporosis. Both the 5 mg/day and weekly 35-mg dosing regimens are available.

Calcitonin

Calcitonin, a naturally occurring peptide hormone, inhibits osteoclast activity and thereby acts as an antiresorptive agent. Calcitonin receptors have been found on osteoblasts and renal cell membranes. Stimulation of these receptors results in a decrease in osteoclast activity and may cause an increase in the production of 1,25-dihydroxyvitamin D with a secondary increase in intestinal calcium absorption. Because it is a polypeptide, calcitonin is not effective when taken by mouth and was initially given by injection. The FDA approved nasal formulations of synthetic salmon calcitonin for the treatment of osteoporosis in women in 1995. Calcitonin inhibits bone resorption and increases BMD in the spine, reducing the incidence of recurrent vertebral fractures by 60% to 66%.[19] One epidemiologic study showed a 31% reduction in the incidence of hip fracture[20]; however, randomized clinical trials have shown little effect on bone density of the femoral neck. A 5-year study revealed that although nasal calcitonin 200 International Units/day only increased spinal BMD by 1.2%, the risk of new vertebral fracture was reduced by 36% compared with patients who received only calcium and vitamin D supplementation.[21] Evidence is accruing to suggest that calcitonin has inherent analgesic properties, making it beneficial for those with osteoporotic vertebral fractures.[22] Women with established osteoporosis and back pain generally experience a decline in back pain and an increase in mobility during the first 6 months of treatment.

The currently available nasal formulation of calcitonin provides a dose of 200 Units, which is to be sprayed in alternating nostrils once per day. Nasal calcitonin is well tolerated; the most common side effects are gastrointestinal upset, facial flushing, rash, and dry nasal mucosa. Flushing and nausea are more closely associated with parenteral administration, but they also occur with larger dosages (400 Units/day) of the intranasal formulation.

Diet and Nutrition

Role of dietary protein. Contrary to popular belief, protein does not reduce bone density, and adequate amounts of protein are needed, as part of a balanced diet, for maintenance of bone health. A 4-year study involving 572 women and 388 men ages 55 to 92 years found that for every 15 g/day of protein consumption, BMD increased by 0.016 g/cm^3 at the hip (P = .005), 0.012 g/cm^3 (P = .005) at the femoral neck, and 0.015 g/cm^3 at the spine (P = .04). The investigators found a negative association between vegetable protein intake and BMD. The association between animal protein intake and increased BMD was statistically significant among the women in the study.[23] Another randomized, controlled study, this one 3 years long, of 342 healthy men and women revealed that BMD was increased with higher protein intake.[24] The negative association between vegetable-protein intake and BMD is interesting, given the research with soy, a rich source of vegetable protein in numerous cultures, and its beneficial effect on bone.

Phytoestrogens. Phytoestrogens, natural plant substances, are broken down into four main classes: phenolic, steroidal, saponin, and terpenoid. Phenolic phytoestrogens, found in the majority of vegetables, fruits, and some grains, are the most heavily researched group. There are seven subfamilies of phenolic phytoestrogens: isoflavones, coumestans, flavones, flavonols, flavonones, lignans, and chalcones. Isoflavones are found mainly in soybeans, chickpeas, and other legumes; lignans are present in cereal bran, seed oils (especially flax), legumes, and some alcohols (beer and bourbon).

Phytoestrogens in the diet may play a role in the modulation of hormone-related diseases, judging from their structural similarity to 17β-estradiol and the weak estrogen/antiestrogen tamoxifen. The presence and position of the hydroxyl groups are considered essential for estrogenic activity.[25] Asian populations with low rates of breast and prostate cancer consume 20 to 80 mg/day genistein, an isoflavone present in many plants, almost entirely derived from soy. Soy is a common source of nutrition in China and a primary source of protein. Dietary intake of genistein in the United States has been estimated to range from 1 to 3 mg/day.[34]

A great deal of research has been conducted on soy, which is a particularly rich source of isoflavones and the major dietary source of phytoestrogens in many populations. Soy is consumed in a variety of forms, including soybeans, tempeh, soy milk, tofu, and soy protein. Foods that were once found only in health food stores, such as soy hot dogs, soy cheese, and soy yogurt, can now be purchased in many mainstream grocery stores. The amount of isoflavones in these soy foods varies considerably, depending on the amount and type of processing they undergo. Soy protein, primarily in the form of nontoasted, defatted soybean flakes, can be isolated from the whole bean and contains up to 50% of the phytoestrogens found in unprocessed soybeans.[25]

A growing body of data suggests that soy consumption has a modest effect on some menopausal symptoms such as hot flashes and night sweats. However, few human clinical trials have been conducted to address the question of whether the consumption of soy or isolated soy isoflavones such as genistein can prevent or ameliorate osteoporosis. Data from in vitro and animal studies modeling postmenopausal osteoporosis demonstrate a significant bone-sparing effect of the soy isoflavones genistein and daidzein (these isoflavones are also present in red clover extract, another popular menopause remedy).

A review of in vitro studies of cultured bone cells, 24 in vivo studies of animal models for postmenopausal osteoporosis, 15 human observational or epidemiologic studies, and 17 dietary intervention studies that focused specifically on the potential influence of phytoestrogens on bone suggest that diets rich in phytoestrogens have bone-sparing effects in the long term.[26] The authors noted that the magnitude of the effect and the exact mechanism(s) of action are speculative or unknown.

Although promising, the data are far from conclusive. Most studies have been of short duration and have involved relatively small sample sizes, making the observation of significant and accurate changes in bone difficult. Intake of soy protein and isoflavones varies, and the optimal isoflavone intake for bone-sparing effects is not known.[27] No studies have been conducted to determine the effects of phytoestrogens on fracture rate. Methodologically rigorous prospective human clinical trials of longer duration are needed for the accurate assessment of the role of phytoestrogens in the prevention and treatment of osteoporosis. However, considering the safety and other beneficial health effects of soy, until more definitive recommendations can be made, it seems reasonable for women to add these foods to their diets if they enjoy them.

Ipriflavone. Ipriflavone, a synthetic derivative of naturally occurring isoflavones, is sold as a dietary supplement in the United States and is commonly recommended by practitioners of integrative medicine for the treatment of osteoporosis and its prevention in those at high risk. Ipriflavone is thought to inhibit osteoclast activity through modulation of intracellular free calcium[28] while stimulating maturation of osteoblasts.[29] More than 60 studies have evaluated the effectiveness of ipriflavone for both the treatment and prevention of osteoporosis. As of 1997, 2769 patients had been treated for a total of 3132 patient years.[30] Five of seven placebo-controlled trials showed that ipriflavone maintains BMD in the spine or distal radius. Two small trials showed an increase in BMD of the distal radius and a reduction in the incidence of spinal fractures. Two problems arise when evaluating most ipriflavone studies. The first is a problem found in many studies of osteoporosis treatments: Fracture is not an endpoint. The second problem is that different BMD measurement techniques were used at different anatomic sites, making comparison difficult.

The largest ipriflavone trial to date is the Ipriflavone Multicenter European Fracture Study, a prospective, randomized, double-blind, placebo-controlled 4-year study conducted in 4 centers in Belgium, Denmark, and Italy between August 1994 and July 1998.[31] Four hundred seventy-four postmenopausal white women, ages 45 to 75 years, with low BMD were randomly assigned to receive ipriflavone 200 mg (n = 234) or matching placebo (n = 240) three times per day; all received 500 mg/day calcium. The primary outcome measure was reduction in fracture incidence. During the study period, no difference was noted in the occurrence of vertebral fractures among women taking ipriflavone compared with those taking placebo. However, only a small number of women in the ipriflavone group sustained vertebral fractures during the 36-month follow-up. One concerning adverse effect noted in this study was significant lymphopenia, which developed in 29 of the 237 women receiving ipriflavone.

Questions have been raised regarding the safety of long-term ipriflavone treatment on breast and uterine tissue. Is ipriflavone estrogenic? Few data exist on this topic at this time. Fifteen postmenopausal women were given 600 or 1000 mg/day ipriflavone or placebo and then evaluated for changes in serum levels of luteinizing hormone, follicle-stimulating hormone, prolactin, and estradiol. No differences were found between the ipriflavone and placebo groups after a single oral dose of 600 or 1000 mg ipriflavone or after 7, 14, or 21 days of treatment.[32] Another study showed that after 21 days of treatment with ipriflavone (600 mg/d), conjugated estrogen (0.625 mg/day), or placebo, vaginal cytologic findings were unchanged in the groups receiving placebo and ipriflavone, compared with a considerable increase in superficial vaginal cells in the group receiving estrogen.[32] Animal studies have shown that ipriflavone inhibits bone resorption in a manner similar to that of estrogen but without uterotropic effects.[33]

Excluding the Ipriflavone Multicenter European Fracture Study, pooled results from 2769 patients participating in small clinical trials revealed adverse effects in 14.5% of patients receiving ipriflavone and in 16.1% of women taking placebo.[31] Complaints in both groups were primarily gastrointestinal: heartburn, vomiting, abdominal pain, constipation, and diarrhea. The largest study, the Ipriflavone Multicenter European Fracture Study, revealed a significant incidence of lymphopenia in the group receiving ipriflavone, compared with placebo.[31] In most cases lymphopenia resolved within 12 to 24 months of discontinuation of the supplement. Dosage reduction is recommended in patients with renal insufficiency. Those with a creatinine clearance of 40 to 80 mL/min should reduce the dosage to 400 mg/d; those with creatinine clearance of less than 40 mL/min should reduce the dosage to 200 mg/day.[34] Reduced theophylline metabolism and elimination were observed in a theophylline-treated patient during ipriflavone administration. After the withdrawal of ipriflavone, the serum theophylline concentration returned to its previous level.[35] In vitro studies indicate a possible inhibitory effect on cytochrome P-450 enzymes.[35]

On the basis of the totality of evidence, ipriflavone (200 mg 3 times daily) may be beneficial in maintaining BMD of the spine in postmenopausal women, although the findings of the largest study to date do not demonstrate a reduction in the incidence of vertebral fractures, at least during the study period. If a patient wishes to use the supplement, monitoring the white blood cell count seems prudent.

Calcium. Calcium intake is positively correlated with bone mass at all ages. A review of 15 trials (comprising 1806 patients) of postmenopausal women randomized to receive calcium supplementation or their usual dietary calcium intake for at least 1 year with recording of BMD of the total body, vertebral spine, hip, or forearm, or the number of fractures, found calcium to be more effective than placebo in reducing the rate of bone loss after 2 or more years of treatment.[36] The data show a trend toward a reduction in the incidence of vertebral fractures but do not meaningfully address the possible effect of calcium on reduction of the incidence of nonvertebral fractures.

Multiple surveys have demonstrated that Americans do not get adequate calcium in their diets, and concern that adolescents are not receiving enough to attain peak bone mass in adulthood is growing. Although calcium intakes of 800 mg/day in children ages 3 to 8 years and 1300 mg/day in children and adolescents ages 9 to 17 years are recommended, only 25% of boys and 10% of girls ages 9 to 17 are estimated to meet this level. Numerous factors contribute to low calcium intake in this population, including restricted intake of dairy products, low consumption of dark green vegetables, and a low intake of calcium-fortified juices in combination with a high intake of low-calcium beverages such as soda. It is not just the young who fail to get enough calcium. In the United States, more than two thirds of women between the ages of 18 and 30 take in less than 800 mg/day calcium, and 75% of women over the age of 35 fail to meet the recommended daily allowance (RDA). The National Health and Nutrition Examination Survey II study found that 50% of older adults consume less than 800 mg of calcium each day.[37] It was noted that in China, where historically no dairy industry exists, calcium intake must come from other dietary sources.

In 1993, the FDA allowed foods and supplements containing at least 200 mg of calcium per serving to include a calcium/osteoporosis health claim on their labels.[38] Low-fat dairy products, tofu, and dark green vegetables are natural sources of calcium, and calcium-fortified foods such as fruit juices, bread, rice, and breakfast cereals can help augment the diet. If the diet is inadequate, however, calcium supplementation should be recommended.

Calcium supplements are available in a variety of forms, including carbonate, gluconate, lactate, phosphate, citrate, malate, and aspartate formulations (Figure 19-1). The bioavailability of calcium supplements differs among preparations because of the low aqueous solubility of some calcium salts (carbonate and phosphate) and the ability of some anionic components (citrate) to form soluble complexes with calcium.[39] Except at high doses, all calcium salts dissolve and become bioavailable in the presence of gastric acid. However, the production of stomach acid is often reduced in older people, individuals with achlorhydria, and patients taking antiulcer medications. The bioavailability of calcium carbonate may be reduced in these individuals as a result of incomplete dissolution.[40]

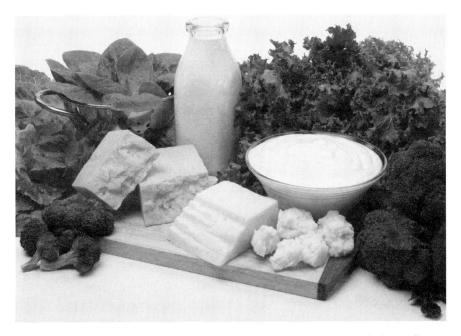

Figure 19-1 Women can find calcium in a variety of foods, including milk (preferably skim), tofu, and yogurt.

Calcium carbonate should be taken with food to improve dissolution and bioavailability. If intestinal colic or constipation occurs, calcium citrate is a useful alternative. Calcium citrate provides excellent calcium bioavailability as a result of its relatively high aqueous solubility. It carries a lower risk of kidney stones than do other calcium supplements and is absorbed well by individuals with digestive disorders.

Absorption of calcium can be affected by a variety of factors. Foods rich in oxalate (spinach, rhubarb, nuts, brewed tea) or phytate (whole wheat) may decrease calcium absorption. Iron absorption is decreased by as much as 50% by some forms of calcium supplementation. Calcium citrate and ascorbic acid enhance iron absorption. Absorption of calcium supplements is most efficient at doses of 500 mg or less.

Dietary constituents, hormones, drugs, age, and genetic factors influence the amount of calcium required for an individual's optimal skeletal health. Guidelines published by the National Osteoporosis Foundation (1999)[41] and the National Institutes of Health Consensus Development Panel on Osteoporosis (2000)[42] recommend 1200 to 1500 mg of elemental calcium and 400 to 800 International Units of vitamin D daily, consumed through a combination of diet and supplementation (Table 19-1).

Table **19-1**

Optimal calcium intake

GROUP	OPTIMAL DAILY INTAKE (mg)
Infant	
Birth-6 mo	400
6 mo-1 yr	600
Children	
1-5 yr	800
6-10 yr	800-1200
Adolescents/Young Adults	
11-24 yr	1200-1500
Men	
25-65 yr	1000
>65 yr	1500
Women	
25-50 yr	1000
>50 yr (postmenopausal)	1500
Those taking estrogens	1000
Those not taking estrogens	1500
>65 yr	1500
Pregnant and nursing	1200-1500

From Brown JP, Josse RG: Scientific Advisory Council of the Osteoporosis Society of Canada. 2002 clinical practice guidelines for the diagnosis and management of osteoporosis in Canada, *CMAJ* 167(suppl 10): S1-S34, 2002.

In conclusion, a lifetime of adequate calcium intake decreases menopause-related bone loss and reduces the incidence of vertebral, and possibly nonvertebral, fractures. Calcium supplementation should be recommended to individuals who do not obtain enough in their diet, which appears to be the majority of Americans. Most experts agree that calcium and vitamin D should not be used as the sole treatment of osteoporosis, but that these nutrients are essential adjuncts to osteoporosis treatment.[43] And they are key tools in prevention.

Vitamin D. Low levels of the activated form of vitamin D are common in the aging population. The vitamin D metabolite calcitriol (1,25-dihydroxyvitamin D) is reportedly decreased in elderly patients, making the need for adequate vitamin D intake or supplementation imperative for women as they age.[44] Significant reductions in hip and other nonvertebral fractures have been observed in patients given calcium and vitamin D_3 in prospective trials. A study of 3270 mobile elderly women living in 180 nursing homes who were assigned to receive placebo or 1200 mg/day elemental calcium in the form of tricalcium phosphate together with 800 International Units/day cholecalciferol (vitamin D_3) revealed a reduction in the rate of incidence of hip fractures. In the 36-month analysis, 138 hip fractures occurred among the 1176 women receiving supplementation; 184 fractures occurred among the 1127 women in the placebo group. The mean duration of treatment was 625.4 days. Adjusted to 1000 women, calcium and vitamin D_3 supplementation prevented 46 hip fractures.[45]

Studies in which only vitamin D_3 was administered have not shown the same benefit. A trial of 2578 elderly men and women receiving 400 International Units/day vitamin D_3 or placebo revealed no protective effect over a 3-year period.[46] Cochrane reviewers concluded that the administration of vitamin D_3 alone, without calcium supplementation, is not associated with any reduction in incidence of hip fracture (relative risk [RR] 1.20, 95% confidence interval [CI] 0.83-1.75) or other nonvertebral fracture. However, the reviewers also found that administration of vitamin D_3 together with calcium supplementation to frail older people in nursing home facilities was associated with significant reduction in the incidence of hip fracture.[47]

Dietary sources of vitamin D are limited. Milk is the most common vitamin D–containing food consumed in the United States. Fish liver oil provides significant amounts of vitamin D in some populations. The majority of vitamin D is obtained through skin exposure to sunlight. The amount of vitamin D produced by the body depends on a variety of factors, including duration of exposure, time of day, season, latitude, and an individual's skin pigmentation. In general, 10 to 15 minutes' exposure of the hands, arms, and face two or three times a week is enough to meet the body's vitamin D requirement. Sunscreen agents dramatically decrease the body's absorption of vitamin D.[48] Although the use of sunscreen is recommended in all age groups for the prevention of skin cancer, patients should also be made aware of the need for some sun exposure to obtain adequate levels of vitamin D.

In conclusion, evidence indicates that calcium and vitamin D are best taken in combination. For some women, especially those who live in northern climates, it may not be possible to obtain adequate amounts of vitamin D through sun exposure. Many experts are recommending 800 International Units/day vitamin D supplementation for postmenopausal women and for everyone over the age of 65.

Vitamin K. Vitamin K occurs naturally in two forms: vitamin K_1 (phylloquinone), which is found in plants; and vitamin K_2 (menaquinone), which is found in meats, cheeses, and fermented products. The K vitamins, a group of napthoquinones, are important in the maintenance of healthy bones. These vitamins are required for the carboxylation of several bone proteins, including the bone matrix protein osteocalcin. High serum concentrations of undercarboxylated osteocalcin and low serum concentrations of vitamin K are associated with lower BMD and increased risk of hip fracture. The Institute of Medicine recently increased the dietary reference intakes of vitamin K to 90 µg/day for adult females and 120 µg/day for adult males, an increase of approximately 50% from previous recommendations.[49]

Epidemiologic studies suggest an association between low vitamin K intake and enhanced risk of osteoporotic fracture. Circulating levels of vitamin K are lower in patients with hip fractures compared with those in controls, and observational studies show that high levels of dietary vitamin K are associated with a lower risk of hip fracture.[50,51] In a 10-year prospective study of women ages 38 to 74 years, an inverse association between dietary vitamin K and the risk of hip fracture was observed.[50] However, this study failed to show a decline in fracture risk with higher vitamin K intake.

Clinical trial data are conflicting with regard to the role of dietary vitamin K intake and BMD. BMD was measured in the hip and spine in 1112 men and 1479 women (age 59 ± 9 years) who participated in the Framingham Heart Study (1996-2000).[52] Dietary and supplemental intake of vitamin K was assessed by a food frequency questionnaire. Additional covariates included age, BMI, smoking status, alcohol use, and physical activity score, as well as menopausal status and current estrogen use among the women. The researchers found that women in the lowest quartile of vitamin K intake (70.2 µg/day) had significantly ($P \leq 0.005$) lower BMD at the femoral neck and spine than did those in the highest quartile of vitamin K intake (309 µg/day). These associations remained after potential confounders were controlled for and after stratification on the basis of age or supplement use. No significant association was found between dietary vitamin K intake and BMD in men. This finding is in contrast to another study in which vitamin K intake was assessed with the use of a food frequency questionnaire in 335 men and 553 women (average age 75.2 years) participating in the Framingham Heart Study in 1988-1989. No association was found between vitamin K intake and BMD in men or women, although the incidence of hip fractures was increased in those in the lowest quartile of vitamin K intake (median 56 µg/day).[53]

In contrast to dietary intake of vitamin K, therapy with very high pharmacologic dosages of vitamin K_2, menatetrenone, has been used to prevent further bone mineral loss and fracture in patients with osteoporosis.[54] Larger, more rigorous studies are needed to determine the absolute risk reduction with the use of menatetrenone for the prevention and treatment of osteoporosis. This product is not available as a dietary supplement in the United States.

On the basis of the data assembled to date, providers should encourage patients to consume healthy amounts of green leafy vegetables and fermented dairy products to achieve adequate dietary levels of vitamin K in their diets.

Fluoride. A meta-analysis of 11 studies examined the efficacy of fluoride therapy on bone loss and vertebral and nonvertebral fractures in postmenopausal women.[55] The duration of treatment varied, and different pharmacologic preparations of fluoride were used, though when viewed in totality, an increase in lumbar spine BMD of 8.1% (95% CI 7.15%-9.09%) after 2 years and 16.1% (95% CI 14.65%-17.5%) after 4 years was demonstrated. The relative risk (RR) for new vertebral fractures was not significant at 2 or 4 years. The RR for new nonvertebral fractures was not significant at 2 years but was significant at 4 years (RR 1.85; 95% CI 1.36%-2.5%) when used at high dosages in a slow-release form.

The toxic effects of fluoride are dose-related, and the prevalence of adverse effects among pharmacologic preparations. Toxicity is particularly associated with plain fluoride and monofluorophosphate; both these formulations can cause gastrointestinal and skeletal side effects. Far fewer gastrointestinal side effects were associated with enteric-coated and slow-release preparations.[43]

Toxicity and adverse effects of fluoride are dose related. Toxicity is particularly associated with plain fluoride and monofluorophosphate; both formulations can cause gastrointestinal and skeletal side effects. Fewer gastrointestinal side effects are associated with enteric-coated and slow-release preparations.[43]

Other micronutrients. The roles of magnesium, zinc, boron, vitamin C, copper, and other micronutrients in bone health are not fully understood. Most research to date has been focused on calcium, with and without vitamin D. Micronutrients are essential to the maintenance of healthy bones. Understanding relationships between and among nutrients beyond calcium and vitamin D may provide important new information for the design and enhancement of therapies to preserve bone density and quality.[56]

Magnesium. When magnesium intake is low, calcium absorption is impaired.[57] Magnesium depletion reduces the sensitivity of the kidneys to parathyroid hormone and reduces the activation of vitamin D[58] and is associated with abnormal calcification of the bone.[59] Animal data demonstrate a profound effect of magnesium depletion on bone, characterized by impaired bone growth, decreased osteoblast numbers, increased osteoclast numbers in young animals, and loss of trabecular bone.[60] Supplementation with magnesium (250 to 750 mg/day) increased bone density and reduced the incidence of fracture in a small 2-year open study of 31 postmenopausal women with documented osteoporosis.[61]

More research is needed to accurately determine the role and optimal dose of magnesium for the prevention of postmenopausal osteoporosis before formal recommendations can be made. Until this information is available, providers should ensure that women are meeting the recommending daily intake for magnesium through diet, supplementation, or both.

The RDA is 280 mg/day for adult women and 350 mg/day for adult men. The average intake for most Americans is 140 to 260 mg/day. Foods high in magnesium include wheat bran, wheat germ, almonds, cashews, Brazil nuts, hazelnuts, peanuts, pecans, walnuts, millet, wheat grain, rye, tofu, and beet greens. Large doses of magnesium cause gastrointestinal upset and diarrhea.

Trace minerals. Manganese, copper, and zinc are important cofactors in enzymatic processes involved in the synthesis of various constituents of bone. Manganese deficiency is known to cause a reduction in the amount of calcium laid down in the bone, thus increasing the risk for fracture.[62] Zinc enhances the activity of vitamin D and is required for the formation of both osteoblasts and osteoclasts. Low serum and bone levels of zinc have been found in elderly people with osteoporosis.[63] Copper deficiency may play a role in the development of osteoporosis.

Rats fed a copper-deficient diet were noted to have reduced BMD and strength.[64] A randomized, placebo-controlled study of 73 women (ages 45 to 56 years) who received 3 mg/day copper or placebo for 2 years found those who took copper supplementation lost an average of 0.64% of their bone density, compared with 6.2% among women in the placebo.[65]

One randomized, placebo-controlled study of trace mineral supplementation in 1137 postmenopausal women was published in 1993. Women received one of four treatments for 2 years:

- 1000 mg/day calcium citrate or malate
- 1000 mg/day calcium citrate or malate plus 15 mg zinc, 5 mg manganese, and 2.5 mg copper
- 15 mg/day zinc, 5 mg/day manganese, and 2.5 mg/day copper
- Placebo

Bone loss in the lumbar spine was measured over a 2-year period. The changes in BMD were as follows: placebo, −2.23%; trace minerals, −1.66%; calcium, −0.50%; and calcium plus trace minerals, +1.28%.[66] These findings suggest a role for trace minerals in the prevention of osteoporosis.

Practitioners should recommend a daily multivitamin/mineral supplement that contains the RDA for zinc, manganese, and copper to ensure adequate intake of these nutrients.

Botanical remedies. A number of herbs are promoted for "bone health" and osteoporosis. Most of these herbal products contain horsetail (*Equisetum arvense*), oatstraw (*Avena sativa*), and nettle (*Urtica dioica*). Herbalists sometimes recommend herbs rich in silica to speed the healing of broken bones and also to prevent or treat osteoporosis. *Silica* refers to naturally occurring materials, mainly silicon dioxide. Horsetail is a rich source of silica and has a strong historical reputation for strengthening the bones. Virtually no research has been conducted to assess the efficacy of this use of horsetail, although supplementation with 500 mg/kg silicon in feed has been shown to prevent the loss of bone mass and reduction in bone growth induced by ovariectomy in weanling rats.[67] The authors of this study suggest that at sufficient dosages, silicon may both inhibit bone resorption and stimulate bone formation. Oats are also a rich source of silica. One would likely be better served by eating a daily bowl of oatmeal porridge than by taking oatstraw in capsule form. Nettles have been consumed as a nutritious form of greens for millennia and are still recommended for "tonic" purposes by herbalists throughout Europe and the United States. Nettle contains calcium, as well as other important nutrients in varying amounts, and can be considered a useful green for the diet; however, calcium supplements provide a more reliable source when the diet is inadequate.

Black cohosh (*Cimicifuga racemosa*) is often recommended for menopausal women who are experiencing hot flashes and night sweats (see Chapter 6). Interest in the herb as a selective estrogen receptor modulator has been growing, and some researchers are exploring whether the herb has any beneficial effect on bone. An animal study demonstrated that an extract of *C. racemosa* (BNO 1055) reduced the loss of BMD in ovariectomized rats.[68] Hydrophilic and lipophilic extracts of *C. heracleifolia* and *C. foetida* have demonstrated inhibition of parathyroid-induced bone resorption in vitro and in ovariectomized rats.[69] It is unclear whether this effect is due to an estrogenic effect, an inhibition of parathyroid hormone, or direct inhibition of bone turnover.

Several Chinese herbs, such as bu gu zhi (*Psoralea corylifolia*, are being studied for the treatment of osteoporosis.[67] At the time of this writing, we have been unable to obtain any detailed information on these Chinese herbs in English, so further comment is not possible.

At this time, no herbs have been clinically shown to effectively treat osteoporosis or prevent bone loss.[70]

Progesterone Cream

Progesterone cream has been heavily touted and marketed for both the prevention and treatment of osteoporosis. Many quote the work of John Lee, MD, and his use of topical progesterone cream for the treatment of osteoporosis. Lee describes an unselected case series of 100 postmenopausal women (ages 38 to 83 years) who were prescribed a 3% progesterone cream, which was applied for 12 consecutive nights each month. Total dose was one half to one third of an ounce of cream per month. The cream was applied to the neck, face, or under the arms; sites of application were rotated. Women were given strict dietary instructions, including an increase in green vegetable intake, avoidance of all carbonated beverages, limitation of alcohol intake, and reduction of red meat consumption to three or fewer times per week. The following supplements were also prescribed: 400 International Units/day vitamin D, 2000 mg/day vitamin C, 25,000 International Units/day β-carotene, and 800 to 1000 mg/day calcium. Conjugated estrogens (0.3 or 0.625 mg/day) were taken for 3 weeks each month unless contraindicated. Women were prescribed exercise for 20 minutes per day or 30 minutes three times a week. Serial bone density assessments were performed at 6- to 12-month intervals. Sixty-three of the 100 women underwent dual-photon absorptimetry. Lee reported an overall increase of more than 15% in BMD over a 3-year period. In one 74-year-old woman, endometrial carcinoma developed.[71]

Problems with this case series include a lack of a placebo arm or control group. Women were prescribed dietary supplements, exercise, and dietary changes, and some were taking estrogen. Patients were not broken down by menopause status, age, risk factors, or diagnosis of osteoporosis in any of the bone density reports. No attempts to record subjects' compliance with dietary, smoking cessation, or exercise prescriptions are included. Little can be concluded from this report about the relationship between progesterone cream and bone density. The development of endometrial carcinoma in one patient raises the question of the safety of using topical creams with exogenous HRT, as a number of women were taking conjugated estrogen with no oral progestogen. A study by Wren et al revealed that progesterone creams providing as much as 64 mg/day, applied on days 15 through 28 for three cycles, failed to achieve a secretory change in proliferative endometrium among 28 women using continuous transdermal estrogen.[72]

A 1999 study addressed the question of bone density and topical progesterone cream. A randomized, placebo-controlled trial was conducted with 102 healthy postmenopausal women who had not taken HRT for at least 1 year. They were given a quarter teaspoon of cream containing 20 mg of progesterone or placebo, to be applied once a day. All women were given multivitamins at 1200 mg/day. The women were evaluated every 4 months for 1 year. BMD (as assessed with the use of DEXA), lipid profiles, and symptoms were followed. No significant difference was found between the treatment and control groups with respect to BMD of the spine and hip.[73]

To date, there is no solid evidence that topical progesterone creams offer protection against bone loss. Progestrone cream should not be relied on to protect the endometrium when oral estrogens are being used.

Exercise and Risk Reduction

Convincing evidence indicates that exercise in elders improves overall function and delays loss of independence, thereby enhancing quality of life. A 1999 meta-analysis of clinical trials of exercise in pre- and postmenopausal women concluded that physical activity prevented or reversed almost 1% of bone loss per year in both the lumbar spine and femoral neck.[74] Another meta-analysis revealed even greater benefit of physical activity, particularly impact exercise, on the spine.[75] BMD of the hip may also benefit from impact exercise, but the effect of nonimpact exercises on hip BMD is not known.[76] Randomized clinical trials of exercise have shown that regular exercise can reduce the risk of falls by approximately 25%. Even in the presence of these data, sadly, exercise is generally low on the list of recommendations made by health care providers when discussing bone health with older individuals.

Tai chi. One type of exercise might be extremely well received by older women: *tai chi*, a meditative, low-impact exercise regimen that has been practiced in Asia for the past 2000 years. It is still common to see elders doing *tai chi* in parks throughout cities of China and Southeast Asia. This "soft" martial art is becoming more popular in the United States as Americans seek exercise routines that both relax and promote strength. The findings of a case-control study suggest that regular *tai chi* exercise helps retard bone loss in the weight-bearing bones of postmenopausal women.[77] A 3-month regimen of twice-weekly 30-minute *tai chi* classes was associated with statistically significant improvements in balance and functional mobility and a reduction in the fear of falling among a sample of older women living in retirement communities.[78] Older women with osteoarthritis who performed *tai chi* exercises for 12 weeks noted a reduction in their arthritis symptoms and improvement in their balance and physical function. In light of the fact that many enjoy this inexpensive, safe, and beneficial exercise, greater emphasis might be placed on offering *tai chi* classes in senior centers around the country.

TOP REASON TO EXERCISE FOR HEALTHY BONES

Among women, bone building peaks during the third decade. Bone density gradually drops off during the thirties and forties, with a sharper loss occurring after menopause. Maintenance of healthy bones is important in preventing osteoporosis, a condition that increases the risk of broken bones. When comparing women assigned to perform either a daily stretching routine or a program of cardiocircuit–weight training, researchers found at the end of 2 years that the women in the cardio–weight training group had a dramatic increase in bone density compared with those performing the stretching regimen. Even though both groups took calcium supplements, only those women who lifted weights had a significant increase in bone density. Weight training gives definition to muscle, increases strength, and revs up the metabolism.

GENERAL RECOMMENDATIONS FOR AVOIDING FRACTURES

Patients should be encouraged to perform appropriate exercise, and information on injury prevention and home safety should be provided. Loose rugs should be removed, adequate lighting should be placed in dark areas and stairways, bathtubs should have safety rails, and floors kept free of clutter to minimize the risks of falls and the fractures that can result. Eliminate or avoid low-built chairs and couches which may cause hips to twist, stress, and break when getting up or sitting down.

SUMMARY

A balanced diet that provides adequate calories and appropriate nutrients is the foundation for the healthy development of all tissues, including bone. An integrated approach that addresses lifestyle, exercise, diet, nutritional supplementation, and pharmacologic interventions, when necessary, can offer women the best opportunity for good bone health through their older years. Alendronate, calcitonin, risedronate, and raloxifene have all been found to reduce the risk of vertebral fractures in clinical trials. Alendronate and risedronate have been shown to reduce the risk of hip fracture in women with osteoporosis, and calcium and vitamin D reduced this risk among institutionalized patients.[79] Exercise is essential and should be encouraged in patients of all ages to maintain strong muscles, improve balance, reduce the risk of falls, and maintain healthy bones. The scientific evidence for botanical remedies is growing but remains too preliminary to support any formal recommendations for these remedies' use in either the prevention or treatment of osteoporosis. In light of the data assembled to date, it seems wise to recommend that both pre- and postmenopausal women take a multivitamin/mineral supplement to ensure adequate intake of nutrients such as magnesium, manganese, zinc, and vitamin C, among others, that play a role in the maintenance of bone density and quality, as well as ensuring adequate calcium intake through diet and supplementation.

References

1. Klibanski A, Adams-Campbell L, Bassford T, et al: Osteoporosis prevention, diagnosis, and therapy. *JAMA* 285:785-795, 2001.
2. Barzel US: Osteoporosis: taking a fresh look, *Hosp Pract* 31:59-68, 1996.
3. *Osteoporosis overview.* National Institutes of Health Osteoporosis and Related Bone Diseases, National Resource Center. Available at www.osteo.org/docs/30.464633275.html. Posted January 2003. Accessed September 2003.
4. Kanis JA, Melton LJ, et al : The diagnosis of osteoporosis, *J Bone Miner Res* 9:1137-1141, 1994.
5. Lindsay R, Hart DM, Clark DM: The minimum effective dose of estrogen for prevention of postmenopausal bone loss, *Obstet Gynecol* 63:759-763, 1984.
6. Filer WD, Filer RB: Transdermal estrogen and prevention of osteoporosis, *Am Fam Phys* 49:1639-1642, 1994.
7. Khosla S, Riggs BL: Treatment options for osteoporosis, *Mayo Clin Proc* 70:978-982, 1985.
8. Riggs BL, Melton LJ: Medical progress series: involutional osteoporosis, *N Engl J Med* 314:1676–1686, 1986.
9. Writing Group for the Women's Health Initiative Investigators: Risks and benefits of estrogen plus progestin in healthy postmenopausal women, *JAMA* 288:321-333, 2002.
10. Cranney A, Wells GA: Hormone replacement therapy for postmenopausal osteoporosis, *Clin Geriatr Med* 19:361-370, 2003.
11. Women's Health Initiative Participant Website: Information for physicians. Available at: http://www.whi.org/updates/advisory_ea_physicians.asp. Accessed on March 18, 2004.
12. Prestwood KM, Kenny AM, Kleppinger A, et al: Ultralow-dose micronized 17beta-estradiol and bone density and bone metabolism in older women: a randomized controlled trial, *JAMA* 290:1042-1048, 2003.

13. Siris E, Adachi JD, Lu Y, et al: Effects of raloxifene on fracture severity in postmenopausal women with osteoporosis: results from the MORE study: Multiple Outcomes of Raloxifene Evaluation, *Osteoporos Int* 13:907-913, 2002.
14. Ettinger B, Black DM, Mitlak BH et al: Reduction of vertebral fracture risk in post-menopausal women with osteoporosis treated with raloxifene. Results from a 3-year randomized clinical trial, *JAMA* 282:637-645, 1999.
15. Russell RG, Rogers MJ: Bisphosphonates: from the laboratory to the clinic and back again, *Bone* 25:97-106, 1999.
16. Black DM, Cummings SR, Karpf DB, et al: Randomized trial of effect of alendronate on risk of fracture in women with existing vertebral fractures, *Lancet* 348:1535-1541, 1996.
17. Harris ST, Watts NB, Genant HK, et al: Effects of risedronate treatment on vertebral and non-vertebral fractures in women with postmenopausal osteoporosis: a randomized, controlled trial, *JAMA* 282:1344-1352, 1999.
18. McClung MR, Geusens P, Miller PD, et al: Effect of risedronate on the risk of hip fracture in elderly women, *N Engl J Med* 344:333-340, 2001.
19. Rico H, Revilla M, Hernandez ER, et al: Total and regional bone mineral content and fracture rate in postmenopausal osteoporosis treated with salmon calcitonin: a prospective study, *Calcif Tiss Int* 56:181-185, 1995.
20. Isenbarger MC, Chapin BL: Osteoporosis: current pharmacologic options for prevention and treatment, *Postgrad Med* 101:129-142, 1997.
21. Chesnut CH III, Silverman S, Andriano K, et al: A randomized trial of nasal spray salmon calcitonin in postmenopausal women with established osteoporosis: the Prevent Recurrence of Osteoporotic Fractures study, *Am J Med* 109:267-276, 2000.
22. Lyritis GP, Tsakalabos S, Magiasis B, et al: Analgesic effect of salmon calcitonin on osteoporotic vertebral fractures. Double-blind, placebo-controlled study, *Calcif Tissue Int* 49:369-372, 1991.
23. Promislow JH, Goodman-Gruen D, Slymen DJ: Protein consumption and bone mineral density in the elderly: the Rancho Bernardo study, *Am J Epidemiol* 155:636-644, 2002.
24. Dawson-Hughes B, Harris SS: Calcium intake influences the association of protein intake with rates of bone loss in elderly men and women, *Am J Clin Nutr* 75:609-610, 2002.
25. Tham DM, Gardner CD, Haskell WL: Clinical review 97: potential health benefits of dietary phytoestrogens: a review of the clinical, epidemiological, and mechanistic evidence, *J Clin Endocrinol Metab* 83:2223-2235, 1998.
26. Setchell KD, Lydeking-Olsen E: Dietary phytoestrogens and their effect on bone: evidence from in vitro and in vivo, human observational, and dietary intervention studies, *Am J Clin Nutr* 78(suppl 3):593S-609S, 2003.
27. Migliaccio S, Anderson JJ: Isoflavones and skeletal health: are these molecules ready for clinical application? *Osteoporos Int* 14:361-368, 2003.
28. Albanese CV, Cudd A, Argentino L, et al: Ipriflavone directly inhibits osteoclastic activity, *Biochem Biophys Res Commun* 199:930-936, 1994.
29. Cheng SL, Zhang SF, Nelson TL, et al: Stimulation of human osteoblast differentiation and function by ipriflavone and its metabolites, *Calcif Tissue Int* 55:356-362, 1994.
30. Agnusdei D, Bufalino L: Efficacy of ipriflavone in established osteoporosis and long term safety, *Calc Tissue Int* 61(suppl):S23-S37, 1999.
31. Alexandersen P, Toussaint A, Christiansen C, et al: Ipriflavone in the treatment of postmenopausal osteoporosis: a randomized controlled trial, *JAMA* 285:1482-1488, 2001.
32. Melis GB, Paoletti AM, Cagnacci L, et al: Lack of any estrogenic effect of ipriflavone in postmenopausal women, *J Endocrinol Invest* 15:755-761, 1992.
33. Cecchini MG, Fleisch H, Muhlbauer RC: Ipriflavone inhibits bone resorption in intact and ovariectomized rats, *Calcif Tissue Int* 61:9-11, 1997.
34. Rondelli I, Acerbi D, Ventura P: Steady-state pharmacokinetics of ipriflavone and its metabolites in patients with renal failure, *Int J Clin Pharmacol Res* 11:183-192, 1991.
35. Monostory K, Vereczky L: Ipriflavone as an inhibitor of human cytochrome P450 enzymes, *Br J Pharmacol* 123:605-610, 1998.
36. Shea B, Wells G, Cranney A, et al: Meta-analysis of calcium supplementation for the prevention of postmenopausal osteoporosis, *Endocrinol Rev* 23:552-559, 2002.

37. Barrett-Conner E: The RDA for calcium in the elderly: too little, too late. *Calcif Tiss Int* 44:303-307, 1989.
38. Health claims: calcium and osteoporosis. Code of Federal Regulations, title 21, vol 2, section 101.72, *Federal Register* 58:2676, January 6, 1993; 58:17101, April 1, 1993; 62:15342, March 31, 1997. Available at: www.cfsan.fda.gov/lrd/cf101–72.html. Accessed September 2003.
39. Pak CYC, Breslau NA, Harvey JA: Nutrition and metabolic bone disease. In: Scarpelli DG, Migaki G, editors. *Nutritional diseases: research directions in comparative pathobiology*, New York, 1986, Alan R Liss, pp 215-240.
40. Recker RR: Calcium absorption and achlorhydria, *N Engl J Med* 313:70-73, 1985.
41. *National Osteoporosis Foundation: physician's guide to prevention and treatment of osteoporosis*, Belle Mead, NJ, 1999, Excerpta Medica.
42. Osteoporosis prevention, diagnosis, and therapy. *National Institutes of Health Consensus Statement* 17:1-36, 2000. Available at: odp.od.nih.gov/consensus/cons/111/osteo_abstract.pdf. Accessed September 2003.
43. Brown JP, Josse RG: Scientific Advisory Council of the Osteoporosis Society of Canada 2002 clinical practice guidelines for the diagnosis and management of osteoporosis in Canada. *CMAJ* 167(suppl 10):S1-S34, 2002.
44. Management of postmenopausal osteoporosis: position statement of the North American Menopause Society, *Menopause* 9:84-101, 2002.
45. Lilliu H, Pamphile R, Chapuy MC, et al: Calcium–vitamin D_3 supplementation is cost-effective in hip fracture prevention, *Maturitas* 44:299-305, 2003.
46. Lips P, Graafmans W, Ooms ME, et al: Vitamin D supplementation and fracture incidence in elderly patients, *Ann Intern Med* 124:400-406, 1996.
47. Gillespie WJ, Avenell A, Henry DA, et al: Vitamin D and vitamin D analogues for preventing fractures associated with involutional and post-menopausal osteoporosis, *Cochrane Database Syst Rev* (1):CD000227, 2001.
48. *Physician's guide to the prevention and treatment of osteoporosis*, Washington, DC, 1998, National Osteoporosis Foundation.
49. Weber P: Vitamin K and bone health, *Nutrition* 17:880-887, 2001.
50. Feskanich D, Weber P, Willett WC, et al: Vitamin K intake and hip fractures in women: a prospective study, *Am J Clin Nutr* 69:74-79, 1999.
51. Hart JP, Catterall A, Dodds RA, et al: Circulating vitamin K_1 levels in fractured neck of femur, *Lancet* 2:283, 1984.
52. Booth SL, Broe KE, Gagnon DR, et al: Vitamin K intake and bone mineral density in women and men, *Am J Clin Nutr* 77:512-516, 2003.
53. Booth SL, Tucker KL, Chen H, et al: Dietary vitamin K intakes are associated with hip fracture but not with bone mineral density in elderly men and women, *Am J Clin Nutr* 71:1201-1208, 2000.
54. Zittermann A: Effects of vitamin K on calcium and bone metabolism, *Curr Opin Clin Nutr Metab Care* 4:483-487, 2001.
55. Haguenauer D, Welch V, Shea B, et al: Fluoride for treating postmenopausal osteoporosis (Cochrane review). In: *The Cochrane Library*, issue 3. Oxford, 2002, Update Software.
56. Ilich JZ, Brownbill RA, Tamborini L: Bone and nutrition in elderly women: protein, energy, and calcium as main determinants of bone mineral density, *Eur J Clin Nutr* 57:554-565, 2003.
57. Sheikh MS, Ramirez A, Emmett M, et al: Role of vitamin D–dependent and vitamin D–independent mechanisms in absorption of food calcium, *J Clin Invest* 81:126-132, 1988.
58. Fatemi S, Ryzen E, Flores J, et al: Effect of experimental human magnesium depletion on parathyroid secretion and 1,25-dihydroxyvitamin D metabolism, *J Clin Endocrinol Metab* 73:1067-1072, 1991.
59. Cohen L, Kitzes R: Infrared spectroscopy and magnesium content of bone mineral in osteoporotic women, *Isr J Med Sci* 17:1123-1125, 1983.
60. Rude RK, Gruber HE, Wei LY, et al: Magnesium deficiency: effect on bone and mineral metabolism in the mouse, *Calcif Tissue Int* 72:32-41, 2003.
61. Sokja JE, Weaver CM: Magnesium supplementation and osteoporosis, *Nutr Rev* 53:71-74, 1995.
62. Leach RM Jr, Meunster AM, Wien EM: I. Studies on the role of manganese in bone formation. II. Effect upon chondroitin sulfate synthesis in chick epiphyseal cartilage, *Arch Biochem Biophys* 133:22-28, 1969.

63. Atik OS: Zinc and senile osteoporosis, *J Am Geriatr Soc* 31:790-791, 1983.
64. Smith RT, Smith JC, Fields M, et al: Mechanical properties of bone from copper deficient rats fed starch or fructose, *Fed Proc* 44:541, 1985.
65. Eaton-Evans J, McIlrath EM, Jackson WE, et al: Copper supplementation and bone-mineral density in middle-aged women, *Proc Nutr Soc* 54:191A, 1995.
66. Saltman PD, Strause LG: The role of trace minerals in osteoporosis, *J Am Coll Nutr* 12:384-389, 1993.
67. Rico H, Gallego-Lago JL, Hernandez ER, et al: Effect of silicon supplement on osteopenia induced by ovariectomy in rats, *Calcif Tiss Int* 66:53-55, 2000.
68. Seidlova-Wuttke D, Jarry H, Becker T, et al: Pharmacology of *Cimicifuga racemosa* extract BNO 1055 in rats: bone, fat and uterus, *Maturitas* 44(suppl 1):S39-S50, 2003.
69. Li JX, Kadota S, Li HY, Miyahara T, et al: Effects of *Cimicifuga* rhizome on serum calcium and phosphate levels in low calcium dietary rats and on bone mineral density in ovariectomized rats, *Phytomedicine* 3:379-385, 1996/97.
70. Micozzi, MS, Fundamentals of complementary and integrative medicine, ed. 3, St. Louis, Elsevier.
71. Lee JR: Osteoporosis reversal: the role of progesterone, *Int Clin Nutr Rev* 10:384-391, 1990.
72. Wren BG, McFarland K, Edwards L, et al: Effect of sequential transdermal progesterone cream on endometrium, bleeding pattern, and plasma progesterone and salivary progesterone levels in postmenopausal women, *Climacteric* 3:155-160, 2000.
73. Leonetti HB, Longa S, Anasti J: Transdermal progesterone cream for vasomotor symptoms and postmenopausal bone loss, *Obstet Gynecol* 94:225-228, 1999.
74. Wolff I, Van Croonenborg JJ, Kemper HCG, et al: The effect of exercise training programs on bone mass: a meta-analysis of published controlled trials in pre- and postmenopausal women, *Osteoporos Int* 9:1-12, 1999.
75. Berard A, Bravo G, Gauthier P: Meta-analysis of the effectiveness of physical activity for the prevention of bone loss in postmenopausal women, *Osteoporos Int* 7:331-337, 1997.
76. Wallace BA, Cumming RG: Systematic review of randomized trials of the effect of exercise on bone mass in pre- and postmenopausal women, *Calcif Tissue Int* 67:10-18, 2000.
77. Qin L, Au S, Choy W, et al: Regular Tai Chi Chuan exercise may retard bone loss in postmenopausal women: a case-control study, *Arch Phys Med Rehabil* 83:1355-1359, 2002.
78. Taggart HM: Effects of Tai Chi exercise on balance, functional mobility, and fear of falling among older women, *Appl Nurs Res* 15:235-242, 2002.
79. Hauselmann HJ, Rizzoli R: A comprehensive review of treatments for postmenopausal osteoporosis, *Osteoporos Int* 14:2-12, 2003.

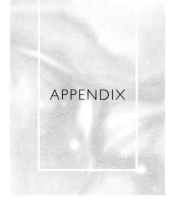

Botanical Products

GENERAL CONSIDERATIONS FOR THE USE OF HERBS

Changes in the practice of medicine are causing a shift to self-care with more benign, less invasive treatments. Practicing clinicians (and, in turn, patients) should be made aware of the indications, actions, and drug interactions of herbal remedies (Appendix Box 1).

The World Health Organization estimates that 80% of the world's population relies on herbal medicine, in part due to the lack of access to conventional care and pharmaceuticals in some geographical areas and a resurgence in use in others, such as Europe, Australia, Canada, and the United States. Today, the use of herbs in the United States is expanding rapidly, to the point that herbal products are found in most pharmacies and supermarkets. From 1990 to 1997, as the use of complementary and alternative medicine by Americans increased from 34% to 42%, the use of herbal preparations quadrupled from 3% to 12%.

These rapid changes have come as a result of popular demand, marketing and the implementation of the Dietary Supplements Health Education Act of 1994. The public has discovered that natural medicines often provide a safe, effective, and economical alternative to mainstream medicine, and research is increasingly validating this finding. Many people who use herbal and high-dose vitamin products fail to tell their physicians that they are doing so. Either they assume that "natural" products are harmless and not worth mentioning, or they fear the reaction of health care professionals who may view the use of such products with skepticism. Health care professionals, however, are beginning to familiarize themselves with the subject. Aside from some advantages of natural products, herb-drug interactions and adverse effects are a growing concern: Almost one in five prescription drug users is also using dietary supplements.[1] In some cases, the use of dietary supplements may help minimize some of the known side effects of prescription medications.

In Europe, the use of herbs poses less of a threat because herbs are classified with other pharmaceutical products and routinely prescribed by physicians. In Germany, prescriptions for St. John's wort outnumber those for all other antidepressants. Most of the research to date originates in Europe, where the phytopharmaceutical industry has had a financial incentive to conduct the necessary research. The United States has recently

Box 1

General guidelines for the use of herbal medicines
■ The clinician should take a careful history of the patient's use of herbs and other supplements.   ■ An accurate medical diagnosis must be made before herbs are prescribed for symptomatic treatment.   ■ Natural is not necessarily safe: Attention should be paid to the quality of a product, its dosage, and potential adverse effects, including interactions with other herbs, foods, and drugs.   ■ Herbal treatments should, for the most part, be avoided by pregnant women (and by those contemplating pregnancy) and those who are lactating.   ■ The prescription of herbs to children should be done with care, with the appropriate dosage based on weight.   ■ Adverse effects should be recorded, and the dosage reduced or the product discontinued. The use of an herb can be carefully restarted in an effort to ascertain whether the herb is the source of the problem.

joined in these efforts, and the National Institutes of Health (NIH) National Center for Complementary and Alternative Medicine and the National Institutes of Mental Health completed a $4.3 million joint clinical trial to determine the efficacy of St. John's wort in the treatment of major depression. At the time of this writing, herbal studies are in progress at several major American medical schools.

HERBS FOR HEALTH

In a Harvard study, two of the top five conditions for which consumers sought alternative treatment were anxiety and depression. In addition to St. John's wort, other herbs are popular remedies for these and related problems: kava for the relief of stress and anxiety (until recently, when concerns about its potential effects on the liver began to emerge), *Ginkgo biloba* for the treatment of senile dementia or benign forgetfulness, and valerian as an aid to sleep. A $20 million NIH trial comparing ginkgo and placebo in the development of dementia in older Americans was initiated in 2000.

Many drugs used in modern medicine are derived from plants. Common examples are morphine, which is derived from the opium poppy; digitalis, which comes from foxglove; and reserpine, which is taken from rauwolfia (Indian snakeroot). In many cases, pharmaceuticals remain the treatment of choice. However, when appropriate, herbs may be preferred, for the following reasons:

■ Herbs are generally less likely to cause side effects. When such effects do occur, they are generally milder than those caused by pharmaceuticals. In fact, in the absence of side effects, patients often do not notice the subtle improvements that occur as these natural medicines begin to take effect. This lack of side effects may also confound double-blind studies. One possible partial explanation for the milder side effects is that the original plant constituents are more compatible with metabolism and body chemistry.

- Although the isolated active ingredient has been assumed to be most effective, using the whole plant also has its advantages. Whereas Western biomedicine seeks to isolate a single active ingredient, herbal medicine relies on the synergistic action of a plant's many constituents.
- These combinations may also yield a variety of effects. For example, through its action on the brain, kava acts as an anxiety-reliever, whereas its relaxant effects are a result of its direct action on both smooth and striated muscle.

SAFETY

Side effects of drugs, the worst being death by overdose, can be quite serious. According to one report, overdoses yielded an annual rate of 30.1 deaths per 1 million prescriptions of antidepressants. On the other hand, to quote Norman Farnsworth, PhD, Professor of Pharmacognosy at the University of Illinois, Chicago: "Based on published reports, side effects or toxic reactions associated with herbal medicines in any form are rare ... In fact, of all classes of substances ... to cause toxicities of sufficient magnitude to be reported in the United States, plants are the least problematic." It is important that patients be told to contact the prescribing practitioner if they feel any ill effects while taking an herbal product. Then, depending on the severity of the reaction, the patient should either reduce the dose or stop taking the herb altogether. Unlike pharmaceuticals, withdrawal reactions are rarely an issue.

It is essential that a complete drug and herbal history be obtained from each patient. Certain combinations are contraindicated and should be covered individually. On the other hand, many combinations work well. For example, an individual taking a drug that may be potentially hepatotoxic may wish to take the liver-supporting herb milk thistle (*Silybum marianum*).

PREGNANCY, BREASTFEEDING, AND CHILDREN

Many herbs have not been approved for use by pregnant and nursing women. Harm from exposure during pregnancy can be difficult to identify, and historical use is not always a reliable source. Alcohol is a useful example. Although women have consumed alcohol during pregnancy for centuries, the association between its use and fetal alcohol syndrome was not recognized until the 1970s. Except for the few herbs normally used in pregnancy— raspberry leaf, ginger, mint, chamomile—it is probably best to avoid medicinal strength botanical medicines during pregnancy and lactation.

Unlike prescription drugs, incentives for the study of dietary supplements/botanicals in general, and particularly in pediatrics, are limited. Research in children brings with it a special set of issues, making many herbal manufacturers reluctant to foot the bill for these trials. The National Center of Complementary and Alternative Medicine at the National Institutes of Health has sponsored studies of chamomile in functional abdominal pain (ages 4 to 16 years), echinacea for acute upper respiratory tract infection (children 2 to 11 years), and echinacea for acute otitis media (ages 1 to 5 years). Studies suggesting beneficial effects for botanicals specifically in pediatrics include ginger for motion sickness, St. John's wort for major depressive disorder; ivy leaf extract for asthma; chamomile cream, evening primrose oil, and borage seed oil for atopic dermatitis; and a combination of chamomile, fennel, balm and vervain for colic, to name a few.

Compared with adverse effects and toxicity arising from pharmaceutical medications, the incidence of harm associated with herbal medicines in the United States is extremely low. Generally, reviews of adverse effects of herbal medicines in children are reassuring. However, given the increasing number of products in the U.S. marketplace specifically targeted at children, knowledgeable practitioners must take an active role in assisting parents to help prevent potentially dangerous consequences from administration of harmful products to young children. Botanical research (pharmacokinetic, pharmacodynamic, reproductive toxicity), basic and continuing education regarding herb use in children, and appropriate monitoring for adverse events are just a few areas that will help ensure the safe use of dietary supplements in children. Finally, caution and common sense should prevail when considering long-term administration of all but the most gentle of herbs (chamomile, catmint, peppermint, lavender, etc.) in children.

> I am sorry to say that Peter was not very well during the evening. His mother put him to bed and made some chamomile tea and she gave a dose of it to Peter, one tablespoon full to be taken at bedtime. — *The Tale of Peter Rabbit* by Beatrix Potter

Aging

Considering the phenomenon of polypharmacy in the elderly and problems of impaired metabolism and clearance, herbs may offer both a safe alternative to some medications and a landmine of potentially dangerous herb-drug interactions and adverse effects. St. John's wort can be quite useful in the treatment of depression in the elderly, ginkgo for the treatment of cognitive decline, and saw palmetto for enlarged prostate. However, St. John's wort may interfere with medications being used by patients, and ginkgo may aggravate bleeding problems in patients taking anticoagulants or large amounts of antiplatelet agents.

SELECTION AND USE OF HERBS
Standardized Extracts

For those new to the medicinal use of herbs, dose selection can be confusing. As noted earlier, herbs often have several different active ingredients, unlike synthetic drugs that contain a single compound. Even these will vary in proportion, depending on such factors as where the plant was grown and when (season or even the time of day) it was harvested. A manufacturer may adjust the mixture to help account for these variations.

To standardize the product—that is, to have a consistent, measured amount of product per unit dose—the manufacturer selects one constituent (or group of constituents) generally thought to play a role in the plant's therapeutic activity.

St. John's wort is standardized to hypericin, the long-accepted active antidepressant ingredient. Further research has shown hyperforin to also be a likely active ingredient. Some St. John's wort products are now standardized for both. In most cases, the standardized product contains the whole plant, although in some very concentrated products, such as ginkgo and milk thistle, not all compounds are present. Standardization of products is useful but limited. In many cases, we simply do not know the active compound(s) for which to set levels.

Herbal Preparations and Dosing

Herbs may be purchased as teas, tinctures, tablets, or capsules. Teas and tinctures, being liquid, are absorbed more rapidly than tablets or capsules. Tinctures are made by soaking one part herbal material (by weight) in 1 to 10 parts (by volume) of an alcohol and water mixture. Echinacea tinctures are typically made with 40% to 60% ethanol; the remaining liquid is water. A 1:5 strength tincture means that there is 1 g of herb in every 5 mL of finished tincture. A 1:10 strength tincture means that there is 1 g of herb in every 10 mL of finished tincture. As a means of removing the alcohol taste, the user can place the tincture in warm water or tea for a few minutes to allow some of the alcohol to evaporate.

Vegetable glycerin may be used instead of alcohol, but the resulting extract is weaker. Capsules and tablets are the most commonly used delivery systems. Gelatin or vegetable-based capsules are filled with powdered dried herb; tablets are powdered herbs compressed into a solid pill, often with a variety of inert ingredients as fillers.

Capsules and tablets are supplied in a variety of sizes and strengths, so reading the label carefully is a matter of importance. The label also usually provides a suggested dose as a guideline to the user. Some of these doses are based on research and clinical findings, but there is very wide variation in the marketplace and it can be very difficult for the average consumer or busy clinician to know how much is an effective and safe dose. For instance, black cohosh, an herb popular for menopause symptom relief, can be found in doses ranging from 40 to 2300 mg/day. Echinacea can be found in standardized and crude forms with doses ranging from 50 to 9000 mg/day. Research should be directed at determining a dose response for the most popular herbs to help patients and providers optimize therapeutic response. In general, it is probably best to start low and gradually increase the dose, as needed.

Regulatory Issues

Most herbal products are regulated as dietary supplements. In 1994, the U.S. Dietary Supplement Health and Education Act (DSHEA) set new guidelines with regard to quality, labeling, packaging, and marketing of supplements. DSHEA allows manufacturers to make "statements of nutritional support for conventional vitamins and minerals." Because herbs are not nutritional in the conventional sense, under DSHEA manufacturers are allowed to make only what they call "structure and function claims," not therapeutic or prevention claims. Therefore the label for a St. John's wort preparation can claim that the product "optimizes mood" but cannot say that it is a "natural antidepressant," which would be a therapeutic claim.

Because by law the labels provide insufficient information, it is particularly important for the health care practitioner to be well educated in this area. Ideally, supplements would be labeled so that the purchaser would know exact indications and possible side effects, as with other over-the-counter medicines.

Quality control is essential, including the assurance that the product contains the ingredients and quantities described on the label and that it does not contain such contaminants as bacteria, mold, or heavy metals. The Food and Drug Administration, in conjunction with the trade and professional organizations, have created a more rigorous and relevant set of standards, called *good manufacturing practices* (GMP), for the industry that will hopefully be released and implemented soon. In general, we recommend buying herbal products from those companies with a U.S. Pharmacopoeia (USP) or National Sanitation Foundation (NSF) quality seal, those that have passed testing by consumerlabs.com, or those that sell clinically tested products. Many companies manufacture high-quality herbal products, but it is virtually impossible for the average consumer to separate the "wheat from the chaff." Several excellent Web sites on this subject are listed below:

- American Botanical Council
  www.herbalgram.org
- Herb Research Foundation
  www.herbs.org
- The Natural Pharmacist
  www.tnp.com
- Consumerlabs
  www.consumerlabs.com

Recommended Reading

Blumenthal M, Goldberg A, Brinckmann J: 2000. *Herbal medicine: expanded Commission E monographs*, Newton, Massachusetts, 2000, Integrated Medicine Communications, p 519.

Bourin M, Bougerol T, Guitton B, et al: A combination of plant extracts in the treatment of outpatients with adjustment disorder with anxious mood: controlled study versus placebo, *Fundam Clin Pharmacol* 11:127-132, 1997.

Ciraulo DA, Shader RI, Greenblatt DJ, editors: *Drug interactions in psychiatry,* edition 2. Baltimore, Md, 1995, Williams and Wilkins.

Cott JM: In vitro receptor binding and enzyme inhibition by *Hypericum perforatum* extract, *Pharmacopsychiatry* 30(suppl II):108-112, 1997.

Davies LP, Drew CA, Duffield P, et al: Kava pyrones and resin: studies on GABAA, GABAB and benzodiazepine binding sites in rodent brain, *Pharmacol Toxicol* 71:120-126, 1992.

Dorn M: Efficacy and tolerability of Baldrian versus oxazepam in non-organic and non-psychiatric insomniacs: a randomized, double-blind, clinical, comparative study [in German], *Forsch Komplementarmed Klass Naturheilkd* 7:79-84, 2000.

Monographs on the medicinal use of plants, European Scientific Cooperative on Phytotherapy, 1997, Exeter, United Kingdom.

Eisenberg DM, Davis RB, Ettner SL, et al: Trends in alternative medicine use in the United States, 1990-1997: results of a follow-up national survey, *JAMA* 280:1569-1575, 1998.

Fontana RJ, Lown KS, Paine MF, et al: Effects of a chargrilled meat diet on expression of CYP3A, CYP1A, and P-glycoprotein levels in healthy volunteers, *Gastroenterology* 117:89-98, 1999.

Fugh-Berman A, Cott JM: Dietary supplements and natural products as psychotherapeutic agents, *Psychosom Med* 61:712-728, 1999.

Garrett BJ, Cheeke PR, Miranda CL, et al: Consumption of poisonous plants by rats, *Toxicol Lett* 10:183-188, 1982.

Hypericum Depression Trial Study Group: Effect of *Hypericum perforatum* (St John's wort) in major depressive disorder: a randomized controlled trial, *JAMA* 287:1807-1814, 2002.

Johne A, Brockmoller J, Bauer S, et al: Pharmacokinetic interaction of digoxin with an herbal extract from St John's wort (*Hypericum perforatum*), *Clin Pharmacol Ther* 66:338-345, 1999.

Landes P: Market report, *HerbalGram* 42:64-65, 1998.

Linde K, Ramirez G, Mulrow CD, et al: St. John's wort for depression: an overview and meta-analysis of randomized clinical trials, *Br Med J* 313:253-258, 1996.

Maurer A, Johne A, Bauer S, et al: Interaction of St. John's wort extract with phenprocoumon (abstract), *Eur J Clin Pharmacol* 55:A22, 1999.

McGuffin M, Hobbs C, Upton R, et al: *Botanical safety handbook*, Boca Raton, Florida, 1997, CRC Press, p 105.

Müller WE, Rolli M, Schäfer C, et al: Effects of *Hypericum* extract (LI 160) in biochemical models of antidepressant activity, *Pharmacopsychiatry* 30(suppl II):102-107, 1997.

Newall CA, Anderson LA, Phillipson JD: *Herbal medicines: a guide for health-care professionals*, London, United Kingdom, 1996, Pharmaceutical Press, pp 239-240.

Ohnishi A, Matsuo H, Yamada S, et al: Effect of furanocoumarin derivatives in grapefruit juice on the uptake of vinblastine by Caco-2 cells and on the activity of cytochrome P450 3A4, *Br J Pharmacol* 130:1369-1371, 2000.

Piscitelli SC, Burstein AH, Chaitt D, et al: Indinavir concentrations and St John's wort, *Lancet* 355:547-548, 2000.

Ruschitzka F, Meier PJ, Turina M, et al: Acute heart transplant rejection due to Saint John's wort, Lancet 355:548-549, 2000.

Santos MS, Ferreira F, Faro C, et al: The amount of GABA present in aqueous extracts of valerian is sufficient to account for [^{3}H]GABA release in synaptosomes, *Planta Med* 60:475-476, 1994.

Schelosky L, Raffauf C, Jendroska K, et al: Letter to the editor, *J Neurol Neurosurg Psychiatr* 45:639-640, 1995.

Shelton RC, Keller MB, Gelenberg A, et al: Effectiveness of St John's wort in major depression: a randomized controlled trial, *JAMA* 285:1978-1986, 2001.

Upton R, Graff A, Williamson E, et al: *American herbal pharmacopoeia and therapeutic compendium on valerian root: analytical, quality control, and therapeutic monograph*, Santa Cruz, Calif, 1999, American Herbal Pharmacopoeia.

Upton R, Graff A, Williamson E, et al: American herbal pharmacopoeia and therapeutic compendium on St. John's wort, *Hypericum perforatum*: quality control, analytical and therapeutic monograph, *HerbalGram* 40(suppl):1-32, 1997.

Vorbach EU: Efficacy and tolerability of St. John's wort extract LI 160 vs. imipramine in patients with severe depressive episodes according to ICD-10, *Pharmacopsychiatry* 30(suppl 2):81-85, 1997.

Welch CA: In: Ciraulo DA, Shader RI, Greenblatt DJ, editors: *Drug interactions in psychiatry*, edition 2. Baltimore, Md, 1995, Williams and Wilkins, p 399.

Wichtl M: In: Bisset NG, Wichtl M, editors: *Herbal drugs and phytopharmaceuticals: a handbook for practice on a scientific basis*, Boca Raton, Fla, 1994, CRC Press, pp 273-275.

Woelk H, Kapoula O, Lehrl S, et al: Behandlung von Angst-Patienten, *Z Allg Med* 69:271-277, 1993.

Wolfman C, Viola H, Paladini A, et al: Possible anxiolytic effects of chrysin, a central benzodiazepine receptor ligand isolated from *Passiflora coerulea*, *Pharmacol Biochem Behav* 47:1-4, 1994.

Yue Q-Y, Bergquist C, Gerdén B: Safety of St John's wort (*Hypericum perforatum*), Lancet 355:576-577, 2000.

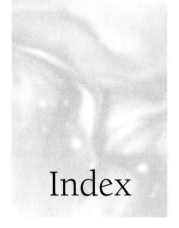

Index

A

Acetylcholine, Alzheimer's disease role of, 201-202, 203-204

Achillea millefolium, herbal use of, 288

Aconitum napellus
toxicity of, 60
Turska's formula containing, 60

Acupuncture, 8-9
breast cancer therapy using, 264-265
menopause treated with, 85
menstrual cramps treated with, 48
migraine treatment using, 166
morning sickness treated with, 99
urinary tract infection and, 104

Age, breast cancer related to, 248t

Agnolyt, PMS treated using, 30-31, 32t-34t

Alcohol
breast cancer odds related to, 248t
heart failure prevention role of, 227

Alendronate, osteoporosis treatment using, 310-311

Allium sativum
cardiovascular effects of, 236-237
vaginal candidiasis treated with, 274

Alternative medicine, 4-5, 5f. *See also* CAM (complementary/alternative medicine).

Althaea officinalis. See Marshmallow.

Alzheimer's disease, 201-215
basic overview of, 201-202
diagnosis of, 202-203
signs and symptoms in, 202-203
treatment strategies for, 203-215
cognitive stimulation in, 203
dietary, 205-207
drug therapy in, 203-205
herbal, 207-215

American mandrake, 284-285, 284f
pregnancy contraindication for, 285
warts treated with, 285

Anagyrine, blue cohosh content of, 111

Analgesics
endometriosis treated with, 52
headache treated with, 148, 150
menstrual cramps treated with, 42-43

Anemone pulsatilla
endometriosis treated with, 56, 59
menstrual cramps treated with, 46

Angelica sinensis. See Dong quai.

Antidepressants
headache treated with, 150-151
PMS treated using, 37-38
postpartum depression treatment using, 136-137

Antifungals, vaginal candidiasis treated with, 272-274, 273b

Page numbers followed by "f" indicate figures; page numbers followed by "t" indicate tables; page numbers followed by "b" indicate boxes.